TREATING

DRUG

PROBLEMS

VOLUME 1

A Study of the Evolution, Effectiveness, and Financing
of Public and Private Drug Treatment Systems

Committee for the Substance Abuse Coverage Study
Division of Health Care Services

INSTITUTE OF MEDICINE

Dean R. Gerstein and Henrick J. Harwood, editors

NATIONAL ACADEMY PRESS
Washington, D.C.   1990

National Academy Press • 2101 Constitution Avenue, N.W. • Washington, D.C. 20418

NOTICE: The project that is the subject of this report was approved by the Governing Board of the National Research Council, whose members are drawn from the councils of the National Academy of Sciences, the National Academy of Engineering, and the Institute of Medicine. The members of the committee responsible for the report were chosen for their competencies and with regard for the appropriate balance.

The report has been reviewed by a group other than the authors according to procedures approved by a Report Review Committee consisting of members of the National Academy of Sciences, the National Academy of Engineering, and the Institute of Medicine.

The Institute of Medicine was chartered in 1970 by the National Academy of Sciences to enlist distinguished members of the appropriate professions in the examination of policy matters pertaining to the health of the public. In this, the Institute acts under both the Academy's 1863 congressional charter responsibility to be an adviser to the federal government and its own initiative in identifying issues of medical care, research, and education. Dr. Samuel O. Thier is president of the Institute of Medicine.

This study was supported by the National Institute on Drug Abuse, U.S. Department of Health and Human Services, under Contract No. 283-88-0009 (SA).

Preface

The committee members and staff appointed in 1988 to conduct the Institute of Medicine's Substance Abuse Coverage Study were given a three-part task:

- investigate the extent of private and public funding of treatment for the chronic, relapsing disorders of drug abuse and dependence;
- evaluate the adequacy of funding patterns to meet the national need for rehabilitation of individuals with these disorders; and
- make recommendations to responsible parties, such as the U.S. Congress, which originally requested the study, regarding what they should do to meet the needs identified by the investigation.

Based on its legislative title, the Substance Abuse Coverage Study seemed destined to focus on the design of health insurance benefits, which had entered the picture of drug treatment financing in a major way in the 1980s. But after carefully reviewing the charge, the character and organization of the treatment system, and the concerns that third-party payers on both the public and private sides persistently voiced about treatment programs and clients, the committee adopted a more comprehensive definition of its task. That definition is suggested by the title and descriptor chosen for this report: *Treating Drug Problems; A study of the evolution, effectiveness, and financing of public and private drug treatment systems*. The various chapters of the report discuss the history of ideas governing drug policy, the nature and extent of the need for treatment, the goals and effectiveness of treatment, the need for research on treatment methods and services, the costs and organization of the two-tiered national treatment system, the scope and organizing principles of public and private coverage, and recommendations tailored to each kind of coverage. Seven papers commissioned to inform and accompany the report are in a companion volume.

Notwithstanding this broad range of issues, there are still some very important constraints and limits on what the committee has done and how this report should be understood. First, the report is about drug treatment and not about drug policy in general. Although the committee is careful to note where treatment fits within the context of prevention and law enforcement approaches to drug problems, it did not study these other approaches comprehensively. Consequently, its recommendations concerning additional resources for treatment do not derive from a systematic comparison of allocations for treatment versus allocations of comparable resources to law enforcement or prevention, but rather from a consideration of treatment needs alone. Comparison of the relative marginal benefits of these different approaches ultimately must be made, based on appropriate studies (which the report calls for), but it was not part of the committee's charge to perform this more encompassing task.

A second limitation is that the committee's recommendations are confined to and reflect drug treatment in the United States. There is relevant scientific literature from other countries pertaining to treatment modalities in the United States, and the committee has explored these important sources. An adequate investigation of treatment systems in other countries, however, would require the same level of historical analysis, expert workshops, intensive site visiting in various localities, and other procedures that the committee employed in the United States. This type of careful international comparative study was beyond the committee's scope and resources.

A third limitation is that the report does not delve into the treatment of alcohol problems. The committee recognizes that alcohol and drug problems overlap in a substantial proportion of the cases now being seen, a fact manifested by the range of problems most programs are willing to treat and the variety of services they provide. The limitation in scope here is largely due to a parallel study of alcohol treatment in the Institute of Medicine, chaired by Robert D. Sparks and directed by Frederick B. Glaser and Herman I. Diesenhaus; their committee's report, *Broadening the Base of Treatment for Alcohol Problems* (1990), is readily available from the National Academy Press.

The alcohol study derived from the same legislation that initiated this study; however, the specific requests proceeded through separate federal channels and followed different timetables. Readers of both reports will easily see that problems associated with the two kinds of substances (legal alcohol and illegal drugs) and their partially divergent treatment systems justify separate investigations, even though the two have much in common. Both committees tried to maintain clear perspectives on each others' work while the studies were in progress. Mark V. Pauly served as a member of both committees, and there was other extensive liaison, including joint staff work. Now that both studies are completed, we are hopeful that a way will be found to draw the results even closer together, perhaps in a future report that focuses on the overlap of alcohol and drug problems.

A fourth limitation is that the committee did not devote major energies to examining the relationship between drug treatment and AIDS (the acquired immune deficiency syndrome). Another committee of the National Academy of Sciences has recently completed two comprehensive studies of AIDS in its behavioral and social contexts, and their reports include a consideration of drug problems from the perspective of AIDS research and policy. We therefore refer the reader to *AIDS: Sexual Behavior and Intravenous Drug Use* (1989) and *AIDS: The Second Decade* (1990), which are both available from the National Academy Press. The latter report is particularly notable for its thorough analysis of women, adolescents, and AIDS.

A final limitation on the scope of the committee's work was imposed by the scarcity of research data since the onset of the crack-cocaine era concerning treatment for drug dependence in women who are pregnant or mothers of young children. Of particular importance here is the question of how such treatment affects not only these women but also the quality of prenatal development, parental care, and environmental conditions in which their children are raised; and how, in turn, the children's health, behavior, and opportunities in life are affected when treatment intervenes. Another disheartening problem is the fragmentary knowledge base underpinning the treatment of drug abuse and dependence among adolescents. The absence of systematic research is perpetuated by excessive barriers to conducting treatment follow-up studies among individuals under 18 years of age. These obstacles arise because of inappropriate and unrealistic requirements at the federal level and in many states to obtain written parental consent for minors to participate (generally, through confidential interviews) in treatment services research.

Although the committee was limited in these respects, we believe the report is fully responsive to its original charge, which expresses a legitimate and urgent national need. Perhaps in part because of the urgency of this need, the committee received willing assistance from many sources. Scores of individuals provided valuable information and trenchant ideas in extensive correspondence with the committee and in the formative workshops it organized during 1988 in Washington, D.C., and Irvine, California. The contributions of M. Douglas Anglin, who took part in both workshops and assisted the committee in other respects, deserve special mention.

The committee is also indebted to programs and agencies that hosted committee site visits in New York, Miami/Dade County, Pittsburgh, St. Louis, the San Francisco Bay area, Los Angeles and Orange Counties, and Portland and Salem, Oregon. Closer to home, James M. Kaple and Albert M. Woodward, the study's project officers at the National Institute on Drug Abuse, were unfailingly helpful, constructive, and circumspect in facilitating the progress of the study. Charles R. Schuster, Salvatore di Menza, Edgar Adams, and other past and present staff of the National Institute on Drug Abuse were also instrumental in the acquisition of important data.

The Research Triangle Institute, which performed the Treatment Outcome Prospective Study and the 1988 National Household Survey on Drug Abuse, among other signal contributions to the field, provided invaluable assistance in developing this report, and its staff, particularly J. Valley Rachal and Lynn E. Guess, have earned the committee's thanks. Two former members of the Lewin/ICF staff, Nina E. Teicholz and Karen F. Monborne, directly assisted the chair, as did Lewin/ICF colleagues Jack Needleman and Robert J. Rubin.

The authors of commissioned papers made major contributions to the committee's thinking and responded graciously to its many requests for more, less, different, or clarifying information. The committee does not necessarily concur with every conclusion drawn by these authors; nevertheless, we learned a great deal from them and are pleased to publish their papers in a second volume of the report.

The committee also benefited from a perceptive and unusually extensive set of review comments solicited by the Institute of Medicine. These reviews stimulated many specific improvements in the draft report, and their contributors represent an admirable tradition of unsung, voluntary professional service to the public interest. We are grateful to be among its beneficiaries.

Speaking for ourselves and for the members of the committee, we cannot praise too highly the quality and dedication of the Institute of Medicine staff. Linda B. Kearney, administrative secretary, and Elaine McGarraugh, research associate, performed coolly and indefatigably in disposing of an unending succession of logistical and technical requirements. The ingenuity, eye for detail, and good judgment of these veterans kept the study on track in the face of numerous complications. Technical editor Leah Mazade carefully graced and polished every line of text in preparing the report for publication. Henrick J. Harwood, associate study director and co-editor of the report, left late in the study to serve in the White

House Office of National Drug Control Policy—but not before organizing and leading several intensely valuable site visits, completing state-of-the-art literature reviews and data analyses, and generally earning the very highest regard of the committee.

Finally, we are fortunate to have a committee whose members are thoroughly distinguished in their professional achievements, demanding in their intellectual standards, congenial and unassuming in person, and thoughtful, persistent, and generous in their abiding commitment to the public good. On behalf of this splendid group, we are pleased to submit the report of the Substance Abuse Coverage Study.

Lawrence S. Lewin, *Chair*
Dean R. Gerstein, *Study Director*

Contents

CONTENTS OF VOLUME 2   xvii

SUMMARY   1
    Questions the Report Answers and Those It Leaves Unresolved, 1
    Ideas Governing Drug Treatment Policy, 2
    Drug Problems and the Need for Treatment, 4
        Patterns of Drug Consumption, 4; Dependence, 5; Recovery and
        Relapse, 5; Determining the Need for Treatment, 7; Estimating
        the Aggregate Need for Treatment, 7
    The Goals of Drug Treatment, 8
        Motivations for Treatment, 9; Treatment and Criminal Justice, 10
    Effectiveness of Treatment, 11
        Methadone Maintenance, 12; Therapeutic Communities, 14;
        Outpatient Nonmethadone Programs, 15; Chemical Dependency
        Programs, 16; Detoxification, 16; Variations in Effectiveness of
        Programs Within Modalities, 17; Treatment in Prisons, 17; Costs
        and Benefits of Treatment, 18; Comparison of Data on
        Effectiveness and Expenditures for the Major Treatment
        Modalities, 18; Needs and Priorities for Research on Treatment
        Services and Methods, 19
    The Two-Tiered Structure of the Treatment System, 21
    Public Financing of Drug Treatment, 22
        The Goals and Priorities of Public Coverage, 22; Federal and
        State Roles, 24; Mechanisms for Providing Public Support, 25;
        Utilization Management, 27

Private Coverage of Drug Treatment, 29
  Extent, Costs, and Trends of Coverage, 29; Mandating Drug
  Treatment Coverage, 30; Optimal Coverage Provisions, 30
Coda, 32

1 INTRODUCTION   33
   The Logic of the Report, 34
   Additional Policy Questions, 37
     Treating Adolescents and Women with Children, 37; The Criminal
     Justice System, 38; The Socioeconomic Environment, 38

2 IDEAS GOVERNING DRUG POLICY   40
   The Character of Governing Ideas, 41
   The Spectrum of Ideas About Drugs, 42
     Libertarian Ideas, 44; Medical and Criminal Ideas, 46; The Classic
     Era of Narcotics Control, 48
   The Rise of Modern Treatment, 49
     Methadone Maintenance, Therapeutic Communities, and
     Outpatient Nonmethadone Programs, 50; Chemical Dependency
     Treatment, 53; The Medical/Criminal Idea of Treatment and the
     Evolution of Governmental Roles, 53
   Conclusion, 56

3 THE NEED FOR TREATMENT   58
   The Individual Drug History: A Model and Overview, 59
     Abstinence, Drug Types, and Normative Attitudes, 62; Learning
     and Drug Experience, 64; Environmental Variations, 66; Age of
     Onset and Drug Sequencing, 68; Diagnosing Dependence and
     Abuse, 69; Recovery and Relapse, 72
   Estimating the Extent of the Need for Treatment, 76
     Household Survey Data, 77; Criminal Justice Populations, 81; The
     Homeless Population, 84; Pregnant Women, 85; Summary, 86
   Quantifying the Consequences, 88
   Conclusion, 90
   Appendix 3A   Estimating the Need for Treatment in the Household
   Population, 92
   Appendix 3B   Estimating the Need for Treatment Among
   Arrestees, 97
   Appendix 3C   Estimating the Costs of Drug Problems, 102
     Drug-related Crime—Victim Losses, 102; Crime Control
     Resources, 102; Employee Productivity Losses, 103; Health Costs,
     104

4 DEFINING THE GOALS OF TREATMENT   105
   Diverse Interests, 106
   Reasons for Seeking Treatment, 109

Criminal Justice Agencies and Treatment, 113
  Court Referral to Treatment, 114; Prison and Parole Referral to
  Treatment, 117; Preliminary Conclusions About "Mandatory
  Treatment," 119
Employers and Treatment, 120
  Employee Assistance Programs, 121; Drug Screening Programs,
  123; How Employers View Drug Treatment, 124
Ambivalence and the Spectrum of Recovery, 125
  Full, Partial, and Nonrecovery from Drug Problems, 126; Setting
  Realistic Goals, 128
Conclusion, 130

5   THE EFFECTIVENESS OF TREATMENT   132
Methadone Maintenance, 136
  What Is Methadone Maintenance?, 136; How Well Does
  Methadone Work?, 142; Why Do the Results of Methadone
  Treatment Vary?, 147; Costs and Benefits of Methadone
  Treatment, 151; Conclusions, 152
Therapeutic Communities, 154
  What Is a Therapeutic Community?, 154; How Well Do
  Therapeutic Communities Work?, 156; Why Do the Results of
  Therapeutic Communities Vary?, 163; Costs and Benefits of
  Therapeutic Community Treatment, 165; Conclusions, 166
Outpatient Nonmethadone Treatment, 167
  What Is Outpatient Nonmethadone Treatment?, 167; How Well
  Does Outpatient Nonmethadone Treatment Work?, 168; Why Do
  the Results of Outpatient Nonmethadone Treatment Vary?, 169;
  Benefits and Costs of Outpatient Nonmethadone Treatment, 170
Chemical Dependency Treatment, 170
  What Is Chemical Dependency Treatment?, 170; How Well Does
  Chemical Dependency Treatment Work?, 172; Why Do the
  Results of Chemical Dependency Treatment Vary?, 173; Benefits
  and Costs of Chemical Dependency Treatment, 174
Detoxification, 174
Correctional Treatment Programs, 176
  Stay'n Out and Cornerstone, 177; The California Civil Addict
  Program, 180; Boot Camps, 183; Conclusions about Prison
  Treatment, 184
Summary and Conclusions about Treatment Effectiveness, 185
  Methadone Maintenance, 187; Therapeutic Communities, 188;
  Outpatient Nonmethadone Programs, 189; Chemical Dependency
  Programs, 190; Detoxification, 190; Correctional Treatment, 191
Recommendations for Research on Treatment Services and
Methods, 192
  Rebuilding the Research Base, 192; Major Research Questions,
  194

6   TWO TIERS: PUBLIC AND PRIVATE SUPPLY   200
    The Two Tiers: An Overview, 201
        Financing Differences, 202; Client Differences, 205; Capacity
        Differences, 206
    The Growth of the National Treatment System, 206
        Trends in Client Numbers and Provider Characteristics, 206;
        Trends in the Funding Base, 210; Sources of Treatment Dollars,
        211; Trends in Federal Funding, 214
    Conclusion, 216

7   PUBLIC COVERAGE   220
    The Principles of Public Intervention, 221
        External Costs, 222; Income Constraints, 225; Positive Response to
        Treatment, 227; Balancing Treatment Needs and Cost Concerns,
        228
    From Principles to Priorities, 230
        Eliminate Waiting Lists, 232; Improve Treatment, 232; Reach
        More Young Mothers, 233; Induce More Criminal Justice Clients
        to Accept Treatment, 235
    Three Strategy Options, 235
        The Core Strategy Option, 237; Comprehensive and Intermediate
        Strategy Options, 238
    Public Intervention in the 1990s, 239
        Federal and State Roles in the 1970s, 240; The 1980s: Block
        Grants, 241; The 1990s: Appropriate Shifts in Federal and State
        Roles, 245; Transitional Steps Toward the Year 2000, 249;
        Utilization Management, 250
    The Special Case of Veterans' Coverage, 252
    Conclusions, 254
    Appendix 7A   Baseline and Strategy Option Calculations, 256
        Baseline Comparison Values, 256; Core Strategy Option, 257;
        Comprehensive Strategy Option, 260; Intermediate Strategy
        Option, 263
    Appendix 7B   Modeling Future Treatment Needs and Effects, 265
    Appendix 7C   Medicaid, 266
        Coverage Policy Determination Under Medicaid, 267; Eligibility,
        268; Coverage Provisions, 270; The Current and Future Status of
        Medicaid Coverage, 271

8   PRIVATE COVERAGE   273
    The Logic of Private Coverage, 276
    The Extent of Private Insurance Coverage, 277
        Employees of Private Companies, 278; State and Local
        Government Employees, 279; Federal Employees, 281; Employers
        and Coverage Decisions, 282
    Trends Affecting Private Coverage: Cost Containment of
    Health Benefits, 283

Private Insurance and State Mandates, 288
    Access to Coverage, 289; Adequacy of Coverage, 290; Cost
    Containment, 291; The Value of Additional Mandates, 292
Conclusions, 293
    Extent, Costs, and Trends of Coverage, 293; Mandating Drug
    Treatment Coverage, 294; Optimal Coverage Provisions, 294

CODA   298

REFERENCES   301

BIOGRAPHICAL SKETCHES OF COMMITTEE MEMBERS
AND STAFF   313

INDEX   321

Contents of Volume 2

COMMISSIONED PAPERS ON HISTORICAL, INSTITUTIONAL, AND ECONOMIC CONTEXTS OF DRUG TREATMENT

A Century of American Narcotic Policy
David T. Courtwright

Federal Leadership in Building the National Drug Treatment System
Karst J. Besteman

Drug Treatment in State Prisons
Gregory P. Falkin, Harry K. Wexler, and Douglas S. Lipton

Employee Assistance and Drug Screening Programs
Paul M. Roman and Terry C. Blum

Markets for Drug Treatment
Richard Steinberg

Cycles of Cocaine
Ronald K. Siegel

Acknowledgments

TREATING
DRUG
PROBLEMS

Summary

QUESTIONS THE REPORT ANSWERS
AND THOSE IT LEAVES UNRESOLVED
(CHAPTER 1)

The Anti-Drug Abuse Act of 1986 called for the Institute of Medicine (IOM) to conduct a study of the extent and adequacy of coverage by public programs, private insurance, and other sources of payment for the treatment and rehabilitation of drug abusers. The act also requested IOM to recommend the means by which the needs identified in the study could be addressed. In responding to this charge, the committee established to conduct the study has covered the following major questions in its report:

- The role of treatment—What is the role of treatment in the ideas that govern and shape drug policy? (Chapter 2)
- The need for treatment—In light of the patterns of drug consumption and consequent problems, what is the estimated extent of the need for drug treatment? (Chapter 3)
- The goals of treatment—What should drug treatment seek to accomplish in the context of treatment seekers' motives and medical-criminal drug policies? (Chapter 4)
- The effects of treatment—What are the available modalities of drug treatment? What are their expected and actual clinical accomplishments? Why do the results of treatment programs vary? What are their respective benefits and costs? (Chapter 5)

1

- The organization of treatment—How, in general, is the supply of treatment organized and financed? (Chapter 6)
- Public coverage—What is the rationale, the priorities, and the optimal level of public coverage of drug treatment? How can public coverage be best arranged and managed? (Chapter 7)
- Private coverage—What are the responsibilities of private coverage for drug treatment in terms of eligibility, benefit and service design, costs, and care management? (Chapter 8)

In answering these questions, and more detailed ones within each chapter, the committee relies on the preponderance of rigorous evidence (where enough evidence is available to be weighed) and judiciously uses expert judgment, including specification of the new knowledge needed to strengthen this judgment, where logic and experience point strongly but rigorous evidence is scant. In view of the severity and complexity of the drug problem and the public's determination to respond, the committee tries to recommend policy decisions regarding drug treatment that are most consistent with the current state of knowledge.

There are three important questions relevant to the drug problem that the committee returned to more than once but could not answer in this study. In one case, neither evidence nor experience were sufficient to counsel a specific judgment; in the other two cases, the questions—and the expertise and evidence needed to answer them—were outside the committee's charge and resources. The most urgent unanswered questions in this regard are the following:

- With sufficient resources and related services, would different drug treatment modalities than the ones now available be more effective for adolescents and mothers of younger children?
- How efficient and effective is the current distribution of criminal justice responses to the drug problem?
- How can society intervene more effectively in socioeconomic environments to prevent drug initiation and discourage rather than facilitate relapse?

IDEAS GOVERNING DRUG TREATMENT POLICY
(CHAPTER 2)

The national response to drugs has always been governed by simple, powerful ideas about the nature of the drug problem and how to control it (see Figure 2-1).[1]

---

[1] The tables and figures referred to in this summary appear in the chapters of the report.

- From Revolutionary times to the Reconstruction era, the drug problem was a minor concern, left at first to the realm of private behavior, and later managed in a loosely enforced regulatory framework; this approach derived from *libertarian* ideas.

- A *medical* conception of opiate and other addictions was formulated in the late 1800s, explaining clinical observations among drug-consuming older women and other groups. Various treatment approaches were devised, including detoxification and, where total abstinence was deemed unachievable, medically supervised maintenance.

- From 1910 to the 1920s, medical approaches were almost wholly swept aside by the rise of a *criminal* conception of the problem focusing on underworld characters who used heroin and other drugs. That conception held sway, with little effective challenge, for 40 years.

In the 1960s and 1970s, medical ideas reappeared in more sophisticated forms, taking much more explicit account of the various criminal contexts of drug use. During 1965–1975, a national medical-criminal treatment policy was made viable chiefly by the emergence of promising new treatment modalities: methadone maintenance and therapeutic communities for heroin and outpatient nonmethadone programs oriented toward nonopiate drugs. In the same period the federal government sponsored the buildup of a substantial public tier of community-based drug treatment programs. This system of programs was the leading edge of national drug policy, complementing criminal justice efforts in responding to drug-related crime.

Other factors that contributed to the reemergence of medical ideas were a shift in attitudes during the "Great Society" period that brought a greater assumption of collective responsibility for the casualties of socioeconomic forces. This shift was followed by the Nixon administration's energetic search for responses to large-scale unrest, particularly the social problems of increasing crime and heroin use.

From 1975 to 1986, federal dollar support for drug treatment eroded, although states moved to replace this support to some degree. The growth of the community-based public tier of treatment stopped while the criminal justice system as a whole entered a period of unprecedented sustained increase. The momentum of medical ideas shifted to a rapidly expanding private tier. In the 1980s, chemical dependency programs, largely comprising hospital-based alcohol treatment providers, began treating growing numbers of heavy alcohol and drug consumers (mostly of cocaine and marijuana) who could afford to pay with private insurance coverage or personal assets.

The public tier of drug treatment has been the neglected front in the drug wars of the 1980s. In formulating the federal anti-drug abuse legislation of 1986 and 1988, the great bulk of the debate and the new sums actually spent were directed toward enforcement against traffickers and prevention among nonusers. Outside of concern with isolating the growing acquired immune deficiency syndrome (AIDS) epidemic, public treatment was all but ignored.

With the rise in alarm about crack-affected children and neighborhoods, however, the pendulum of public policy is once again moving. Modalities of treatment attuned to medical-criminal ideas again seem increasingly attractive. It is becoming widely appreciated that the drug problem does not lend itself to simple characterization or solution, that a combination of ideas and policies is the most fruitful way to respond to it, and that treatment programs can and should reflect this principle of combination.

DRUG PROBLEMS AND THE NEED FOR DRUG TREATMENT (CHAPTER 3)

Patterns of Drug Consumption

The nation's drug problem is a complicated evolving composite of millions of individual patterns of drug-consuming behavior and consequences that may differ according to time and place and that change as the marketing, technology, and reputations of drugs evolve. Crack-cocaine, heroin, marijuana, amphetamines, and all other illicit drugs are consumed in patterns that range from experimental use to dependence. To determine the extent of need for treatment in the population, drug consumers must be categorized based on the frequency and amount of their drug consumption and the severity of associated problems and consequences.

A conceptual paradigm of individual drug consumption, consequences, and societal responses is presented in Figure 3-1. Although individual patterns are not always so orderly, patterns or types of drug taking in this simplified scheme occur in progressive stages of use, abuse, and dependence, each more hazardous and intrusive than the one before. Each stage entails the risk of further progression, but progression is not inevitable. A minority of experimental users reach the stage of abuse, fewer yet the stage of dependence.

The bulk of initial, experimental drug use occurs during the teenage years. Very few children aged 10 or younger have begun to use drugs. Nearly as few people begin using drugs—or even any particular type of drug, unless it was never previously available—after reaching 25 years of age.

For many years, the introduction to drugs in the great majority of cases that go on to further stages has proceeded in a general cumulative sequence: alcohol and tobacco, to marijuana, to other inhalable or orally ingestible substances, to hypodermic injection of opiates or powerful stimulants (cocaine, amphetamines). This sequence is almost always initiated between the ages of 12 and 15, and the injection phase, when reached, generally begins between the ages of 17 and 20. The sequencing phenomenon is thought to reflect drug availability and the degree of opprobrium attached to respective types of drugs. However, as the marketing of cocaine continues to expand and that of marijuana diminishes, the sequence of introduction to these drugs may become less uniform.

The mixture of drug effects that consumers seek or are satisfied with tends to change subtly over time, moving *typically* from just "getting high" or being sociable in the early stage of use to the achievement of temporary relief from the persistent desire or learned need for a drug (which persists even after short-term withdrawal is completed) in the stage of dependence. Drug-seeking behavior is highly volitional during initiation and continuation of use, although profoundly influenced by the environment. But the initial voluntary component of drug-seeking behavior is typically compromised by the psychological, physiological, and social aspects of the dependence process, which dramatically increases the probability that treatment will be needed to extinguish drug-seeking behavior.

Dependence

Dependence (not only on illicit substances but also on such licit agents as alcohol and tobacco) is the most extreme pattern of drug consumption. It is the persistent seeking and consumption of one or more types of drugs in excessive amounts, despite such high costs as the accumulation of harm to health and functioning, viewed broadly by social standards and judged specifically according to clinical diagnostic criteria. The most severely drug-impaired individuals are dependent on one drug and make heavy use of one or more others (including alcohol), perhaps to the point of multiple dependencies. Many such individuals also have serious mental illnesses and medical complications.

There is a range of individual vulnerability to drug dependence when environmental conditions are held constant. But social environments are not constant, and variation in environmental conditions correlates strongly with ecological variation in drug dependence rates.

Recovery and Relapse

Drug dependence is characteristically a chronic, relapsing disorder. Drug abuse often assumes this character as well, but not as often. Dependent drug-seeking behavior and the strong desire or craving for drugs that is its subjective aspect are difficult to lose completely, or extinguish, once they have been established. It is easier to complete detoxification (the short-term transition from being acutely dependent to being free of dependence symptoms) than it is to sustain that asymptomatic state beyond the short term—that is, to avoid relapse. Nevertheless, individuals can successfully put a complete stop to an established pattern of chronic dependent behavior. Not only can they safely stop using drugs in the short term, with or without formal assistance, but they can also avoid the recurrence of drug seeking that ends in relapse. This extinguishing of individual drug-seeking behavior is the most fundamental element in the recovery process.

Studies of the life history of dependent individuals indicate that there is usually a complicated path to recovery. Individuals with severe problems (including deficits in their social environment) that precede their drug dependence or abuse—for example, family disintegration, lack of legitimate job skills or opportunities, illiteracy, or psychiatric disorders—will probably continue to have these problems unless specific services are available to deal with them. These individuals are also at intrinsically high risk of relapse.

Many individuals are too damaged by the consequences of drug dependence or other factors, too bereft of alternative behavioral skills and supports, to complete (sometimes even to begin) the recovery process without lengthy or continuing help in coping with psychological, social, economic, or pharmacological problems. For these individuals, recovery is not only a matter of extinguishing drug-seeking behavior but also of addressing directly a range of functional impairments that usually preceded drug seeking and were worsened by it. Recovering functionality in society to whatever degree is possible is a more comprehensive definition of recovery.

Treatment of drug problems, therefore, often addresses itself not only to drug consumption as such but also to the chronic personal impairments and social and economic deficits that often characterize those who enter treatment. Individuals without accompanying problems, who have long-term assets such as a stable job and supportive family, are not likely to need specific adjunctive services and have been found to be intrinsically less likely to relapse.

It is characteristic of recovery processes from any type of drug dependence that, although many people do recover, recovery is seldom achieved, or even begun, before the individual recognizes that he or she has suffered and caused significant personal and social harm—an understanding that often requires overcoming a strong tendency to denial. The more severe and prolonged the periods of dependence or severe abuse, the greater the need for help in extinguishing drug-consuming behavior.

Autonomous cessation, or self-recovery, although not uncommon, is not universal. Many, probably the majority, of those who are dependent or severe abusers relapse after their first (and later) attempts at self-recovery. Most people who enter drug treatment have tried self-recovery previously but did not succeed. Most people who recover after treatment do so after more than one treatment episode.

Determining the Need for Treatment

Drug treatment is (or in most cases should be) an intensive, personalized intervention. Treatment is not an appropriate or efficient response to the most common patterns of drug consumption, namely, experimental and occasional use, and may not be needed in cases of abuse in which impairment is slight or the pattern of abuse is new. Other interventions, such as brief preventive counseling, educational services, and disciplinary sanctions, may be legitimate, useful, or effective in promoting cessation and abstinence in these instances.

Formal diagnostic criteria for determining the appropriateness of treatment have evolved over the years and now encompass a constellation of drug-related problems rather than focusing exclusively on classical signs such as tolerance and withdrawal symptoms. Practice in diagnosis is highly variable; nevertheless, the majority of individuals entering drug treatment programs are dependent or severe abusers by any reasonably discriminating criteria.

In the committee's judgment, drug treatment is justified and appropriate for an individual if there are clinically significant signs of dependence or chronic abuse. Assessment of individual problem severity and the degree of help needed for recovery is thus exceedingly important. These factors are usually but not always taken into account in matching individual treatment seekers with appropriate modalities and in "fine-tuning" treatment by choosing among specific therapeutic components.

Estimating the Aggregate Need for Treatment

An estimated 5.5 million Americans clearly or probably need treatment at this time, which is somewhat more than 2 percent of the total population over 12 years of age. About one-fifth of the estimated population needing treatment—and two-fifths of those who clearly need it—are under the supervision of the criminal justice system as parolees, probationers, or inmates (see Table 3-4).

In the household population not under criminal justice supervision, those clearly or probably needing drug treatment are two-thirds male and heavily concentrated among adults aged 18 to 34. Youths under the age of 18 make up about 9 percent (about 400,000 persons) of the total household group needing treatment, and adults over 34 account for about 16 percent (roughly, 725,000 persons). Most of the household adults—75 percent—hold some type of job at least part of the time, 10 percent are unemployed (twice the national average), and 15 percent are in school, retired, disabled, or carrying household responsibilities.

Current survey and surveillance data indicate that, although lighter drug consumption—experimental and occasional use—is becoming less prevalent, the problem of severe drug abuse and dependence is growing larger, more difficult, and more costly. The difficulties are due both to the expanded menu of drugs that are now widely consumed—most prominently, marijuana and cocaine, barbiturates and other depressants, amphetamines and PCP in some parts of the country, and heroin—and to the complications induced by AIDS, chronic unemployment, and extended family disintegration in the inner cities. Because of the complex, protean, time-extended character of the drug problem, aggregate treatment needs are not necessarily closely linked to the current overall societal prevalence of drug involvement. Total social costs are especially difficult to estimate, being subject to many uncertainties of measurement. The costs of drug problems in the form of treatment for AIDS, prevention programs, and drug treatment programs are not insubstantial, but they are clearly much smaller than the costs incurred as a result of drug-related crime.

THE GOALS OF DRUG TREATMENT
(CHAPTER 4)

To know whether treatment is appropriate and whether the money it costs is well spent, the goals of treatment need to be made explicit. Lifetime abstinence from all illicit drug consumption is the central goal of drug treatment. However, in light of the chronic, complex nature of drug problems, the more pragmatic day-to-day objective is to reduce illicit drug consumption by as large a fraction as possible relative to the consumption one might expect in the absence of treatment. Reduction of illicit drug consumption produces socially and personally valuable results and may serve as a critical intermediate step to lifetime abstinence. A useful shorthand for the pragmatic goal of drug treatment is that it tries to initiate, accelerate, and help sustain the recovery process.

The goals of the treatment delivery system are not confined to reducing the drug consumption of specific individuals. These goals, assigned overtly or implicitly by public policy or private payers, are multiple and may include the following:

- reduce the overall demand for illicit drugs;
- reduce street crime;
- change users' personal values;
- develop educational or vocational capabilities;

- restore or increase employment or productivity;
- improve the user's overall health, psychological functioning, and family life; and
- reduce fetal exposure to drug dependence.

Success in achieving one set of these goals may be related to but is not equal to success in achieving the others. Generally, the more severely the user is impaired with respect to these various goals when he or she enters treatment, the more services will be needed for drug treatment to be effective.

Motivations for Treatment

The nature and success of drug treatment is complicated by the typical reluctance of dependent or abusing individuals to seek treatment or stay in it. The main reason for this reluctance is that drug consumers like drugs; drugs "work" for them and provide the effects they seek, which vary from pleasure to relief. Drug dependence or abuse, in and of itself, is often not what sends people to treatment, at least, not initially. Individuals often enter treatment as a strategy of partial rather than full recovery—that is, to help manage serious problems with the law, their family, their mental or physical health, other drug consumers or dealers, a threat involving criminal justice supervision, or an abrupt loss of customary income. In other words, they may enter treatment to establish better control over their drug behavior or its consequences but not necessarily to extinguish the behavior entirely. Another factor that contributes to some individuals' reluctance to enter or stay in treatment is that drug treatment is often demanding, imposing schedules and controls and requiring extensive work on the part of the client to overcome social deficits and heal psychological impairments.

Overall, because of the inherent disinclination toward drug treatment, some form of perceived threat or pressure is nearly always present as a triggering element when treatment is sought. The pressure can derive from an internal or an external problem, which is usually but not necessarily a direct consequence of drugs. The most common internal pressure is the cumulative and demoralizing realization that the increasing trouble that comes with sustained drug abuse or dependence leads to a dead end.

Clients formulate exterior motives for entering treatment as "to get [someone] off my case." External pushes are usually allied to some degree of positive pull or motivation to change. The positive motives are often not strong enough in themselves to initiate or sustain recovery, but reinforcement though external pushes into treatment and therapeutic pressure within treatment can be effective in doing so. The specific mixture and source of motives vary with the circumstances. For someone with a high-paying, prestigious job, the direct threat of losing that livelihood and position can carry a great deal of weight. For someone who is unemployed and unskilled, no threat short of a long prison sentence may carry a comparable degree of weight or pressure. The civil liberties implications of this inequity are troubling, but such is currently the state of affairs.

Treatment and Criminal Justice

The treatment system and crime control systems in this country share important goals—especially, the attainment of less criminal and drug-involved lives by their clientele. On a given day, out of 1 million persons in confinement, there are probably 40,000 individuals in jail or prison custody who are also in drug treatment programs. More broadly, many courts and correctional systems use commitment or referral to community-based treatment programs, usually ones involving close supervision, as alternatives or adjuncts to probation or parole status. Half or more of the admissions to typical community-based residential and outpatient drug treatment programs (except perhaps for methadone) are on probation or parole when they enter treatment. These statistics are a direct manifestation of the criminal-medical policy idea regarding the drug problem.

The criminal justice system is already the largest single source of external pressure on individuals leading them to enter drug treatment. In most cases, the court (or another criminal justice agency) has simply ordered the individual to stay free of drugs and crime or else be remanded to custody. In this instance the individual chooses to seek treatment under the assumption that avoiding drug use (or at least avoiding abuse or dependence, which are far more troublesome and difficult to conceal) will be facilitated by treatment. In more direct cases the court or other agency offers the client a choice, generally between a term in prison and a period of probation or parole with treatment.

Criminal justice referral to treatment occurs for several reasons, including relief of court and prison overcrowding. Treatment takes responsibility for a case somewhat out of the criminal justice system, reduces the high cost of continuing incarceration, and assures a degree of supervision beyond what probation or parole offices may be able to afford. When referral occurs to relieve overcrowding, however, the stipulation "go to treatment and comply with the program *or risk being returned to custody*" loses its credibility. The more overcrowded and strained the criminal justice system, the less pressure it can muster to help push any particular individual into seeking and complying with treatment.

There is frequent favorable reference today to "mandatory," "compulsory," or "required" treatment. Contrary to earlier fears among clinicians, criminal justice pressure does not necessarily vitiate treatment effectiveness and probably improves retention. Yet the most important reason to consider these or related schemes to compel more of the criminal justice population to seek treatment is not that coercion may improve the results of treatment but that treatment may improve the rather dismal record of plain coercion—particularly imprisonment—in reducing the level of intensively criminal behavior that ensues when the coercive grip is relaxed.

EFFECTIVENESS OF TREATMENT
(CHAPTER 5)

In the context of a medical-criminal policy, the practical objective of treatment at present is primarily to reduce illicit drug consumption and other criminal activity, secondarily to increase success in conventional activities such as employment and child rearing, and to improve health status, including, most recently, reducing AIDS risk behavior among clients. The standard for success is whether behavior during and after treatment is appreciably better than what would probably occur in the absence of treatment.

Does drug treatment achieve these goals? It varies; for a more discriminating answer, it is necessary to pose a more sophisticated set of questions.

• *What are the basic concepts or modalities of treatment*? That is, what are the underlying designs or theories of treatment, what specific types of drug problems or population groups are being addressed by each design, and what are the best results that have been obtained under ideal conditions?

• *How well does each modality work in practice? If a modality works less well than might be expected, what are the reasons for this variance*? For example, is the implementation or replication of the modality flawed or incomplete? Are the wrong kinds of clients being treated? Are there unexpected side effects? Does the environment neutralize the effectiveness of the treatment?

• *Do the benefits of treatment justify the costs*? In other words, is treatment a good investment?

• In addition to the above questions about treatment as it exists: *How might further research help to improve treatment*?

All of these questions must be asked, but they cannot all be answered at present. There are four major modalities of drug treatment for which answers of varying confidence can be supplied: methadone maintenance clinics, residential therapeutic communities, outpatient nonmethadone treatment, and chemical dependency units. The most extensive and scientifically best-developed evidence concerns methadone maintenance. A lower although still suggestive level of evidence is available for therapeutic communities and outpatient nonmethadone programs. An even lower level of evidence is available for drug treatment in the chemical dependency modality. Except for a description of the model, there are virtually no data to answer any of the critical questions for the quasi-treatment modality of mutual self-help groups, such as Narcotics Anonymous.

The most extensive usable results of research on the effectiveness of drug treatment are from several planned experiments and natural or quasi-experiments and from prospective longitudinal studies involving thousands of clients. There have been two large-scale, multisite, federally sponsored studies: the Drug Abuse Reporting Program (DARP), a 12-year follow-up of a 1969–1971 national admission sample cohort, and the Treatment Outcome Prospective Study (TOPS), which involved a 10,000-person national sample of 1979–1981 admissions to 41 drug treatment programs in 10 cities, followed for up to 5 years. DATOS (the Drug Abuse Treatment Outcome Study), a third large-scale national prospective study, is scheduled to begin in 1990; important related studies are under way.

Drug users and treatment programs do a substantial amount of selection according to client characteristics and modality. The modalities were designed for different types and severities of problems, and prospective clients often have very set ideas about what type of treatment they want. As a result, the profiles of clients admitted to the major modalities are quite different, and one cannot compare the performance or results of each modality with the others as if they were all simply interchangeable.

Methadone Maintenance

Methadone maintenance is a treatment for extended dependence on opiate drugs (usually heroin). A sufficient daily oral dose of methadone hydrochloride, which is a relatively long-acting narcotic analgesic, yields a very stable metabolic level of the drug. Once a newly admitted client has reached a stable, comfortable, noneuphoric state, without the psychophysiological cues that precipitate opiate craving, he or she is amenable to counseling, environmental changes, and other social services that can help shift his or her orientation and lifestyle away from drug seeking and related crime toward more socially acceptable behaviors.

Methadone programs are nearly always ambulatory, with daily visits to swallow the methadone dose under observation in the clinic, except for traditional Sunday take-home doses. After several months in the program with a "clean" drug testing record and good compliance with other program requirements, one or more daily doses may be regularly taken home between less-than-daily visits; however, this convenience is a revocable privilege. Some methadone clients voluntarily reduce their doses to abstinence and conclude treatment after some time, whereas others remain on methadone indefinitely, particularly if earlier attempts to leave methadone have ended in relapse.

Methadone maintenance has been the most rigorously studied modality and has yielded the most positive results for those who seek it. Yet it is also the most controversial treatment, largely based on the judgmental grounds that methadone clients have "merely" switched their dependence to a legal narcotic and that many clients continue to use heroin and other drugs intermittently and to commit crimes, including the sale of their take-home methadone.

In the committee's judgment, these controversies and reservations are neither trivial nor in themselves compelling. Methadone is an opiate drug, but consumption of a stable, clinically appropriate oral methadone dose is not behaviorally or subjectively intoxicating and does not impair functioning in clinically detectable ways. Toxic side effects during long-term treatment are extremely rare, and the general health of methadone clients improves markedly compared with their status when using heroin. Prior to admission, the great majority of methadone clients had been consuming high levels of illicit drugs and committing other crimes (including drug selling) on a daily basis. Some programs have very good and others very poor client compliance with rules against illicit drug use and criminal activity.

The issues are to what extent undesirable behaviors are reduced and positive behaviors increased as a result of methadone maintenance, in comparison to no treatment or to alternative measures, and whether poorly performing programs can be improved. Regarding behavior and treatment, the extensive evaluation literature on methadone maintenance yields firm conclusions as follows:

- There is strong evidence from clinical trials and similar study designs that opiate-dependent individuals have better outcomes on average in terms of illicit drug consumption and other criminal behavior when maintained on methadone than when not treated at all, when simply detoxified and released, or when methadone is tapered down and terminated as a result of client request, program expulsion, or program closure.
- Methadone clinics have significantly higher retention rates for opiate-dependent populations than do other treatment modalities for similar clients.

• Although methadone dosages need to be clinically monitored and individually optimized, clients have better outcomes when stabilized on higher rather than lower doses within the typical ranges currently prescribed (30 to 100 milligrams per day).

• Following discharge from methadone treatment, clients who stayed in treatment longer have better outcomes than clients with shorter treatment courses.

It is important to note that most of these results date from the 1970s to the early 1980s. Since then, the expanding cocaine market has created additional strains on many methadone programs. Methadone has no direct pharmacological bearing on the metabolism of cocaine (as it does on that of opiates); in addition, most methadone programs' counseling and other clinical resources have been substantially eroded or limited as a result of fiscal constraints. Moreover, the high seroprevalence of human immunodeficiency virus (HIV), which is generally acquired long before program admission, and the prevalence of AIDS symptoms and deaths create a heavy medical and psychological burden on methadone programs (and others, such as therapeutic communities, which serve the most severely impaired drug-using groups) in cities in which the AIDS epidemic is far advanced.

Therapeutic Communities

Therapeutic communities (TCs) are residential programs with expected stays generally of 9 to 12 months, phasing into independent residence with continuing contact for a variable period. TC programs are highly structured blends of resocialization, milieu therapy, behavioral modification practices, progression through a hierarchy of occupational training and responsibility within the TC, community reentry, and a variety of social services. TCs originally used very rigid program models and relied extensively on recovering "graduates" as program staff. They have become more flexible in program design and more multidisciplinary in staffing over time while retaining their core features, including an absolute prohibition on any drug use or violent behavior by clients during treatment.

Therapeutic community clients are more diverse in their drug use patterns than methadone clients because the modality is not specific to any particular class of drugs. From the 1960s to the early 1980s, a majority of TC clients were primarily dependent on heroin. In the later 1980s, cocaine dependence began to predominate in many programs. Therapeutic communities are designed for individuals with major impairments and social deficits, including histories of serious criminal behavior.

The primary conclusions on therapeutic communities are as follows:

- TC clients demonstrate better behavior (drug use, criminal activity, social productivity) during treatment and after discharge than before admission.
- The minimum retention necessary to yield posttreatment improvement in long-term users seems to be at least 3 months, with further improvement continuing to be evident for full-time treatment of up to 12 to 18 months.
- TC clients demonstrate better outcomes at follow-up than individuals who contacted but did not enter the same treatment programs.
- Graduates of TCs have better outcomes at follow-up than dropouts from the same programs.
- The length of stay in a TC is the strongest predictor of outcomes at follow-up.
- Attrition from TCs is typically high—above the rates for methadone maintenance but below the rates for outpatient nonmethadone treatment.

Outpatient Nonmethadone Programs

Outpatient nonmethadone programs display a great deal of heterogeneity in their treatment processes, philosophies, and staffing. The clients are generally not opiate dependent but otherwise vary across all types of drugs. They also tend to have less serious criminal histories than methadone or TC clients and to include more nondependent individuals. Outpatient nonmethadone programs generally provide one or two visits per week for individual or group psychotherapy/counseling, with an expected course averaging about six months.

Despite the heterogeneity of programs and their clients, the limited number of outcome evaluations of outpatient nonmethadone programs have generated conclusions qualitatively similar to those from studies of TCs:

- Outpatient nonmethadone clients during and following treatment show better performance than before treatment.
- Those clients actually admitted to programs have better outcomes than clients contacting but not entering programs (and clients only undergoing detoxification).
- Graduates have better outcomes than dropouts.
- Outcome at follow-up is positively related to length of stay in treatment.
- Retention in nonmethadone outpatient programs tends to be poorer than for methadone maintenance or therapeutic communities.

Chemical Dependency Programs

Chemical dependency (CD) programs generally are residential or in-patient, with a three- to six-week duration, followed by up to two years of attending self-help groups or a weekly outpatient therapy group. CD programs are based on an Alcoholics Anonymous (12-step) model of personal change and the belief that vulnerability to dependence is a permanent but controllable disability. Its goals are those of total abstinence and lifestyle alteration.

Chemical dependency programs largely treat primary alcoholism, and they have not been carefully evaluated for treatment of drug problems. A few follow-up studies of individuals who have completed CD treatment indicate that clients whose primary problem is drugs have poorer outcomes than clients whose primary problem involves alcohol.

CD programs are often located in hospitals. In the committee's judgment, none of the model therapeutic core elements of this modality require the presence of acute care hospital services. There is no evidence that hospital-based CD programs are either more or less effective for drug problems than CD programs not sited in hospitals.

Detoxification

Detoxification is therapeutically supervised withdrawal to abstinence over a short term, that is, up to 21 days but usually 5 to 7 days, often using pharmacological agents to reduce client discomfort or the likelihood of medical complications. Detoxification is seldom effective in itself as a modality for bringing about recovery from dependence, although it can be used as a gateway to other treatment modalities. Detoxification episodes are often hospital based and may begin with emergency treatment of an overdose. However, clinicians generally advocate that, because of the narrow and short-term focus and very poor outcomes in terms of relapse to drug dependence, detoxification not be considered a modality of treatment in the same sense as methadone, TCs, outpatient nonmethadone, and CD programs.

Much drug detoxification (an estimated 100,000 admissions annually) is now taking place in hospital beds. It is doubtful that hospitalization (especially beyond the first day or two) is necessary in most cases, except for the special problems of addicted neonates, serious sedative dependence, and concurrent medical or severe psychiatric problems, and for clients with a documented history of complications or flight. In this committee's judgment, detoxification may be undertaken successfully in most cases on a nonhospital residential, partial day care, or ambulatory basis.

Variations in Effectiveness of Programs Within Modalities

Effectiveness measurement was a critical early issue in the development of the drug treatment system. Data from the 1970s indicated that client retention and discharge status varied significantly across geographic areas. Aside from methadone studies, however, there is no published literature examining whether these differences were systematically related to client characteristics or to differences in the therapeutic process—or, indeed, whether such variations might be expected to occur as a result of chance.

Studies of methadone treatment indicate that program characteristics such as inadequate methadone dosage levels, staff turnover rates, and differences among counselors (which are not fully defined) are significantly related to differences in client performance while in treatment. Currently, however, program effectiveness measures are virtually unused in the management of the treatment system.

Treatment in Prisons

About 30 percent of state prison inmates report drug consumption patterns serious enough to indicate a need for treatment. According to the most recent (1986) sample survey of state penitentiaries, 15 percent of all inmates reported some episode of voluntary drug treatment *while in prison* (during the individual's current or previous confinement). At least two-thirds of prison treatment episodes are probably equivalent to the outpatient nonmethadone modality—periodic individual or group therapy sessions. The other episodes are similar to stays in a therapeutic community, including separation from the general prison population for the expected 6 to 12 months until graduation from the program.

Because the correctional system has custody of so many individuals in need of treatment, it would seem to be an important site for drug treatment programs, and numerous such programs have been established at various times over the years. Most prison drug treatment programs studied, including specialized "boot camp" or "shock incarceration" facilities, have not reduced the typically high postrelease rates of recidivism (return to criminal behavior) among untreated prisoners. However, a small number of controlled prospective studies of well-established prison TCs with strong linkages to community-based treatment programs indicate that prison TCs can reduce the treated group's rate of *rearrest* by a worthwhile margin. These studies also yield, within the treated group, the strong correlations between outcome and length of retention in treatment that are found in studies of community-based modalities.

Costs and Benefits of Treatment

There is qualified evidence that methadone maintenance, therapeutic communities, and outpatient nonmethadone treatment are cost-beneficial. The qualification is necessary because, first, there have been very few cost/benefit studies; second, although those performed have been consistent in finding positive results, they have not been derived from fully controlled clinical trials but rather from controlled observational studies.

Methadone treatment, when implemented at the resource levels observed in the late 1970s, provides individual and social benefits over a term of at least several years that are substantially higher than the costs of delivering this treatment. The benefits of TC treatment are also substantial, but the short-term costs are higher than those of methadone treatment, yielding generally somewhat lower benefit/cost ratios but ones that still favor the use of this treatment. The benefits of outpatient treatment are smaller than those of methadone or TC treatment, but the cost of the treatment is low and the yields thus are favorable. There are no cost/benefit analyses for chemical dependency programs, detoxification, or prison-based treatment.

Comparison of Data on Effectiveness and Expenditures for the Major Treatment Modalities

Table 5-6 summarizes, for the four principal treatment modalities, the type and amount of available treatment effectiveness data, from the most rigorously conducted randomized clinical trials,[2] to natural experiments, to controlled observation studies using multivariate analysis (the DARP and TOPS), to simple studies of treatment cohorts with limited comparisons and analyses. Methadone has received far more analysis than any other modality, followed by therapeutic communities and outpatient nonmethadone. Chemical dependency programs have had by far the least study.

In contrast to the weight of the effectiveness data are the numbers of clients treated by different modalities and the annual revenues (discussed more extensively in Chapter 6). Chemical dependency is the treatment modality with the highest revenues, probably the second largest number of clients, and the smallest scientific basis for assessing its effectiveness. Outpatient nonmethadone programs treat more clients than all other modalities

---

[2] The scientific attractiveness of clinical trials of a treatment versus a placebo or of treatment A versus treatment B is clear in principle, but such trials have proven very difficult to conduct with the major modalities of drug treatment. The modalities are quite different (and therefore hard to make "blind" to clients or clinicians), require extended duration (creating attrition problems), involve reluctant and socially troubled clients (leading to difficulties in achieving random assignment, compliance, and retention), and deal with complicated prognoses, especially owing to the chronic, relapsing nature of the problem (creating problems of participant selection, measurement, and comparability).

combined, and although there have been two major studies (DARP and TOPS) that examined the effectiveness of multiple programs, the literature on this modality does not adequately deal with the diversity of treatments and client differences subsumed in this category. Methadone maintenance has been studied much more extensively than any other modality, has the smallest annual revenues of the four major modalities, and is appropriate only for long-term treatment of opiate-dependent individuals. Therapeutic communities have been studied much more than outpatient nonmethadone programs but substantially less than methadone programs.

Needs and Priorities for Research on Treatment Services and Methods

Research on drug treatment is a core responsibility of the National Institute on Drug Abuse (NIDA) and has been a roughly constant proportion of NIDA's program for a number of years. NIDA's total research funding declined by nearly half in real terms from 1974 to 1983, but it has greatly increased since then and is projected to reach triple the 1983 level in 1990.

Major treatment research questions that need to be addressed for the major modalities of public treatment are the following: What client and program factors influence treatment-seeking behavior, treatment retention and efficacy, and relapse after treatment? How can these factors be better managed? Treatment-seeking factors include community outreach, family and employer interventions, and program intake and triage procedures. Retention and efficacy factors include optimal durations and schedules, pretreatment motivations, counselor or therapist behavior, incentives and conditions of employment, clinic procedures, criminal justice contingencies, and ancillary services. Posttreatment factors include relapse prevention interventions, abstinence monitoring, and environmental reinforcement.

Despite the difficulties of maintaining the integrity of controlled experiments in treatment programs, these studies provide the most incontrovertible evidence about comparative treatment effects, and efforts to conduct them should be strongly encouraged. A more detailed understanding of treatment processes through ethnographic and case study methods is also badly needed. This work is the basis for the design and interpretation of survey instruments.

Studies should be initiated within as well as across each major treatment modality to answer the following question: What are the relations of treatment performance (that is, differential outcomes, taking initial client characteristics into account), the content and organization of treatment (specific site arrangements, service offerings, therapeutic approaches, staffing practices), and the costs of treatment?

Health services research is a critical element in building treatment systems. An important foundation for services research as well as program accountability is the development, maintenance, and analysis of a system of data acquisition on treatment programs and client performance. Results from these kinds of studies will permit more fully optimal, cost-effective selection of facility quality, staff salary and training levels, services coordination methods, intensity of services, and other components.

Systems of this sort were established in the 1970s but were effectively disassembled as a matter of federal policy in the 1980s. **Treatment data acquisition systems must be rebuilt and effectively managed and utilized if the improvement of treatment knowledge and practice is to be evaluated and facilitated in the 1990s. Data on treatment effectiveness and costs should become the cornerstone of decisions about treatment coverage by public and private programs.**

Chemical dependency programs are the least well studied of the drug treatment modalities. The aggressive marketing that many such programs have deployed has created suspicion about these programs in many quarters that cannot be allayed without investment in objective treatment research and evaluation. The optimal site of delivery and length of programming, including the duration of intensive treatment and aftercare periods, and the inclusion of specific therapeutic elements need to be more closely investigated.

Only a few chemical dependency treatment providers have played positive roles in providing data and research opportunities for effectiveness studies; many more need to do so in order to answer these questions: What is the effectiveness of chemical dependency treatment for drug-impaired clients of varying characteristics? Are there variations in program effectiveness, and if so, why? What are the actual costs and benefits of the most effective components of chemical dependency treatment?

The major efforts to date to investigate treatment efficacy occurred prior to the epidemiological reemergence of cocaine in the 1980s. There is reason to believe that some findings about treatment modalities—such as the importance of time in treatment—will prove robust in the face of changing drug markets, but others may not. **The infrastructure of treatment research centers decayed during the stagnation of drug research funding, and as this capability is rebuilt, it should specifically address the following questions about cocaine treatment: What are the most effective treatment elements for cocaine dependence and abuse? To what degree can current modalities be effective for crack-cocaine? What new or existing pharmacological and nonpharmacological treatment elements can improve the clinical picture?**

The majority of individuals in treatment are young adult males (20 to 40 years old), and their responses dominate treatment research statistics. The major findings of research to date on the effectiveness of different modalities and elements of treatment seem to apply roughly as well to adolescents and women with young children (including pregnant women) as to the more prevalent demographic groups. However, the potential significance of child-rearing/child-bearing women and young clients in terms of the future benefits of present treatment (or future costs of present nontreatment) is great. Research plans in all areas need to devote special attention to differentiated knowledge about these populations. The committee recommends that a special study initiative be undertaken by the National Institute on Drug Abuse, in conjunction with other relevant agencies of the Public Health Service, on the treatment of drug abuse and dependence among adolescents and women who are pregnant or rearing young children.

THE TWO-TIERED STRUCTURE OF THE TREATMENT SYSTEM (CHAPTER 6)

There are two highly contrasting tiers of treatment programs—a public and a private—distinguished fundamentally by their mode of financing. This distinction generates and sustains differences in clientele, services offered, and current readiness to accommodate new admissions.

As reported in a 1987 survey, the public tier supplied 636,000 treatment episodes with revenues of $791 million, about four-fifths financed by public funds; it comprised largely not-for-profit and some publicly owned outpatient clinics (2,434 nonmethadone and 267 methadone), more than 900 residential programs, 159 public hospitals, and 72 prison programs (see Table 6-1). This tier served mostly indigent clients, and in high-prevalence parts of the country it was at or above effective capacity.

The public tier was developed about 20 years ago with federal leadership, a role that has largely shifted to the states, few of which have come close to covering the big reductions in federal contributions that have taken place since 1975. This tier continues to treat as many individuals as in the past but with less adequate facilities, services, and personnel. It is operating short of current demand in some but not all parts of the country.

The private tier in 1987 supplied 212,000 drug treatment episodes with revenues of $521 million, three-fourths from privately paid fees and reimbursements; it comprised 801 proprietary and not-for-profit hospital programs (offering in almost all cases chemical dependency treatment), 331 for-profit outpatient programs, 76 proprietary residential programs, and 67 methadone programs.

The private tier treats mainly insured working-class, middle-class, and upper class cocaine and marijuana clients (within a larger program serving mostly alcohol clients); in most instances it has been treating drug cases for less than 10 years and has grown very rapidly. Per diem charges in private-tier outpatient programs (methadone and nonmethadone) appear similar to those in the public tier, but residential and hospital per diem charges are three to four times greater. The private tier reports abundant reserve capacity.

In 1987, reports of reserve treatment capacity were highest (more than 50 percent above the current census) in private and public hospitals and in private-tier residential facilities; reserve capacity was lowest in public-tier methadone and outpatient facilities. There were substantial regional differences in public-tier availability; when these are taken into account, it appears that some areas of the country are sorely pressed for public residential treatment as well.

There is a need to selectively expand the public tier—but with a very important reservation. The current resource intensity of the public-tier programs is marginal at best. Expansion will almost certainly reduce and dilute this intensity unless aggressive measures are instituted. The need for more resource-intensive treatment appears equal in importance to the need for increases in capacity. Research data on returns to more intensive resources per patient are scarce, but the most sensible course is to increase public resources to restore earlier levels of service intensity, facility quality, and staff skills, as well as to increase the capacity for new admissions.

In selected regions, the public tier needs greater investments in both intensity and capacity. The private tier appears at this time to be heavily committed to acute care hospital treatment for cocaine and marijuana problems and may benefit most from either a shift toward greater use of nonhospital residential and outpatient modalities or, if such a shift cannot be effected, a move toward cost or charge structures that will permit and encourage the more extended periods of care typical of these modalities, in contrast to the short stays and high per diem charges now characteristic of hospital-based chemical dependency treatment.

PUBLIC FINANCING OF DRUG TREATMENT
(CHAPTER 7)

The Goals and Priorities of Public Coverage

Two basic principles justify public coverage of drug treatment, and these principles in turn suggest specific priorities for the expansion of the public tier that is now under way largely as a result of the recent federal anti-drug legislation. The first principle is that public coverage should seek to reduce external social costs—in particular those relating to crime and family role dysfunctions. The second principle is that public coverage should remedy constraints arising from inadequate income. Based on these principles, **the general goal of public coverage should be to provide adequate support for appropriate and timely admission, as well as completion or maintenance, of good-quality treatment for individuals who cannot pay for it (fully or partly) whenever such individuals** *need* **treatment, according to the best professional judgment, and** *seek* **treatment or can be** *induced* **through acceptable means to pursue it, assuming there is some probability of positive response.**

The committee estimates that 35 million individuals qualify as indigent with regard to private purchase of any form of drug treatment; that is, they are neither adequately insured nor able to pay out of pocket for appropriate forms of specialized treatment if needed and thus would have to rely on public services. For residential drug treatment, the committee's estimate of those who are unable to afford it if needed rises to 60 million.

The resources still needed to achieve the general goal of public coverage represent a major increase in public support for treatment, and even under the current conditions of extraordinary public concern about the drug problem and the possibility of commensurate appropriations, everything cannot be done at once. Priorities for treatment thus need to be defined. **The committee recommends the following priorities for public-tier expansion:**

- **end delays in admission when treatment is appropriate, as evidenced by waiting lists;**
- **improve treatment (by raising the levels of service intensity, personnel quality and experience, and retention rates of existing modalities; by having programs assume more integrative roles with respect to related services; and by instituting systematic performance monitoring and follow-up);**
- **expand treatment through more aggressive outreach to pregnant women and young mothers; and**
- **further expand community-based and institutionally based treatment of criminal justice clients.**

The upgrading of performance and quality levels is intrinsic to the other three priorities and would be needed even if expanded treatment admissions were not an objective. The recent decade-long hollowing-out of treatment programs through resource attrition, together with research findings about substantial variations in program performance, and the consistent importance of retention in predicting outcome all support the need for restoration of funding and quality levels in treatment.

The upgrading of staff capabilities and morale and modest but critically needed renovation of decrepit facilities and furnishings have multiple significance. Good staff morale and decent facilities increase the attractiveness of treatment programs and thus their ability to recruit and retain staff.

These factors also affect client interest in program admission and retention. Most critically, the competence, quality, and continuity of care givers may well be a critical element in explaining the differential effectiveness of treatment programs.

It is possible to estimate the amount of new public financing needed to meet these priority objectives, although to do so, key assumptions must be made about such parameters as capital costs, training expenses, and the number of individuals who could be induced to enter treatment at various levels of effort. **The committee judges that the amount needed to upgrade and expand the drug treatment system, beyond current spending rates, is $2.2 billion in annual operating costs (plus $1.1 billion in one-time costs) for a comprehensive plan, $1 billion annually (plus $0.5 billion up front) for a core plan, or $1.6 billion annually (plus $0.8 billion in up-front costs) for an intermediate plan.** Details are provided in Table 7-1. Because data supporting the costs of the recommended strategies are uncertain, it is essential that relevant data collection be developed very quickly and its products analyzed as soon as possible.

The committee's recommended strategies lead to a consideration of needed changes in how to manage the public tier. These issues divide into the following: the roles and interrelations of the states, the federal government, and public-tier providers; the most appropriate shorter and longer term financing mechanisms for providing public support (direct service programs versus public insurance); and the controls needed to make the most effective and efficient use of public funds.

Federal and State Roles

State governments have played the major role in financial administration and quality control of drug treatment programs in recent years, but there has also been cyclical movement between state and federal leadership. The federal government originally built most of the public tier of providers and then transferred responsibility for regulating and supporting this tier largely to the states; it is now moving back into the lead role. This expansion of federal support should be accompanied by more active, centralized direction and control of treatment resources.

States will continue to have the major operational responsibility for implementing new drug treatment priorities and standards. The increasing streams of federal monies must be allocated so as to help support the critical data collection, training, and technical assistance functions to be deployed through state offices. In the recommended expansion of support, it is appropriate for the federal government to take the lead in the short term in upgrading program quality and extending outreach to critical populations. In so doing, there are two important near-term management objectives. One objective is to ensure the most efficient and effective expenditure of existing and incremental funds, preserving as much discretion as possible on the federal level so that federal agencies have the flexibility to encourage states to reach the new goals. The second objective is to maximize coordination with other anti-drug abuse activities (including public safety, justice, and correctional institutions) and other social welfare and health services.

In lieu of fixed formulas for the allocation of funds received by the states (which, as most recently revised, are based on population weighted somewhat by degree of urbanization), **the committee recommends that state agencies be required to submit plans that analyze the conjunctions and mismatches among the most current epidemiological information and known treatment capabilities; it further recommends that the states be required to propose annual spending patterns that reflect this information.** In addition, a portion of the federal dollars must go into technical assistance and data system building to ensure at the state, local, and program levels that this planning effort will have a factual basis.

One other notable element of the federal role is support for veterans. The Veterans Administration has previously targeted drug programs for drastic budget reductions in order to meet overall fiscal limitations. At the very least, outpatient or residential drug treatment services—furnished directly or by contract—should be made available to meet the needs of former inpatients.

Mechanisms for Providing Public Support

At present, the public sector provides access to drug treatment through two distinctly different financial mechanisms: direct program financing through service contracts and grants to formally defined and certified addiction treatment programs, versus individual insurance financing through Medicaid and similar programs. The largest and most important guarantee of access to drug treatment is the program of public grants or contracts with public-tier treatment providers, who serve virtually all of the medically indigent population (the poor, uninsured, or underinsured) needing drug treatment. Continued expansion of the dollar level of this form of support is the primary means recommended by the committee to address public coverage goals and priorities over the next 5 years.

Emphasis on direct service is an appropriate model for directed system building, but long-term system maintenance may be better served by a proportionately greater use of public insurance financing, supplemented by direct service grants to ensure critical program elements such as outreach and other important services to the many individuals for whom low income is not the only barrier to seeking and responding well to treatment. The ground should be prepared to "mainstream" drug treatment more fully in the next 5 to 10 years, incorporating it as much as possible into public health care insurance for the poor, that is, the set of state programs presently gathered under the tent of federal Medicaid.

Currently, eligibility for Medicaid among poor people is sharply circumscribed for those between the ages of 18 and 65 who are not permanently disabled. There are large gaps in eligibility in the health insurance programs of the 50 states and the District of Columbia, all of which participate in the federal Medicaid matching program. Medicaid does provide significant health care coverage for low-income women (especially if they are pregnant) and their children who are less than 18 years old (especially if the children are less than 6 years old). All states, however, exclude nondisabled single men from coverage, and there is great variation across states in the family income ceilings for Medicaid eligibility, which can be and often are well below the federal "poverty line."

Fewer than a handful of states with the broadest eligibility and benefits now account for a large majority of all Medicaid support for drug treatment. Yet even in these states, the programs cover only some of the services needed in—or adjoined with—drug abuse treatment (e.g., medical examination at intake, visits for methadone dispensing, hospital-based services), and payment levels are often much lower than the cost of covered services.

There are five steps that would be particularly useful as incentives toward a larger role for Medicaid in treating drug problems and that would not compromise the efficiency of the direct service support mechanism. The first step is to require all parties to cooperative agreements, grants, or contracts involving federal funds to develop and display evidence of progress toward the long-term goal of increasing the receipt of funds from the Medicaid system. Examples of potential strategies include facilitating the registration of clients eligible for Medicaid benefits and meeting relevant accreditation standards familiar to Medicaid, such as those of the Joint Commission on Accreditation of Healthcare Organizations or the Commission on Accreditation of Rehabilitation Facilities.

The second useful step is to begin stipulating matching requirements rather than maintenance-of-effort requirements for increases in grant support to the states. By determining the matching ratio with the same formula used to determine Medicaid matching, the incentive to states to use Medicaid structures will be increased, and the disincentive—states must match every new Medicaid dollar but can get more block grant dollars without increasing state appropriations—will be removed.

The third step is for the federal government to require state Medicaid programs to include drug treatment as part of the standard package of benefits offered to all current (and any newly added) Medicaid-eligible per-

sons. The drug benefit package should cover methadone treatment, outpatient nonmethadone treatment, and residential treatment in state-accredited freestanding (nonhospital) as well as hospital-affiliated residential facilities and outpatient programs. No special copayments or limitations—that is, no copayments or limits not generally applicable to medical/surgical benefits—should be applied to drug treatment. For those states with private insurance mandates for drug treatment insurance coverage, the Medicaid drug treatment benefit should be at least as comprehensive as (which does not mean identical with) the mandated private insurance benefit.

The fourth step is to reduce gross inconsistencies in the way drug problems are handled in eligibility determinations for Medicaid, Aid to Families with Dependent Children, Medicare, Supplemental Security Income, and other income maintenance, education, and housing assistance entitlement programs. These inconsistencies create a bureaucratic nightmare for the drug treatment programs and state agencies that draw on more than one such source of funds—which most of them try to do. The Office of National Drug Control Policy should analyze definitional inconsistencies among federal programs and lay out a plan to minimize resulting problems.

The fifth step is to develop a thoroughgoing system of public utilization management (a term describing arrangements to define access to effective treatment while keeping costs at efficient levels). Good utilization management works to ensure that a fully appropriate and needed range of services is used and that different service components are coordinated. Many of the components of such a system were developed in the early 1970s but subsequently disestablished. These components are described in the next section.

Utilization Management

The most fundamental principle of utilization management is that access to and utilization of care should be controlled and managed on a case basis by "neutral gatekeepers" or central intake personnel (although this triage or central intake function may need to be dispersed geographically). These personnel should be regulated by certification standards and undergirded by time-limited, performance-accounted licenses and contracts. Client assessment, referral, and monitoring of progress in treatment should be reviewed (or performed) independently of the treatment provider. These personnel should have appropriate clinical credentials that include the understanding that longer residential and outpatient durations are strongly correlated with beneficial results among public clients. **Effective utilization management should recognize that drug abuse and dependence are chronic, relapsing disorders and that for any one client, more than one** treatment episode may be needed and different types of treatment may need to be tried. "Gatekeepers" should have access to ongoing performance evaluation results and responsibility for implementing cost-control objectives.

There should be rigorous preadmission and concurrent review of all residential drug treatment admissions, and especially of hospital admissions, and concurrent review of outpatient treatment. Unlike the objective in utilization management of acute hospital care for most medical conditions, which is basically to hold inpatient lengths of stay to a minimum, the objective for drug treatment services should be to increase client retention in appropriate, cost-efficient treatment settings.

The major cost-control concern in this area is the use of high-cost treatment when lower cost alternatives could be as effective. This hazard attaches principally to acute care hospital inpatient services for detoxification or rehabilitation treatment. The public tier generally has not been heavily invested in hospital-based drug treatment, and this should continue to be the case—but not as a matter of rigid exclusion. **The committee recommends that hospital-based drug services be reimbursed at the same level as nonhospital residential treatment rates, unless there is evidence that a client specifically requires continuing acute care hospital services. Hospital-based drug detoxification should only be covered in the event of medical complications such as those noted below or the lack of appropriate residential or outpatient facilities nearby. Indications for hospital-based inpatient drug detoxification are the following:**

- **serious concurrent medical illness such as tuberculosis, pneumonia, or acute hepatitis;**
- **history of medical complications such as seizures in previous detoxification episodes;**
- **evidence of suicidal ideation;**
- **dependence on sedative-hypnotic drugs as validated by tolerance testing (therapeutic challenge) to determine the appropriate length of stay; and**
- **history of failure to complete earlier ambulatory or residential detoxification versus completion in inpatient settings.**

As perhaps the most important and immediately needed utilization management requirement, the committee recommends that all drug treatment programs receiving public support be required to participate in a client-oriented data system that reports client characteristics, retention, and progress indicators at admission, during treatment, at discharge, and (on a reasonable sampling basis) at one or more follow-up points. There should be periodic, independent investigation on a sampling basis of the quality and accuracy of the data system or systems, and the systems should be designed to dovetail or link with ongoing services research and data collection in other government agencies and units concerned with drug problems (see the discussion of research needs in Chapter 5). Certification for public support should be time limited and based on performance—especially client retention and improvement—rather than on process standards. Performance is to be demonstrated by outcome evaluation, and the standards of performance adequacy should be informed by past and ongoing treatment effectiveness research on retention and outcomes.

PRIVATE COVERAGE OF DRUG TREATMENT (CHAPTER 8)

Extent, Costs, and Trends of Coverage

The private tier of drug treatment providers is largely oriented toward treating the employed population and their family members. The majority of this population, about 140 million individuals, have specifically defined coverage for drug treatment in their health insurance plans. About 48 million others who are privately insured do not have specifically defined coverage for drug treatment, although coverage may occur de facto under general medical or psychiatric provisions. As of 1988, the health plans of about 67 percent of full-time employees of firms with 100 or more employees offered specifically defined coverage for some types of drug treatment, although the actual extent of benefits under these defined coverage provisions is uncertain.

Actuarial studies of claims experience yield rather modest estimates for the overall cost of covering drug treatment. Drug treatment expenditures tend to be buried under more inclusive headings and behind "horror stories" involving troubled adolescents with multiple diagnoses spending months in psychiatric facilities. Nevertheless, the committee estimates that a health plan with typical coverage now spends 1 percent or less of its total outlays for explicit drug treatment, most of it for hospital inpatient charges—with a large fraction of that cost devoted to detoxification. There has been a substantial apparent growth in the rate of drug treatment claims in recent years, although it is unclear how much of this increase is due to more revealing or accurate drug problem diagnoses versus increased demand for drug treatment.

Although this growth is disturbing to the degree it increases the aggregate cost of health insurance premiums, it is desirable if it means that more of those who need treatment are seeking and receiving it, particularly if the treatment delivered is appropriate, effective, and reasonable in cost. Some payers, however, reacting in part to the high costs of a small number of cases and the high incidence of recidivism, have strongly questioned the value of drug treatment episodes, and they have moved to differentially limit reimbursement of drug treatment to help trim increasing overall costs.

Mandating Drug Treatment Coverage

There are legislative mandates in 18 states plus the District of Columbia requiring that certain categories of employer-supplied group health plans specifically cover—or offer optional coverage for—drug and alcohol treatment. (Another 19 states require some degree of coverage for alcohol treatment only.) In the committee's judgment, private coverage of drug treatment is beneficial to individuals and employers and should be included in every health package; however, legislative mandates at the state level have not necessarily proved to be an effective way, and are clearly not the only way, to induce adequate coverage. Most insured individuals whose plans include explicitly defined coverage for drug treatment reside in states that do not have legislative mandates for such coverage. Moreover, the political process has often produced less-than-optimal mandatory provisions that are difficult to adjust, overly rigid, and pay too much attention to limits on the length of stay and the number of visits rather than to the cost and effectiveness of treatment. Most mandatory provisions have the constraining effect of funneling people toward one particular modality of treatment by favoring inpatient stays of prespecified lengths.

The committee believes that the development of soundly derived standards for admission, care, and program performance will do more at this time to generate appropriate coverage than a further set of mandates. If mandates are to be used, efficiency and fairness dictate that they be applied to all competing insurers. Yet if the private market leaves large numbers of the insured population without coverage for drug treatment, it may be necessary for government to intervene. Such action could involve subsidies for drug treatment coverage, tax preferences for certain kinds of coverage, or mandates, with the choice dependent on judgments about the incidence, efficiency, and equity of alternative ways of financing coverage.

Optimal Coverage Provisions

Private insurance provisions (including most legislatively mandated benefits) often include financial incentives for beneficiaries to seek more expensive hospital or residential treatment. Although residential drug treatment, including hospital treatment, often serves clinically important functions such as permitting intensive therapy and isolating the patient from an adverse environment or treating concurrent psychiatric or medical complications, hospital-specific components (e.g., 24-hour onsite medical coverage) do not seem to be the therapeutically important elements in drug treatment programs that are sited there, even though the availability of these components is used to justify charging acute care hospital rates for all clients.

The committee recommends that curbs on unit-of-service costs for

inpatient care be strengthened and that payers insist on the generation of reliable performance/outcome data. Drug treatment services at hospital sites should be reimbursed separately from other diagnoses or hospital services; there appears to be no compelling reason why these services for most drug treatment patients should routinely command fees comparable to acute care rates rather than to reasonably competitive residential treatment rates.

Insurers and employers need to become better informed about drug treatment and to structure their benefits to support controlled access to a broad range of the most appropriate, effective, and efficiently priced treatments rather than to a narrow (and expensive) band of options that are similar in form to the treatment of acute medical conditions. Private plans should cover appropriate, adequate, cost-effective drug treatment and not reimburse the cost of excessive, inappropriate treatments or charges (see Table 8-2 for placement guidelines).

The committee recommends that private risk bearers, in lieu of arbitrary payment caps or exclusions, institute rigorous, independent preadmission review (where possible) and concurrent review of all hospital and residential admissions as a way to control access and utilization, ensure appropriate placement, and manage costs. Preadmission review may not be necessary for such admissions, but early concurrent utilization review is important for such treatment to ensure that diagnostic criteria are observed and charges are reasonable. Employee assistance programs can serve as utilization managers in cases in which their personnel have appropriate training for matching patients to treatment. Hospital utilization should be managed under the same terms as those recommended for public coverage (see the section on utilization management in Chapter 7).

The committee further recommends that private payers insist that providers participate in and agree to the publication of regular, independent follow-up surveys to determine client outcomes, taking into account data on admission characteristics such as problem severity. Providers and payers should be able to compare treatment results with overall program norms to ensure the maintenance of good performance and the identification of poor performance when it occurs.

The committee recommends that the provisions of drug treatment benefits, including deductibles, copayments, stop-loss measures, and scheduled caps, be similar to provisions for treatment of other chronic, relapsing health problems. Except in terms of limitations on the length of stay and number of visits, such provisions are mostly the rule today. Sound utilization management that includes reliable performance and outcome measurements is likely to obviate the need for separate length-of-stay and dollar caps on coverage. Nonhospital residential and outpatient treatment delivered in state-certified treatment programs should be covered. Coverage limitations, charge schedules, and cost-containment incentives (e.g., copayment schedules) should be adjusted to reflect the findings of research on appropriate models, lengths, and costs of drug treatment—especially the recognition that longer residential and outpatient stays are strongly correlated with more beneficial results.

CODA

The drug problem is not a fixed constellation but a restless, ever-changing composite. Within this pharmacological and sociological diversity, treatment addresses the chronic, relapsing disorders of drug dependence and abuse. The best treatment interventions have been shown to "work"—reversing drug-seeking behavior, related criminal activity, and other dysfunctions—only partially; that is, the different treatment methods encourage recovery from these imperfectly understood disorders to a greater or lesser degree. Moreover, each modality of treatment can attract and affect only some of the people in need.

Success in treatment is not guaranteed and is often not complete, but even if it managed to be both, there would still be a major problem: most people who need treatment seek it only reluctantly, after failing at self-help, after much harm has been done, and after much pressure—interior and exterior—has been brought to bear. However, as with heart disease and cancer in the health domain, theft and assaultive behavior in the realm of violent crime, or homelessness and family dissolution in the area of social welfare, the lack of a panacea does not excuse society from responding to the best of its ability. The overall costs of drug problems are so high that reducing them even modestly is worthwhile. The committee is persuaded that the treatment methods available today can at least potentially realize benefits that well exceed the costs of delivering these services. Treatment makes sense on the grounds of utility as well as humanity.

The treatment system should do a better job of knowing itself and acting on that knowledge. Much of the knowledge gained in the past about the elements and optimal costs of effective treatment was brushed aside in the 1980s in the zeal to cut public spending and increase private revenues. In the 1990s, a different perspective seems to be gaining ground. Solutions to the challenge of improving drug treatment can be achieved if current financial trends continue and if leaders of the public and private tiers of drug treatment bend their efforts to the modest but necessary task of making the system learn its lessons.

1

Introduction

A provision in the Anti-Drug Abuse Act of 1986 instructed the secretary of health and human services to seek an independent study of substance abuse treatment coverage. The study was mandated to report on the extent and adequacy of financing—public and private—for treating and rehabilitating drug abusers and to make recommendations as needed.[1] It seemed likely that the study might identify unmet needs for new federal action. For example, the state-level components of the national drug treatment system had been cast adrift in the 1980s from earlier, more restrictive federal controls, and the system's ability to help communities respond to new challenges, such as the crack-cocaine epidemic, the acquired immune deficiency syndrome (AIDS) epidemic, and the growing violence of drug markets, appeared tenuous. What was not clear was what to do about the situation.

This volume is the response to the congressional charge, fulfilling an agreement, finalized in December 1987, between the National Institute on Drug Abuse and the Institute of Medicine. It is the outcome of an Institute of Medicine/National Academy of Sciences committee process that included reviews of the scientific literature, specially commissioned

---

[1] The operative language of the law (P.L. 99-555, section 6005) reads: "...the Institute of Medicine of the National Academy of Sciences [is] to conduct a study of (1) the extent to which the cost of drug abuse treatment is covered by private insurance, public programs, and other sources of payment, and (2) the adequacy of such coverage for the rehabilitation of drug abusers. ... The report shall include recommendations of means to meet the needs identified in such study."

papers (to be published in a separate volume), field visits to cities around the country, conferences and correspondence with experts in many relevant fields, and application of the expertise accumulated by committee members and staff in their own professional work.

The operational questions the committee has tried to answer are tempered versions of the congressional mandate: Is it good policy to invest as much—or as little—of society's pooled resources (basically, public programs and private insurance) in drug treatment as is now being invested? And if this much expenditure—or more—is truly necessary and worthwhile, how can these dollars be spent most prudently and equitably, with the highest likelihood of yielding good results?

The committee's overall conclusion is that it is a "good bet" to put more resources into drug treatment. Public expenditures should be increased, especially at the federal level, to support the most carefully validated treatment modalities, as well as to improve clinical training and facilities, treatment research activities, and program evaluation and management systems. Public funding should focus on boosting the average quality of treatment as well as the number of program admissions, with special emphasis on increasing treatment opportunities for those under criminal justice supervision and for pregnant women or women who care for young children. In the private sector, coverage policies should be revised. Insurers should institute better control over tendencies toward preferential reimbursement of an increasing number of high-cost treatment episodes. They should also encourage more widespread reimbursement and utilization of less expensive facilities and programs, under comprehensive systems of utilization review based on performance evaluation.

These conclusions appear straightforward, but they did not in fact come quickly or easily. The controversies that have surrounded drug treatment stem as much from the sheer complexity of the drug problem— and the resulting potential for misconception and confusion—as from any other factor. The series of investigations and arguments that led to the committee's conclusions are logically retraced and presented in the chapters that follow. The report's organization is described briefly in the sections below.

THE LOGIC OF THE REPORT

Chapters 2, 3, and 4 set the stage for analyzing the clinical effectiveness and organizational features of drug treatment coverage. Because it is critical to understand how drug treatment fits into and is shaped by drug policy as a whole, the committee undertook a general review of the historical and contemporary dimensions of drug policy, commissioning original analyses by Karst Besteman and committee member David Courtwright. Based on these and other sources, Chapter 2 assesses the role assigned to treatment in the ideas that govern drug policy, emphasizing the combination of medical and criminal conceptions of the problem that dominate current thinking.

Chapter 3 focuses on epidemiological research knowledge and clinical experience regarding patterns of drug consumption behavior, the individual and social consequences of drug patterns, and the extent of the need for treatment. The special concerns of this chapter are drug abuse and dependence, recovery, and relapse—the behavior patterns that have the greatest significance for treatment programs. A special analysis of data from the Research Triangle Institute/National Institute on Drug Abuse (RTI/NIDA) 1988 National Household Survey and analysis of U.S. Bureau of Justice Statistics reports provide important reference points for this chapter.

Given the policy contexts and the extent and character of the problems that require attention, what can treatment for drug problems be expected to achieve? Chapter 4 takes up the issue of defining a realistic set of treatment goals, particularly in terms of reducing illicit drug consumption and other criminal behavior. It notes the reluctance many individuals express about entering and complying with treatment, as well as the close association between the objectives of criminal justice agencies and drug treatment programs. This chapter draws on commissioned papers by Mary Dana Phillips and Gregory Falkin and colleagues.

With the parameters of policy, epidemiology, and treatment objectives in place, it is possible to review efficiently the literature on clinical modalities of treatment and characterize the state of knowledge about their results under controlled conditions and in the field. Chapter 5 thus surveys the available evidence on "what works" among the handful of conventional modalities of drug treatment. Discussing such aspects as how effective a treatment modality is, for whom, why or why not, at what cost, and with what level of benefits, the chapter draws heavily on analyses of the large-scale Treatment Outcome Prospective Study, a NIDA/RTI project. The chapter is equally concerned with what is *not* known about treatment modalities and results and leads finally to recommendations for improving the knowledge base about treatment.

In analyzing the treatment literature, reviewing submitted evidence, and visiting treatment programs in the field, committee members were struck by differences between programs that principally served privately insured clients and programs that did not. These differences became dramatically evident in detailed analyses of data collected in the 1987 National Drug and Alcoholism Treatment Utilization Survey. The differentiation of treatment providers into public and private tiers and the effects of this structure on treatment provision and accessibility in this country are discussed in Chapter 6.

Chapter 7 considers the public tier of treatment delivery, which is largely supported by federal, state, and local funds and in the main comprises nonprofit treatment programs that hold contracts with government agencies. To achieve the general goal of public coverage—ensuring that appropriate treatment is available to those who cannot afford it themselves—the committee offers a plan, complete with breakdowns of estimated costs, for three alternatives: a $2.2 billion comprehensive program, a $1 billion core program, and a $1.6 billion intermediate program of expanded public support. The plan relies in the near term on direct program financing, with a longer term goal of incorporating drug treatment support more systematically into Medicaid and other mainstream health care payment mechanisms. Important components of the plan are more extensive outreach to mothers and criminal justice populations in need of treatment, well-developed systems of performance assessment, and better utilization review and control, particularly of high-cost elements.

Private coverage for drug treatment is a result of decisions and negotiations by individuals, employers, insurers, care managers, and providers. Chapter 8 considers private coverage in terms of eligibility, benefit design, costs, and provisions for the management of care. Drug treatment is a relatively small but fast-growing element among private health insurance claims, and it is difficult to titrate precisely the factors that have led to this growth. Mandates for specific coverage have played some role but do not appear to be the most important factors at this time. The committee's major recommendation in this area is to broaden the scope of covered treatment while instituting better cost management and accountability. Commissioned papers by Richard Steinberg and by Paul Roman and Terry Blum were particularly useful in shaping the committee's analysis of private coverage.

In reaching conclusions and formulating recommendations, the committee has relied wherever possible on rigorous evidence. On many issues, however, there is no such evidence by the usual standards of the scientific community. Consequently, the committee made judicious use of its best expert judgment in cases in which logic and experience pointed strongly but good evidence was scant. The grounds for this course lie in the complexity and severity of the nation's drug problem, the congressional charge to provide recommendations, and the public's underlying determination to respond. These conclusions are clearly signaled by explicit use of the formula, "in the committee's judgment." In virtually every such instance, the committee also specifies the new knowledge that needs to be generated to test and strengthen such judgments.

ADDITIONAL POLICY QUESTIONS

There are several issues bearing on drug treatment to which the committee members returned again and again during their deliberations but that they could not satisfactorily address because there was no clear basis from which to draw firm conclusions. In some cases, the issues involved large amounts of unanalyzed data and conceptual problems that extended beyond the sphere of treatment coverage. It was impossible to pursue in depth those matters that were centered far outside the study's mandate, however revealing the inquiries might eventually be. Nevertheless, the committee resolved to highlight here those issues it considered the most important: drug treatment specifically for adolescents and younger children, including drug-affected babies; the operations of the criminal justice system in relation to the drug consumer; and modification of the socio-economic environment that conditions drug use, especially in impoverished neighborhoods.

Treating Adolescents and Women with Children

Most of the findings and recommendations in this report are based on and pertain directly to the treatment of adults, especially those aged 18 to 40 years old. Juvenile drug problems rightfully capture a great deal of attention, but in terms of sheer demographic mass, the drug problems of major concern today occur principally in adult populations. The overwhelming majority of drug transactions are between adults, the social costs of their problems clearly predominate, and most identified drug treatment resources are directed toward them. Moreover, in comparison to juveniles, treatment research and evaluation data for adults are richer, the criteria for differential diagnoses are clearer, and typical adult treatment modalities are more sharply distinguished (for better or worse) from other mental and physical health care, education, criminal justice, and social/rehabilitative services.

Unfortunately, much evidence suggests that juveniles who are directly or proximally involved in drug problems today are the source of tomorrow's pool of more severe adult drug problems. The committee consequently reviewed the scattered literature and discussed some of the problems encountered in treating adolescents, women with children, and drug-exposed infants. However, no conclusions could be drawn from these investigations, although some substantive possibilities were derived and are discussed in the report. Of principal concern is the extent of the limitations of the knowledge base on whether treatment of the young has requirements different from those for treatment of adults. Also at issue are the changes in outcome that might be produced by variations in services.

Considering the importance of treatment for juveniles and the paucity of necessary knowledge, the committee urges that drug treatment of the young—adolescents, drug-exposed infants, and the ages in between—be subjected to intensive study. Investigations must be designed to plumb the reservoir of practical clinical experience and research knowledge as deeply and systematically as possible to stimulate development of the kind of foundation and synthesis for policy purposes that is not yet at hand. The National Forum on the Future of Children and Families, a joint effort of the Institute of Medicine and the National Research Council, has recently conducted the first in a series of workshops and panel meetings to address some of these issues.

The Criminal Justice System

The criminal justice system at present is the first line of societal response to drugs, absorbing about 90 percent of the public expenditures allocated to this problem. In fact, much of the nation's current drug treatment strategy and system was designed to allay public concern about street crime engendered and aggravated by drugs. This report examines the effectiveness of community-based treatment programs in terms of how well those concerns about drugs and crime are being satisfied. In addition, it presents conclusions about the legitimacy and effectiveness of correctional treatment and treatment of individuals on probation and parole and identifies ways in which treatment programs can and should relate to the criminal justice system.

Beyond these issues, however, lie a range of critical questions about how the law enforcement and criminal justice systems are organized to deal with drug-related crime and how they distribute attention and resources to address its various manifestations—possession, trafficking, and other serious crimes. There is a crowded field of opinion and vested interest about these questions, as well as some relevant research. But there is no objective, comprehensive, up-to-date analysis of the criminal justice response to the drug problem, and the committee doubts whether any current efforts, including those of the Office of National Drug Control Policy, even aspire to develop one. This issue is a rapidly growing, multi-billion-dollar vacuum that demands to be filled.

The Socioeconomic Environment

It is difficult to overstate the critical importance of the socioeconomic environment. Individuals make choices, but they always do so in a social and economic environment, and there is ample evidence that such environments exercise great influence over drug consumption. They can promote the initiation of drug use, aggravate and amplify drug effects, and counteract the process of recovery from drug dependence. The capabilities necessary to change socioeconomic factors must be developed so that these environments will help channel more individuals away from rather than toward drug problems.

The report covers some aspects of drug etiology and relapse that are relevant to environmental dimensions. Nevertheless, a comprehensive assessment of the extent and adequacy of preventive interventions in this domain was beyond the purview of this study. The committee looks toward investigations, such as the study of drug abuse prevention research now being conducted by the National Research Council, to address these issues and work toward comprehensive recommendations regarding appropriate environmental interventions to prevent drug problems.

2

Ideas Governing Drug Policy

Three fundamental ideas about drugs, the people who use them, and ways to respond to them lie behind drug treatment and virtually all other instruments of drug policy in the United States. Embodied in criminal, medical, and libertarian approaches, these governing ideas have dominated the terms of public discussion and the gross allocation of public and private funds. As a result, there can be no detailed analysis of drug treatment without first understanding what these ideas are, where they come from, how they relate to each other, and how they have shaped the role and functions of treatment.

That the governing ideas are plural reflects two underlying realities concerning drugs and society. The first is that psychoactive drugs have a multiplicity of medical and social uses and consequences. Some of the uses are clearly beneficial, others are clearly pernicious, and still others are a complex mixture. Moreover, the pharmacopoeia is not static but growing. New drugs and innovative technologies to administer them are constantly arising from scientific research and folk-pharmaceutical explorations.

The second reality is the persistence of social change, including the dialectic of political parties and philosophies and the continuous renegotiation of relationships between different institutions of government. Such change ensures the potential for different ideas to gain or lose potency. Therefore, if the social arrangements supporting policies associated with one fundamental idea turn unfavorable, the programs arising from those policies may wither only to revive again if conditions change.

The climate surrounding drug problems appears to be changing in the

United States, but its future direction is uncertain. A complex balance of ideas and policies led to the current forms of drug treatment and treatment delivery. The major lesson of this chapter's analysis of historical ideas and their social roots is that a re-tuning of that policy balance appears to be in order. Such a re-tuning is, moreover, a prerequisite to ensuring that these programs—and perhaps other instruments of drug policy—will be able to function at the most humane and effective level possible.

THE CHARACTER OF GOVERNING IDEAS

> In a democracy, government policy is inevitably guided by commonly shared simplifications. This is true because the political dialogue that authorizes and animates government policy can rarely support ideas that are very complex or entirely novel. There are too many people with diverse perceptions and interests and too little time and inclination to create a shared perception of a complex structure. Consequently, influential policy ideas are typically formulated at a quite general level and borrow heavily from commonly shared understanding and conventional opinions. (Moore and Gerstein, 1981:6)

Drug policy is no exception to the rule of simple ideas. For much of this century, drug policies were—and still are—profoundly affected by a body of conventional wisdom. Especially influential has been the belief that drug problems are largely attributable to morally compromised or pathological individuals who were not properly inculcated in childhood with normal American values such as self-control and respect for the law. These individuals must be disciplined and punished by authorities to deter them from involvement (for pleasure or profit) with inherently dangerous, addicting drugs. The power of ideas like these is apparent in that they are widely treated as obvious facts that any well-intentioned, intelligent participant in drug policy formation either subscribes to or treats very seriously.

Much can be said for the wisdom of governance through shared ideas. If many people understand and agree with an idea, its prima facie legitimacy is established. Moreover, widespread understanding and acceptance of an idea establishes a necessary condition for effective policy implementation in any society in which governmental power is broadly dispersed. Although shared simplifications generally fail to reflect or capture all the important aspects of a problem, they at least focus attention on some of the more significant dimensions. Thus, simplified conceptions help to concert social attention and action—something that more complicated ideas usually cannot achieve.

Yet there is also a price to be paid for simple ideas. Simplification inevitably distorts one's perception of a problem. Although some important features may be enhanced, others that could plausibly claim equal significance are subordinated. In turn, some avenues for social intervention may be brightly illuminated, whereas others that could well be as effective are obscured or condemned to obscurity.

Such limiting approaches can be of two sorts. One simplifying strategy is to select a narrow set of *effects or objectives*. One could then focus on adverse health effects, for example, and promote policies that would best reduce overdoses, withdrawal, and diseases such as AIDS that may be associated with drugs, taking everything else as of secondary importance. Alternatively, one might consider drug-induced crime to be of overriding importance and concentrate on policies that would effectively punish and isolate the drug user from society.

A different simplifying approach is to decide which *causes* are most important in generating the adverse effects of drug use and then choose policy instruments that operate most directly on these causes. One might judge (on the basis of available evidence) that the total quantity of drugs used is the main determinant of the observed pattern of effects and try to develop policies that reduce overall drug consumption. Alternatively, one might determine that drug problems are mainly due to a relatively small number of unusually feckless or vulnerable users and tailor policies specifically to keep such people away from drugs (or treat or pretreat them in some fashion that would make them more problem resistant).

The most successful simplifications combine both kinds of limitations: the major effect or objective of the policy and the judgment about what causes it are tied together into a neat conceptual bundle. A few such bundles have had widespread, durable appeal in U.S. society because they proved compatible with common social views, evolving social experience, and the interests and purposes of organized groups. These cognitive bundles are referred to here as *governing ideas*. Each has had considerable intellectual appeal and at some point succeeded in capturing the attention, imagination, and actions of the broad population. They provide the crucial context for understanding the nature of the drug treatment system, as well as the goals set for it and the financial arrangements that underlie it.

THE SPECTRUM OF IDEAS ABOUT DRUGS

The evolution of drug policy in the United States can be concisely and usefully described in terms of a simple spectrum or continuum of concepts that ranges from the least restrictive in approach to the most restrictive (Figure 2-1). Of course, reducing ideas to a one-dimensional continuum distorts them somewhat, stripping them of nuances and cross-fertilizations. Furthermore, the placement of ideas along this continuum does not necessarily refer to the actual consequences of policies but only to the character of the ideas that inform them. The determinants of policy consequences are more complex than ideas alone, embracing economic

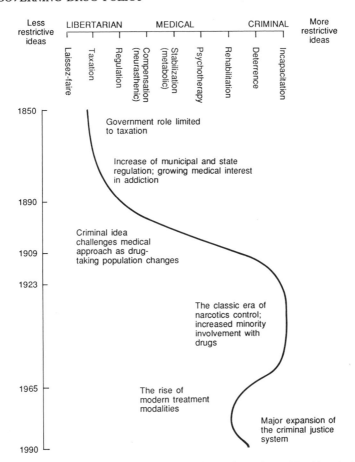

FIGURE 2-1 A simplified spectrum of governing ideas about drugs. The historical changes represented in this figure by a continuous trend line constitute the committee's summary judgments about the ideological "center of gravity" in the country from 1850 to 1990, based on the evidence reviewed by Courtwright and Besteman (both 1990) and elsewhere in the report, particularly Chapters 4 and 6.

conditions, political mobilization, religious movements, and the educational level and degree of alienation or frustration of the population.

Although the spectrum is continuous and shows that ideas shade into one another at their edges, simplification demands that sharper boundaries be drawn. Three main parts of the spectrum are thus distinguished, constituting the three major governing ideas that underlie the historical evolution of drug policy in the United States. As little as 100 years ago the left side of the spectrum was mainly in evidence. Only after the middle and right side had developed could drug policy be compared across the broad range of options.

Libertarian Ideas

Libertarian approaches to the drug problem are the oldest of the three sets of governing ideas. Until after the Civil War, imported drugs such as opium were relatively cheap and available without much restriction to those whose cultural customs, personal tastes, or medical needs motivated their use. This state of affairs was less a reflection of positive ideas about drugs than an outcome of the methods of governance in the new nation. American constitutionalism prescribed a weak, rather minimal federal government whose attentions had to be concentrated on a few matters where they could have an impact. The libertarian ideal is Jeffersonian at its heart, advocating minimal interference by government in private affairs or political expression. It envisions a relatively small government apparatus concerned for the most part on the national level with foreign affairs, national security, and the currency, and on the local level with protecting property rights and maintaining civil order. Libertarian ideas were, and still are, the default value in American political life; thus, minimal policy, expressed as a practical lack of interest in the actual or potential significance of drugs in society, was the reality for much of the nineteenth century.

Only from the middle to the late 1800s, as the country's concern with the problem of alcohol was culminating in major legislative measures, did the libertarian approach (or nonapproach) to drugs begin to lose ground. This decline coincided with the growth of two other governing ideas: the criminal—that drug abuse is a problem of shiftless living closely associated with crime and violence—and the medical—that drug abuse is a medical problem arising from a misguided but understandable search for relief from painful or oppressive circumstances.

Yet even before these newer ideas were articulated, libertarian thinking itself had begun to respond to shifts of several kinds that were stirring in the mid-nineteenth century. First among these currents of change were social and political developments. The abolition of slavery by the Union during and after the Civil War was a clear signal that the boundaries of political permissiveness were contracting. The spread of industrialization, the growth of American military (especially naval) power to world-class status, and the immigration of Asians and eastern and southern Europeans in unprecedented numbers from 1880 to 1920 remade the face of the country that the Jeffersonians had fashioned. In the end, the libertarian ideal of minimal government was shattered by the pressures of a growing and increasingly diverse population and especially by conflicts over the proper role of the national state—the federal government—in organizing economic life and aligning local political culture with a national vision.

The libertarian view of drug use was further assaulted by a second, technological line of development. Modern chemistry and metallurgy isolated psychoactive botanical alkaloids such as morphine and cocaine and made their injection possible. The twentieth century saw the creation of exotic, mood-altering drugs, although these substances were not fundamentally different in effect from the nonsynthetics. Nevertheless, these new, more concentrated products altered the drug picture in numerous ways that included increasing the potential of drugs to induce addiction and a variety of unanticipated disease implications. (In the same way, the invention of shredded-leaf, flue-cured, machine-made tobacco cigarettes greatly changed the economic and epidemiological significance of tobacco products.)

The third development was the increasing concern about a new type of drug user: the "pleasure user," for whom drugs were neither bound to tradition or custom nor a source of relief from physical pain. Although the pleasure user was sometimes stereotyped in racial terms—associated originally with Chinese immigrants, later with African and Mexican Americans—the model was just as often the European American urban criminal, a member of the underworld linked to prostitution, thievery, and saloon-going.

The libertarian indifference to drugs was challenged by these developments and began to give way before pressure for some kind of governmental action. Early legislation tried to discourage opium smoking by outlawing opium dens or levying high taxes on imports of opium prepared for smoking. In 1906 the federal government passed legislation that required nostrum makers to list all ingredients, including narcotics, on the label. A number of states also passed laws requiring that narcotics be sold only by prescription and that pharmacists record all transactions. Ultimately, the U.S. Congress passed legislation to ban imports of opium prepared for smoking and attempted to confine other narcotics transactions entirely to medical channels.

Today, there are still some adherents to libertarian views regarding the problem of drugs, particularly in regulatory approaches, and these ideas have experienced something of a renaissance in the past several years. Yet the actual policy contributions of this idea are now largely constraining rather than leading. For example, libertarian ideas have limited the spread and influenced the character of employee drug testing (see Roman and Blum, 1990). On only one issue, the reduction of statutory penalties from the felony level to misdemeanors or infractions for the possession or transfer of small amounts of marijuana, has the libertarian idea attained a semblance of governing force in recent years—an effect that reached its current perimeter of authority in 1973 with the last of 11 state decriminalizations.

On a more abstract level, the decision-making logic characteristic of libertarian thought—namely, its calculus of utility—has retained some influence. In this theory of action, an individual, operating within the bounds of law and civility (noninfringement of others' fundamental rights), makes those expenditures—which may include the purchase of treatment— that in the individual's view will provide benefits that most exceed the cost of purchase. On an aggregate level, the polity, in its collective decisions, should at the least permit (if not encourage outright or, under appropriate circumstances, spend collective funds for) the supply of those goods or services whose aggregate benefits most exceed their costs. This logic implies an economic cost/benefit standard by which to measure the worth of public or private purchases of drug treatment. It has been used in some analyses, although it has not played a primary role in treatment policy.

Medical and Criminal Ideas

The medical idea arose in the 1870s and 1880s as physicians began to realize that a significant number of citizens, mostly middle-class, "respectable" women, were addicted to powdered morphine sulphate and other opiates. (The number was later estimated at several hundred thousand, but lower figures were actually more realistic [Courtwright, 1982, 1990].) Many of these individuals began to use these drugs on the advice of physicians to deal with a physical problem or a "nervous" complaint. There was widespread medical prescription, promotion, and sale of opiates and other substances for a variety of ailments and as routine "tonics." It gradually became clear to observant practitioners that individuals who had become accustomed to using these compounds became ill, agitated, and despondent if they tried to do without them; yet these same individuals functioned reasonably well with continued regular doses, even though these doses often reached high levels.

Opiates were very much a staple of nineteenth-century medical practice—one of the few truly effective medicines of the day, capable of reducing the suffering of many patients for whom no other useful medical intervention was known. As a result, this observation of the addictive effects of chronic use was viewed as regrettable but not catastrophic, particularly because so many of those affected were older women, many of whom had begun using the habit-forming drugs under medical or pharmaceutical advice or supervision and who on the whole seemed harmless. One standard medical response to this problem was maintenance on a prescribed dose, with the goal of continuing the patient on a course of normal, comfortable functioning. A variety of detoxification therapies, some sensible and some quite exotic, were also attempted, but relapse to habitual use was common, making maintenance appear even more reasonable as an alternative.

Of much greater concern were "opium habitués" of the lower social classes whose lives centered around multiple, daily periods of intoxication achieved through the opium pipe, the needle, or tinctures of high opiate (and alcohol) content. These individuals were quite different from respectable middle-class users—but their agitated responses to a threatened loss of access to the drug were quite similar. From these observations, physicians formulated the medical view of narcotic drugs: whatever the origins of opiate use or the prevailing moral judgment regarding it, individuals invariably display an addiction withdrawal syndrome if they have consumed powerful intoxicants such as narcotics for a long enough period. This syndrome involves physical distress when the drug is withdrawn, which is relieved when it is taken, and craving for the drug when the individual is abstinent. The similarity between the alcohol and narcotic addiction and withdrawal syndromes was recognized in many quarters.

The initial explanation developed for these phenomena was an extension of psychiatric theory of the period. The middle-class people who sought opiates seemed to belong to the "neurasthenic" personality type—people of weakened and unstable temperament who needed pharmacological assistance to endure the rigors of modern life. In the 1920s, as physicians saw more and more urban "pleasure users," a darker assessment arose: these users seemed more and more to be afflicted not with temperamental weakness but with psychopathic dispositions.

This darker medical assessment of the drug problem began to resemble the view taking shape as modern "scientific" police forces were organized in the rapidly growing cities of the late nineteenth and early twentieth centuries. Formulators of a view of drug use as a criminal matter were more impressed with the criminal associations and irresponsibility of disreputable drug users than with the commonalities in symptomatology with respectable users. The criminal view held that narcotic drug use was fundamentally immoral, ruinous behavior. The lower class user was seen not only as self-destructive but also as someone who might encourage and lure others into drug use and who could be emboldened by drugs to commit more and graver crimes.

In the criminal view of the drug problem, families, with churches and schools as social backstops, are fundamentally responsible for teaching children to behave responsibly and morally, behavior that includes shunning intoxicating drugs. The presence of moral anchors—most generally, the capacity for self-control in the face of temptation and a generalized respect for the law—is the vital element that separates the good citizen from the pleasure-seeking drug user. If the family or school, for whatever reason, fails in its responsibility to provide moral education, the problem must be dealt with by another authority. The main such agencies are the police, the courts, and prisons; there may, however, be room for intermediate socializing agencies (guidance counseling or social work) to supplement or substitute for the family, especially in cooperation with the juvenile justice system.

The criminal and medical views of the U.S. drug problem during the late nineteenth and early twentieth centuries had two rather different perceptions of drug users. The medical observers who originally developed the idea of addiction viewed the user population largely as members of the middle class and majority ethnic groups who were unfortunates worthy of help. But increasingly, from 1895 to 1920, the medical profession, the police, lawmakers, and the public in general saw the ranks of users as predominantly lower class in income and occupation and often of minority ethnic composition (that is, minorities not originating in northern and western Europe). The association of pleasure drug use with poor Chinese, Italians, slavic Jews, Mexicans, and African Americans deepened the rift of censure that divided official community moral guardians from drug users; the compassionate impulse to comfort the wretched became more and more a determination to administer a good swift kick to the wayward.

The Classic Era of Narcotics Control

The mixture of the two competing views, medical and criminal, was an uneasy one. The Harrison Act of 1914, aimed at controlling the distribution of narcotics, skirted the question of indefinite drug prescription for an addict's personal use. In 1919, however, a critical court case, decided by a Supreme Court vote of 5 to 4, firmly established the legal basis for prosecuting addicts and physicians who maintained them. Once this bridge was crossed, the criminal view quickly gained ascendancy in the debates surrounding drug policy formulation.

The medical view, on the other hand, was set back dramatically during the prohibitionist and xenophobic 1920s, as many physicians who prescribed opiates to addicts were visited by federal agents, and several efforts to treat addicts in morphine or heroin maintenance clinics were abruptly terminated. Addicts were sought, prosecuted, and jailed in unprecedented numbers— so many were imprisoned, in fact, that they strained the capacities of the federal prison system. In response to this overcrowding, federal prison wardens made a pact with advocates of the medical approach (represented by the U.S. Public Health Service), and the U.S. Congress agreed to fund two massive new "farms" for narcotics addicts—federal prison-hospitals that would accept both inmates and voluntarily committed patients. These facilities were opened near Lexington, Kentucky, and Fort Worth, Texas, in 1935 and 1938.

The criminal view dominated the nation's drug control efforts for more than 40 years, during most of which Federal Narcotics Bureau Director Harry Anslinger was the leading figure of narcotics policy and dealers and nonmedical users were arrested at virtually every opportunity. Nevertheless, the criminal view of drug problems was affected by changing times and changing ideas about controlling criminal behavior. Within this fundamental view of drug use as a criminal problem and users as moral derelicts deserving of retribution, several variants have arisen that correspond to philosophies reflected in the broad streams of modern criminological thought. The idea of *rehabilitation*—criminals may be redeemed by appropriate arrangements, incentives, and lessons fashioned within the penal environment—is the basis of prison as a place of penitence, or "penitentiary"; it is explicit as well in the term "corrections." Evidence of its diffusion is also found in widespread acceptance of probation—a period of testing to discover the true character of the offender—as an appropriate response to first or minor offenses. The concept of *deterrence* draws a sharper line: the lesson conveyed by punishment is intended not only for the individual but also for the community as a whole, or at least for all others who might consider similar deeds. Finally, *incapacitation* takes the bleakest view of the criminal, putting little stock in the possibility of redeeming or deterring criminal behavior. Instead, this school of thought calls for protecting society by isolating the criminally inclined for the longest period consistent with community standards of "just deserts" for the crime, or crimes, committed (in the extreme, a sentence of life—or death).

THE RISE OF MODERN TREATMENT

The nation's drug problem seemed to diminish slowly but steadily during the Depression and World War II. The number of underworld addicts did not change much during this period, but as the cohort of more "respectable" medical addicts aged and died, they were not replaced. By the turn of the century, the health professions had become more sophisticated and scientific regarding the use of narcotic medications, cautions about patent medicines had increased, and nonnarcotic analgesics such as aspirin had come into widespread use. As effective medical therapies multiplied, the use of narcotics for the symptomatic treatment of pain in a wide range of illnesses declined.

Around 1948, however, active heroin markets began to resurface in American cities. A wave of "drug epidemics" began, which continued into the 1950s and early 1960s despite increasing criminal penalties. Dismayed by the escalation of seemingly fruitless criminal sanctions, a series of blue-ribbon government and private panels began urging a reconsideration of the national commitment to a nearly exclusive criminal approach.

The beginnings of the national treatment effort lay within the federal prison-hospitals at Lexington, Kentucky, and Fort Worth, Texas. These facilities not only incarcerated criminals on narcotics convictions but also provided therapeutic services for their drug addiction. In addition, the two facilities served as sites for fundamental research on the course of drug dependence, the behavioral and physiological processes related to drug use, and the properties of narcotics. The benefits of the programs, however, proved elusive: evaluations indicated that the detoxification and unstructured psychotherapy delivered at these hospitals probably had limited if any long-term effectiveness (e.g., Hunt and Odoroff, 1962; Vaillant, 1966a,b,c).

Still, the federal hospitals were pivotal in three respects in the evolution of the community-based treatment system. First, the narcotics "farms" preserved the pre-control-era right of access that enabled addicts to commit or admit themselves voluntarily to treatment for addiction without being convicted of a criminal act. Second, the prison-hospitals established the precedent of direct federal provision of specialized treatment. Finally, through Public Health Service research programs and psychiatric residencies, Lexington and Fort Worth exposed a cadre of researchers and psychiatric clinicians to the challenges of treating drug-dependent individuals. When the new community-based treatment modalities of therapeutic communities and methadone maintenance were introduced and disseminated, this group of clinicians and researchers, whose careers had dispersed them across the country, were of critical importance in implementing and evaluating the new programs and organizing training initiatives.

Methadone Maintenance, Therapeutic Communities, and Outpatient Nonmethadone Programs

Methadone maintenance, a treatment modality first formally described in the *Journal of the American Medical Association* (Dole and Nyswander, 1965), was originally based on an explicitly medical concept that substantial heroin use created a persistent if not permanent imbalance of brain metabolism, which could be stabilized by the right pharmacological treatment. This notion was a more sophisticated version of the physiological ideas current among some of the physicians who, for a short period after 1919, operated medical maintenance clinics using morphine in a number of American cities—until federal agents shut them all down by 1923. Federal agents also wanted to stop methadone maintenance at its inception but backed down from openly challenging its determined originators in court.

Vincent Dole and Marie Nyswander, a distinguished research endocrinologist and a Lexington-trained psychiatrist, respectively, discovered during hospital studies of the effects of different opiates that giving heroin addicts an appropriately adjusted, daily oral dose of a relatively long-acting, synthetic opiate called methadone led to quite different effects than those resulting from other opiates. (Methadone was invented by German chemists as a morphine substitute during World War II; its addiction liability and acute effects had been further studied at Lexington.) Heroin addicts who were maintained on oral methadone experienced neither euphoria nor withdrawal, rarely displayed any toxicological side effects, and thus were able, if so motivated, to begin or resume more conventional lives—and with Dole and Nyswander's therapeutic assistance, most of the early patients were so motivated.

Dole and Nyswander were mainly concerned with individual patients who could now forego their obsession with acquiring drugs, an obsession that had led many of them to crime. But they and others saw broader implications to their work for the entire community, which might be spared thousands of criminal acts, once such obsessions ended. Thus, as the Kennedy-Johnson era "War on Poverty" gave way to the Nixon era "War on Crime," a rapid expansion of the methadone treatment program begun by the city of New York in the wake of the Dole-Nyswander research was underwritten by the federal government and implemented nationally. The goal of the expanded treatment was to take crime-committing addicts off the streets and out of the jails, on the theory, buttressed by substantial amounts of evidence, that a large proportion of these addicts' crimes were committed to support their addiction.

The Dole-Nyswander model soon evolved to a different stage as a result of regulatory conditions imposed by the Food and Drug Administration at the behest of the Bureau of Narcotics and Dangerous Drugs. These regulations, which were "interpreted" still further by the state inspectors who enforced them, reflected major concerns about the diversion of methadone from closely supervised pharmaceutical administration to street drug markets. Although these concerns were well grounded in evidence, the possibility of such diversion was viewed with little alarm by some clinicians who considered diverted, street-purchased methadone a less dangerous substance than injectable heroin and who saw the street methadone market as a potential step toward clinic admission. The regulations also incorporated biases against indefinite maintenance, toward low dose levels (of arguable efficacy), and toward certain therapeutic rigidities, including specific staffing and facility parameters.

A completely different treatment approach originated in California with Synanon, the original therapeutic community for drug addiction. Charles Dederich, founder of Synanon, drew some of its central treatment concepts from psychiatric therapeutic community in military medicine (Jones, 1953) and from the fellowship of Alcoholics Anonymous. But the therapeutic community was most clearly compatible with the psychological rehabilitation concepts of the criminal view of the drug problem—except that it was devoted to building a *self-policing community* as a path toward redeeming addicts. In a move symbolic of this linkage with criminal justice concepts, an important second-generation therapeutic community, Daytop Village, was founded directly under the auspices of the Brooklyn probation department with a community-based board of trustees (Joseph,

1988), and therapeutic communities were soon implemented in numerous prisons, including the Fort Worth facility (Maddux, 1988). Over time, the more rigidly punitive dimensions of the early therapeutic communities were softened as clinical experience became more sophisticated and additional professional components were integrated into the concept. Nevertheless, the therapeutic community remains a remarkable merger of the therapeutic optimism of psychiatric medicine and the disciplinary moralism of the criminal perspective.

The third locus of expansion of the treatment network in the early and mid-1970s, and the backbone of treatment efforts in most of the country today, was outpatient nonmethadone treatment. Comprising various forms of counseling, psychotherapy, and supervision, this branch of the treatment network developed originally in the 1960s in the matrix of federally supported community rehabilitation and community mental health services. Outpatient nonmethadone programs were the most diversified of the treatment approaches, both institutionally and therapeutically.

The Narcotic Addiction Rehabilitation Act (NARA) of 1966 was the first major federal acknowledgment of the reemergence of the medical perspective. Building on the examples of earlier California and New York civil commitment initiatives, NARA took the significant step of authorizing community-based supervision and treatment of addicts *after* release from incarceration (on parole). The authority of NARA was used to provide grants-in-aid and contracts to community programs delivering treatment and supervision. By 1970, roughly 150 local NARA programs were in operation (Besteman, 1990).

The next breakthrough for the application of medical ideas came with a 1968 amendment to the Community Mental Health Centers Act. This law mandated and supported the provision of treatment for drug abuse and alcoholism within community mental health centers, a major health policy initiative that originated during the Kennedy administration.

At roughly the same time as the 1968 amendment, the Office of Economic Opportunity began to support community-based drug and alcohol treatment programs, particularly those that offered a variety of treatment alternatives. A model program in this respect was the Illinois Drug Abuse Program in Chicago, which pioneered the "multimodality" approach. It was characterized by a central point of program entry to assess the patient's needs and living situation, followed by assignment to whichever of several modalities within the program seemed appropriate. In addition, each patient received an individualized treatment plan that called for gradually decreasing program services as rehabilitative milestones were achieved. The director of the Illinois program, Jerome Jaffe (a psychiatrist and alumnus of Lexington), later became the first head of the White House Special Action Office for Drug Abuse Prevention—the first national "drug czar."

Chemical Dependency Treatment

The final significant phase of the application of the medical idea to drug use since the mid-1970s has occurred largely outside the public system of drug treatment. The 1980s have seen the rapid expansion of a privately financed network of programs providing chemical dependency treatment, a derivation of ideas associated with a neighboring but generally autonomous domain: the treatment of alcoholism using the 12-step recovery concepts of Alcoholics Anonymous but operating under the umbrella of the health professions. The idea of bringing recovered alcoholics into the hospital setting as part of a therapeutic alliance was developed at Willmar State Hospital in Minnesota; it was further extended and refined (to include, for example, family therapy where indicated and a two-year ambulatory aftercare phase) at the Hazelden Foundation and the Johnson Institute, nonprofit treatment agencies in that state. In consequence, this modality is often called the "Minnesota model," and units implementing the modality are often called "28-day programs," based on a figure for an average length of inpatient stay reported at one time by the Hazelden center.

Although its origins were in the public sector, the chemical dependency modality is now most widely provided by private for-profit and not-for-profit hospitals and rehabilitation facilities that draw most of their revenues from third-party insurance payments. The typical client in this system is not the convicted criminal or sometime blue-collar worker generally found in the public system, whose drug use frequently involves a combination of heroin, cocaine, and amphetamines along with heavy alcohol consumption. Instead, the typical client here is steadily employed, often a white-collar professional, who is abusing or dependent on cocaine and alcohol. Alternatively, he or she may be a marijuana-dependent middle-class teenager who is failing school and is finally sent to treatment by worried parents. A third staple client is the counterpart of the middle-class neurasthenic of days gone by— an older, female, nonworking user of depressants, including barbiturates, tranquilizers, and alcohol.

The Medical/Criminal Idea of Treatment
and the Evolution of Governmental Roles

The most important single federal treatment initiative since the founding of the Lexington and Fort Worth facilities was the "War on Drugs" of the Nixon administration. This effort directly enlisted community-based drug treatment in the task of decreasing criminal activity on the streets of the nation's big cities. The concept of treatment as visualized in the national strategy merged the criminal and medical ideas in a single framework. It drew on the popular impression that heroin addiction, because of its great expense, motivated addicts to take up criminal careers. Police estimated that half of all major urban crimes were committed by addicts. If the new forms of treatment were successful in eliminating the desire or need for heroin, the criminal chain would be broken; if enough addicts were treated, national crime rates would be dramatically reduced.

President Nixon, who had already made the war on street crime a centerpiece of his domestic policy, became convinced that attacking the drug problem would be the key to winning that war. By massively increasing the number of both correctional and community-based treatment program "slots" available to criminal addicts, it was felt that increased street-level police activity (supported by a new federal Law Enforcement Assistance Administration and Office of Drug Abuse Law Enforcement) could not only incapacitate but also rehabilitate. Through an Executive Order in 1971 and subsequent legislation, the Special Action Office for Drug Abuse Prevention (SAODAP) was created in the Executive Office of the President; it was given an unusually broad mandate and the authority to organize, direct, and evaluate the federally supported drug treatment effort.

The high point of federal commitment to drug treatment occurred when the Special Action Office negotiated directly with local treatment providers to "buy" their waiting lists (i.e., provide sufficient new funding to admit these individuals for treatment). The Special Action Office also required that preexisting levels of local funding be maintained and specified the nature of treatment to be delivered. Moreover, it set reimbursement rates prospectively on the basis of those specifications, monitored treatment program performance in terms of both enrollment and patient status at discharge, provided technical assistance to program managers, and organized and delivered staff training.

Although this initiative marked the fullest commitment of the federal government to building a national drug treatment system, it also laid the groundwork for its dismemberment and subsequent parceling out to the states. Under this initiative, the first grant program was established to deliver funding to states instead of directly to communities or providers. For the first time, states were required to designate a lead agency and develop and submit to the federal government their own plan for establishing and operating a treatment system. Furthermore, the contracts being made with community treatment agencies at this time had explicit provisions for progressive cost sharing, with the federal contribution to be reduced over the life of the contract. The program or community was required to make up the declining federal share from state or local appropriations or other sources (including client fees).

In 1973 the narcotic drug abuse branch of the National Institute of Mental Health was separated and elevated to become the National Institute on Drug Abuse (NIDA), collecting from across a number of government departments all of the major treatment and prevention services and drug abuse research programs. Although an Office of Drug Abuse Policy continued to exist in the White House, NIDA assumed SAODAP's responsibility for the national treatment system; Robert DuPont, the head of SAODAP following Jerome Jaffe's departure, became NIDA's first director. Responsibility and authority were given to state agencies progressively, leading to the institution of relatively unfettered block grants to the states in 1981 for allocation among alcohol, drug, and mental health programs. Since 1981 the federal share of payment for drug treatment programs has dropped well below the state share, and federal activities in the treatment field, particularly the mission of NIDA, have concentrated on biomedical and, to a lesser degree, behavioral and social sciences research.

More broadly, drug policy at the federal level has shifted its focus to direct an increasingly greater proportion of attention and resources toward enforcement and interdiction. This emphasis was apparent throughout the Reagan administration and in the provisions of the 1986 Anti-Drug Abuse Act. Passed in the wake of the deaths of several prominent athletes from cocaine overdose, this bill symbolized heightened public and governmental concern about the drug problem, particularly cocaine, and translated that symbolism into large sums of federal dollars—far more of which were assigned to enforcement and prevention services than to treatment.

The 1988 Anti-Drug Abuse Act and 1989 emergency supplemental appropriation for treatment and prevention signaled a reconsideration of the balance of federal attention, driven by concern about the startling increase in gunshot deaths in crack-selling areas in and around Washington, New York, and Los Angeles, and by the steep incidence of AIDS connected with drug use in these and other areas. Along with continued large sums for enforcement, the 1988 act authorized significantly increased funding commitments to the alcohol/drug/mental health block grant, together with higher "set-asides" (funds specifically earmarked) for drug treatment. The act also initiated a new temporary program specifically to reduce treatment waiting lists through grants to providers (reminiscent of the approach of SAODAP). However, as a consequence of Congress's deficit-driven spending limits, not much of the authorized increase was appropriated.

The 1988 act also created a new Office of National Drug Control Policy in the White House. The office is directed by a quasi-Cabinet-level "drug czar," who is assisted by respective deputies for supply and demand reduction; it has unusual budget control authority, high visibility, and a statutory requirement to develop an annual National Drug Control Strategy. The first director was appointed in 1989: William Bennett, a lawyer and trained philosopher who previously headed the U.S. Department of Education.

The new office is a chrysalis of the ideological elements of national drug policy. The first national strategy document (issued in September 1989) sweepingly rejected libertarian ideas and argued for much tougher criminal approaches to drug users. Medical ideas were drawn upon in two contexts: the public health argument that the casual or regular (nonaddict) user is *"highly* contagious . . . a potential agent of infection" and that drug addiction is a chronic disease with no permanent cure, thus presenting the continuing possibility of relapse. The document defined treatment's role in terms of the medical/criminal idea, leavened with additional concerns characteristic of America in the 1980s, such as danger to the lives of unborn children, AIDS, and the economy. In line with the overall stress on a stronger criminal view, the document argued for a reexamination of the effectiveness of voluntary (versus enforced) drug treatment. The second document, which was released in January 1990, was more sophisticated in its analysis of the treatment system, but it continued the major strategic emphases of the initial edition.

CONCLUSION

It would be natural to assume that drug treatment is the kept creature of medical approaches to the drug problem, that treatment programs are compatible only with medical ideas and must stand in a relationship of contradiction or antagonism to both libertarian and criminal ideas and institutions. Nevertheless, both in principle and in practice, drug treatment is a flexible set of instruments capable of achieving several socially desirable objectives and of serving more than one ideological master without necessarily losing its essential rehabilitative character. Because of the complex and constantly changing character of the drug problem, practical policies to deal with it will always need to meld the fundamental ideas in some way; as a result, policy differences over treatment are more often matters of emphasis, priority, and allocation than of rigid ideological exclusion. Each major governing idea is influential in determining the policy role of treatment and what it should be expected to contribute.

In the case of each idea, the implicit standard of treatment success looks to serve both the individual and the collective interest. Libertarian ideas argue that, for the individual, treatment should maintain or increase the individual's privacy and independence, which may have been diminished by drugs; for the society, treatment should reduce net social costs (such as public medical and criminal justice expenses) and increase productivity (job earnings and tax receipts). Medical ideas also imply two standards: for the individual, response to therapy is measured in terms of reduced morbidity and mortality, that is, relief of suffering from somatic illnesses and psychological distortions and compulsions, and greater longevity. For the society, the public health should benefit through an overall reduction in the prevalence of drug morbidity and mortality, which have a disproportionate effect among the young, and perhaps through reductions in incidence or further transmission *to the degree that drug problems are communicable from the treatable population.*

The criminal view focuses on the reduction of illegal conduct—not only drug offenses per se but also associated personal, property, and public-order crimes. The collective counterpart to individual treatment effects would be a reduction in overall rates of criminal victimizations, prosecutions, and incarcerations.

Libertarian, criminal, and medical goals overlap in practice. For example, the calculus of social benefit and cost includes the costs of illness and criminality. The therapeutic objectives of drug treatment include social adjustment and satisfaction (including reduced criminal involvement); in the prevention-oriented disciplines of mental health and public health, the damaging effects of individual behavior on others through criminal activity are important concerns. Finally, the missions of probation, corrections, and parole authorities with regard to their supervisees often extend beyond the prevention of criminal behavior to imparting legitimate job skills and improving the fulfillment of family and community obligations.

The treatment system that was built under federal direction in the early 1970s and that continues today is based on a balance of ideological concerns. The national policies of the early 1970s concentrated criminal justice efforts on the drug judged most dangerous—heroin—while expanding the options for treatment programs that could work cooperatively with criminal justice institutions. Since 1975 the balance of public policy has moved steadily back toward the criminal idea, while the momentum of the medical idea has shifted into the private realm and led to increasing treatment of a segment of drug problems in private hospitals and clinics. The movement on the public side has been heavily responsive to larger political currents that have favored security interests over other welfare concerns. There continue to be strongly expressed as well as inchoate sentiments favoring libertarian approaches, but the net movement has been a massive transfer of public emphasis to enforcement and incarceration at the expense of the public treatment sector. That pendulum appears to have swung to its limit, and the opportunity for explicit reconsideration of the role, extent, and financing of public and private drug treatment is greater now than at any point since the mid-1970s. This is the context in which the following chapters describe the problems that treatment can address, examine where and how the treatment supply system has changed, present plans to restructure it where needed, and define the costs and benefits that may accrue.

3

The Need for Treatment

The history of drug policy provides evidence on the role of treatment programs in the array of policy responses to the drug problem. But what exactly needs to be treated? And how widespread is it? These questions are addressed in this chapter, which specifies the current need for treatment in terms of objective criteria based on scientific research and clinical experience. This is not the same as determining who wants treatment. Subjective motives or desires to seek help are not necessarily consistent with objective evaluation or practicality. Assessing need is also different from measuring the actual demand for treatment, which is critically bound up with treatment cost and the ability and willingness of someone—the individual, a charitable provider, a third party, or some combination of these—to cover that cost. The issues of wants/motives and demand/cost are covered in subsequent chapters; the focus here is on scientific and clinical understanding of the drug problem, which enables a definition and measurement of treatment needs.

In clinical applications, diagnostic criteria can be used to determine, within an accepted range of precision and replicability, whether treatment is needed in an individual case. By appropriate methodological extension, these criteria can provide a probabilistic estimate of the aggregate need for treatment in the population as a whole. Refined diagnostic tools, in combination with treatment effectiveness studies, might further indicate not only whether treatment is needed but also what type is most likely to be beneficial.

Diagnostic criteria, which are discussed in detail below, distinguish drug use—for which no treatment is called for, although other responses may be—from drug abuse and dependence. The criteria are based on *the level and pattern of drug consumption* and *the severity and persistence of functional problems* resulting from these consumption patterns. Their development has been an evolutionary process, and consensus is not yet total. Reasons for this gradual rate of progress are not hard to locate. Drug consumption patterns and their consequences are extremely complicated and continually changing. The modalities and philosophies of treatment are diverse. And as new drugs and ways of administering them appear, the applicability of even well-tested diagnostic criteria must be reestablished.

As a basis for understanding the need for treatment, the committee first outlines a conceptual model of the different types and stages of individual drug consumption and its consequences: use, abuse, dependence, recovery, and relapse. The major factors that are thought to propel this model are then summarized, namely, individual learning processes that lead to the modification, persistence, or extinction of drug consumption. Learning is contingent on drug effects, socially conditioned reinforcers, and, to some degree, personal characteristics. In turn, the availability of drugs and other reinforcers and of good opportunities for character development are strongly shaped by economic, political, and cultural factors that vary through time and across different geographic locations.

Treatment focuses largely on ending or at least reducing the severity of an individual's dependence or abuse and associated problems—that is, on initiating and maintaining recovery and averting relapse. In the sections that follow, the committee analyzes a number of general and special-population surveys that include items approximating the diagnostic criteria for dependence and abuse. These analyses yield new estimates of the need for treatment in the population at a fixed point in time. Yet these estimates are simple approximations only. Individuals continually move into and out of dependence and abuse. Although these movements can be understood qualitatively, quantitative data at the national level lack the necessary density and precision for a full-scale dynamic analysis. Nevertheless, when joined with calculations of the social costs associated with drug problems, these population estimates provide a basis for further analysis of the drug treatment system and its adequacy.

THE INDIVIDUAL DRUG HISTORY:
A MODEL AND OVERVIEW

During any given month in the past 20 years, at least 14 million (in the peak months, more than 25 million) individuals in the United States consumed some kind of illicit drug. Each of these individuals had a specific history of drug experience, in the context of unique biographical circumstances, yielding millions of different patterns of risks and consequences. To some degree, these patterns of drug behavior, context, and risk can be grouped according to familiar stereotypes. But even the stereotypes are highly diversified. For example, consider the differences among the following:

- a young teenager who lives in a welfare-supported, innercity household with no adult male relatives present, sporadically attends junior high school but appears daily at a street venue to deliver crack-cocaine to customers (mostly adults) of an older gang member, and feels superior to these customers but has recently smoked some crack and marijuana laced with phencyclidine (PCP) several times with another young "dealer";
- an adolescent college student from an affluent two-parent family, whose illicit drug experience is taking amphetamine pills to stay awake and cram for final exams and smoking marijuana with friends at house parties a few times during a semester;
- a single person in the mid-20s, steadily employed as an office manager, who takes amphetamines for weeks at a time as an appetite suppressant and uses marijuana or cocaine several weekend nights a month on dates or at parties;
- a divorced woman in her early 20s with two pre-school-age children, who supports herself mostly through welfare, intermittent prostitution, and larceny, which has led to several misdemeanor convictions and investigations by the family protective services office; she is currently pregnant and using crack-cocaine, marijuana, alcohol, and/or mood-lifting pills nearly every day by herself and with customers or boyfriends;
- a white-collar professional about 30 years old with a working spouse and no children, who has been snorting progressively larger quantities of powdered cocaine night after night (and increasingly, during the day) for several months—abstaining and crashing for a few days occasionally with larger than usual doses of alcohol; and
- a man in his mid-30s who was a childhood immigrant to the United States and has no fixed address or occupation, irregular contact with a common-law wife and children, and a 20-year criminal record that includes burglary, armed robbery, assault, and drug sales convictions leading to extensive prison time; he is currently injecting heroin several times a day and supplementing that with cocaine, PCP, amphetamines, alcohol, and whatever else comes to hand; he is also seropositive for the AIDS virus.

The treatment implications of these drug consumption patterns are quite different, and many individual variations cut across these stereotypes. To clarify clinical decisions and permit intelligible estimation of the overall need for treatment in the population, it is necessary to categorize drug

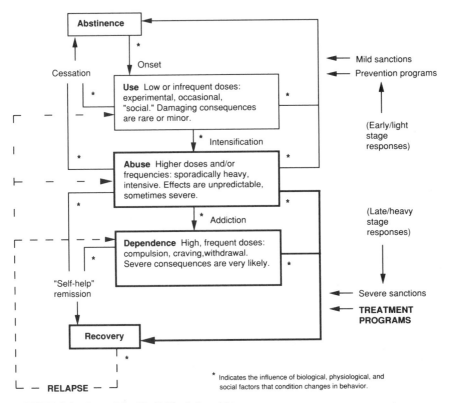

FIGURE 3-1 A model of individual drug history.

consumers based on their current dose, frequency, and method of drug consumption, taking into account their past consumption patterns and weighing the severity of associated problems and consequences—including physical, emotional, and social problems. A conceptual paradigm of illicit drug consumption and responses is presented in Figure 3-1.

This scheme depicts the principal patterns or types of drug-taking behavior and orders them into common stages that, taken together, constitute a developmental pathway for individuals. Across large numbers of people, transitions from one stage to another can be summarized as risks or probabilities. These transition probabilities are heavily influenced by the interaction of two elements: the specific pattern of drug consumption and the presence of other biological, psychological, and social factors.

Drug consumption is divided into three levels or stages commonly distinguished by clinicians and researchers: *use*, *abuse*, and *dependence*. (Other terms—for example, those used by the National Commission on Marijuana and Drug Abuse [1973] and Siegel [1990]—are related to this triad: experimental, occasional, or social/recreational *use*; intensified, regular, sporadically heavy or "binge" *abuse*; and compulsive or addictive behavior, which is *dependence*.) Each of these stages is, on average, more hazardous, more obtrusive, and more likely to provoke or induce social interventions (e.g., punitive sanctions, attention by prevention programs, admission to treatment) than the one before.

Abstinence, Drug Types, and Normative Attitudes

Prior to drug consumption, there is abstinence. Abstinence here is defined behaviorally and means not seeking out, not consuming, and not being impaired as a result of having consumed psychoactive drugs. Abstinence so defined is usually but not necessarily the same as being physiologically "drug-free," which refers strictly to the absence of pharmacological effects or traces of drugs or their metabolites. Taking psychoactive drugs under legitimate medical supervision at prescribed doses for generally recognized therapeutic purposes does not in itself violate abstinence.

Federal and state codes define specific psychoactive drugs by their chemical names, dividing them into several classes of controlled and proscribed substances (Table 3-1). Some drugs, such as the volatile solvents in model airplane glue, are virtually uncontrolled. Others, such as nicotine (in tobacco) and alcohol, are legally available to those above certain ages but only under circumscribed terms and conditions, including various situational prohibitions (e.g., tobacco smoking is prohibited in many public and commercial locations, drinking of alcohol is prohibited while driving). Because of the partial legality of alcohol and tobacco, little attention is paid in this report to their use, abuse, or dependence except in conjunction with illicit drug consumption.

Abstinence from illicit psychoactive drugs is normative—that is, legally and morally unquestioned by most people most of the time. But social norms are much less homogeneous across social groups or situations than are legal definitions, and they are subject to change across time. The shifting normative status of marijuana among young middle-class Americans over the past 25 years is a good illustration. The overall degree of normative chill attached to illicit drug consumption varies from slight to grave depending on the details, gradations similar to the moral index applied to other classes of illegal acts ranging from traffic infractions through mass murder. For example, when a public sample was asked about the severity of crimes, only homicide/manslaughter and forcible rape were rated as worse offenses than selling cocaine (Jacoby and Dunn, 1987, cited in Flanagan and Jamieson, 1988). Using cocaine, however, was seen as comparable in severity to drunk driving without an accident or thefts or burglaries of moderate amounts of goods—serious crimes but much lower on the scale. In a 1986 opinion

TABLE 3-1 Classification of Psychoactive Drugs

Class	Examples	Effects for Which Used	Other Possible Effects
Opiates	Heroin, morphine, methadone, codeine	Euphoria, relaxation, mood elevation (reduction of pain, anxiety, aggressive or sexual drives)	Drowsiness, respiratory depression, nausea
Depressants	Barbiturates, methaqualone (Quaalude), diazepam (Valium)	Like alcohol: euphoria, relaxation, mood elevation	Drowsiness, mood volatility, respiratory depression, nausea, impaired coordination
Stimulants	Cocaine, amphetamine, nicotine, methylphenidate	Euphoria, alertness, sense of well-being, suppression of fatigue and hunger, increased sexual arousal	Increased pulse and blood pressure, tremor, insomnia, paranoia, psychosis, cardiac arrest
Hallucinogens	LSD, mescaline, psilocybin, MDA	Vividly altered perception, detachment from self	Increased blood pressure, tremor, impaired judgment and perceptions of time and distance, panic reaction
Phencyclidines	PCP, ketamine	Detachment from surroundings, numbness, distorted perceptions, illusions of strength	Anxiety, impaired coordination, paranoid delusions
Cannabinoids	Marijuana, hashish	Euphoria, relaxation, altered perceptions, increased sexual arousal	Increased appetite, disorientation, impaired judgment and coordination, paranoia, headaches
Inhalants	Acetone, benzene, nitrous oxide, butyl nitrate	Euphoria, giddiness, illusions of strength, distortions of visual perception	Hallucinations, slurred speech, drowsiness, headache, nausea, respiratory depression, cardiac arrest

NOTE: The effects of different compounds within each drug class differ in duration and in the specific combination of effects. In addition, the responses to a drug vary according to the dose level, the drug taker's prior experience with the drug, including current tolerance, the drug taker's prior mental and physical condition, and the situation. The effects of a drug change from immediate reaction across time to the clearing of extended responses, which may involve withdrawal symptoms after chronic use.

survey in which 96 percent of respondents disagreed with the statement that all illicit drugs should be made legal, 85 percent agreed that "the best place for most drug abusers is a drug treatment program and not jail" (Flanagan and Jamieson, 1988:194).

Learning and Drug Experience

An individual drug history is most readily understood as a sequential learning experience. An individual cannot know beforehand exactly how a drug will affect him or her because there is great variability in this response, depending on the drug and the specific dose exposure, the individual's biological and psychological state, and the social circumstances (Levison et al., 1983). Every naturally occurring or synthetic psychoactive drug affects the brain and other nervous tissue by mimicking, displacing, blocking, or depleting specific chemical messengers between nerve cells, called endogenous neurotransmitters. Most drugs directly affect one or several of the numerous neurotransmitter systems, but the brain is so complex and interlinked that many functions may be significantly affected by action on a single type of messenger/receptor system. These dose-dependent metabolic effects are responsible for a number of phenomena: immediate changes in mood, thinking, and physiological states; medium and longer term neuroadaptation such as increased tolerance to some (but not all) drug effects; and, in some cases, persistent or irreversible changes in brain functioning or memory. (Such changes are not necessarily strange or ominous; strong memories of any kind produce persistent changes in the brain.)

Some drug effects are hard to duplicate without the drug's presence; other effects differ, if at all, only quantitatively (that is, in how rapid, long-lasting, or uniform the effects are across individuals) from the way other kinds of stimuli can affect the brain (e.g., motion, touch, sights and sounds, including human communication). Drug effects depend heavily on the dose, the route of administration (smoking and intravenous [IV] injection are very fast; snorting, chewing, drinking, or eating, rather slow), previous exposure, and other characteristics of the individual consumer, including what he or she expects the drug to do. The metabolic mechanisms of drug action in humans are shared with some other mammalian species, which has been a basis for developing animal models that have been important sources of scientific insight and testing.

Some individuals respond quite positively to their initial drug experience;[1] others react quite negatively (experiencing nausea, paranoia, or a

---

[1] In dramatic terms: "It's so good, don't even try it once." Although this exhortation mimics current beliefs about crack-cocaine, it is actually a quotation about heroin (Smith and Gay, 1972).

painful drug hangover). Still others react with puzzlement: "Well, that's different—but what's all the fuss about?" There are various reasons for these different responses, but their relative importance is uncertain. Not only the drug's metabolic effects, modulated by the individual's chemistry, but also the associated circumstances and activities, filtered through the individual's personality, shape the initial response to drugs, creating different degrees of satisfaction or discomfort. If the individual continues to use drugs—which may occur even if the initial trial is not rewarding, as a consequence of continued curiosity, local custom, or peer pressure—a history of experience is built up, a learning curve, in effect, that can lead in different directions depending on the specifics of the individual's experience.

The balancing of pleasurable or rewarding experiences and punishing or unpleasant experiences that occurs during the early weeks or months of drug involvement may be of critical importance. If the net impact of those experiences is highly positive, the effect or memory of that "honeymoon" can remain remarkably strong over time, even as continuing reward diminishes and punishment increases, especially if alternative competitive behaviors are not exercised or reinforced as strongly. Social interventions directed toward the individual—criminal penalties, job-related or family sanctions, prevention programs, and treatment programs—contribute to the learning history, but precisely how depends on the details of that individual's experience (Ray, 1988).

Added to the specific hazards associated with each stage of drug use are the risks of transition to further stages. Each stage entails some chance of progression to the next, although progression is not inevitable. A minority of experimental users intensify their consumption to the level of abuse; fewer yet advance into dependence. Nevertheless, the entire U.S. population, even abstainers, can be viewed as incurring some risk from drug consumption: even those who have never used drugs are slightly at risk by virtue of drugs being available to them (in an ever-active market) and by virtue of the behavior of drug users in their environment.

What the drug consumer learns through drug experience takes the specific form of tendencies to seek drugs. That pattern, at least, is what the observer sees; the consumer often defines this "tendency" as something else—a habit, interest, hunger, or craving. These drug-seeking tendencies vary in when they are expressed as well as how forcefully—that is, how effectively the tendency to seek drugs competes with other behaviors. The tendency may be entirely dormant unless some condition or cue evokes it. Cues may be purely internal or set off by external contingencies. Purely internal cues could be physiological sensations owing to earlier drug exposure—for example, immediate or delayed withdrawal syndromes—or they may be moods, thoughts, or sensations that were associated in time or meaning with taking drugs. These phenomena are as varied as individual biography: for one person, pain, distress, or sadness may lead to drug craving; for another, feelings of pleasure, including the pleasure of certain company, may evoke the response; for yet another, waking up in the morning and going to bed at night may produce this effect. Times, places, people, objects—any association with earlier drug taking may evoke drug craving, and the closer the link, the stronger the cue.

The mixture of drug effects that consumers seek, or are satisfied with, tends to change subtly over time, moving *typically* from just "getting high" or being sociable in the early stage of use to the achievement of temporary relief from the persistent desire or learned need for a drug (a desire that persists even after short-term withdrawal is completed) in the stage of dependence. From a subjective point of view, drug-seeking behavior seems highly volitional during initiation and early use; this voluntary period, however, is profoundly influenced by the conditions and responses of other people in the immediate vicinity and by individual variation in how drugs affect the brain and personality.

Environmental Variations

There is a range of individual susceptibility to the learning of drug-seeking behavior that would be seen clearly if environmental conditions were held constant. But social environments are not constant; indeed, variation in social environmental conditions correlates strongly with demographic and geographic variations in drug use, abuse, and dependence rates. Other factors that affect drug-seeking behavior are the contexts and conditions of availability of different drugs (e.g., cocaine, heroin, marijuana, and amphetamines) as well as the new technologies and marketing organizations that are periodically introduced.

Cocaine is a good example. Cocaine is a chemical in the leaf of the coca plant that functions for the plant as a pest repellent. Human societies in the Andean region have used the coca leaf as a stimulant in low but effective oral doses (often by chewing the leaf, although there are a variety of preparations) for about 5,000 years, both as an ordinary tonic and in various medicinal and ceremonial applications. By 1860 the cocaine alkaloid (base, or free-base) had been isolated and extracted; a few decades later, its water-soluble salt, cocaine hydrochloride, became widely popular in Europe and the United States. Cocaine hydrochloride was offered in a variety of commercial preparations, including cocaine snuffing powder, coca cigars, coca wines, Coca-Cola, and injectable solutions. This epidemic of popular use ended with the onset of better medical knowledge regarding the substance, pharmaceutical regulation, and criminal sumptuary laws motivated by strong racial fears. Cocaine was confined to the underworld, where it was used mostly by injection along with heroin.

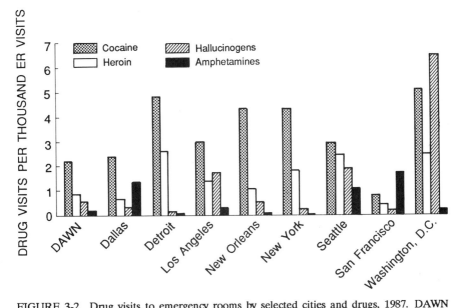

FIGURE 3-2 Drug visits to emergency rooms by selected cities and drugs, 1987. DAWN = all cities reporting to the Drug Abuse Warning Network. Source: National Institute on Drug Abuse (1988a).

Cocaine reemerged in the 1970s, mainly as an expensive snuffing powder. There was also a brief vogue of desalting the powder to return it to the free-base, heating it to vaporization, and inhaling the vapor (smoking it). More recently, cocaine base has been brought directly to market as "rock" or "crack." As a result of large-scale investments in cultivation, manufacture, and smuggling protection in the early 1980s, the product became widely available, packaged for street sale in a number of large urban areas in as small as single-dose amounts.

The drifting of cocaine consumption between popularity and insularity, and through different technologies and recipes, is not atypical of ethnopharmaceuticals, although every drug has its own particular industrial and epidemiological history. As well as differences across time, there are differences from place to place at the same time. The Drug Abuse Warning Network (DAWN), which has tracked the ebb and flow of different drugs in the United States for approximately the past 15 years, reveals very different comparative levels of severe drug reactions, and, by implication, of abuse and dependence patterns, in large U.S. cities (Figure 3-2). Although there are relatively small differences among Hispanic, white, and black U.S. population groups in the overall use of illicit drugs, these differences are much larger for the consumption of specific drugs.

Age of Onset and Drug Sequencing

The onset of drug use has been studied fairly extensively. Two salient findings common to surveys of youth, the general population, treatment enrollees, and prison populations involve the age of onset of use and the sequence of drug involvement. The bulk of initial, experimental drug usage occurs during the teenage years. Very few children aged 10 or younger have begun to use drugs. Nearly as few people begin using drugs—or even any particular type of drug, unless it was never previously available—after reaching 25 years of age. (There is increasing concern about abuse and dependence syndromes among elderly individuals, but those conditions are largely the result of the escalated use of alcohol and prescription drugs.)

Most new users of any drug do not progress very far, and there are often shifts from intermittent use back to abstinence. The use stage may continue for a long period, or it may be transitory; the individual may return to long-term abstinence either in response to some form of intervention or direct persuasion or on his or her own initiative. The earlier drug use begins, however, the more likely it is to progress to abuse or dependence; the later it begins, the more likely it is to "tail off" into renewed abstinence without further progression or, if progression occurs, to yield to earlier, more sustained recovery.

Cessation without intervention does not necessarily imply a self-contained decision that "drugs are bad." A convenient source of a favored drug may disappear, and new sources may prove undesirable or too costly. Alternatively, an individual may cease drug use as a result of social circumstances (changing friends, falling in love with someone who does not use or approve of drugs, marriage, child-raising, and job responsibilities; Schasre, 1966; Waldorf, 1973; Eldred and Washington, 1976; Robins, 1980; Kandel and Maloff, 1983) that leave little time for evening bar-hopping and party-going. Another incentive for cessation may be learning about previously unsuspected hazards through news stories or by personal observation (Johnston, 1985). For many years, introduction to drugs in the majority of cases has proceeded in a general, cumulative sequence: tobacco and alcohol, to marijuana, to other inhalable or orally ingested substances, to hypodermic injection of opiates or powerful stimulants (cocaine, amphetamines).[2] This sequence is almost always initiated between the ages of 12 and 15; the injection phase, when reached, generally begins between the ages of 17 and 20. The sequencing phenomenon is thought to reflect two factors: drug availability and the degree of opprobrium attached to

---

[2] Drug preparations are often contaminated with biologics or adulterants. When the needle route is used and injection equipment is reused without thorough cleaning, transmission of infectious diseases is common. AIDS is the best known and most feared of such diseases, although hepatitis and heart infections are very commonly transmitted.

the respective drug types. As cocaine's marketing expands and marijuana's diminishes, the sequence of introduction to these drugs may become less uniform.

There are multiple theoretical reasons for these age and sequential uniformities, but the data are insufficient to scale these reasons precisely according to strength, distribution, or importance. The most frequently advanced explanations for the uniformity of adolescent onset are sociological and biological: adolescence is a period of transition between childhood dependency and adult self-responsibility; in many cases, the continuous adult supervision characteristic of childhood diminishes substantially; errors in newly enfranchised judgment—exercised as "trying out identities," "testing limits," and "rebelling"—are more widely tolerated or permitted among adolescents than among children or adults; adolescents grow quickly to nearly adult size and mobility, experiencing strong passions and desires ("raging hormones") that they are slow to learn how to channel and control. Whatever the reasons, a variety of mildly to seriously deviant behaviors (e.g., sexual profligacy, suicide attempts, assaultive behavior with weapons, thievery for profit) begin to occur at these ages.

If progression occurs (from use to abuse to dependence), it generally takes from 5 to 10 years following the first experimental use of any drug—in the late teens or early 20s—and from 1 to 4 years following the experimental use of the particular drug that is being consumed in a dependent manner (Brown et al., 1971; Robins, 1980; Kandel and Maloff, 1983; White, 1988; Kozel and Adams, 1985). Progression seems to be more rapid with stimulants such as cocaine and amphetamines than with other types of drugs.

Typically, the initial voluntary component of drug-seeking behavior is compromised by the cumulative physiological, psychological, and social effects of the dependence process. The conditioning of behavior by physiological and psychological drug effects and by the distribution of rewards and punishments in the proximate social environment can conspire to steadily undermine the individual's ability to control the level and timing of drug consumption. Eventually, continued high-frequency drug consumption behavior becomes so ingrained that the individual must explicitly *unlearn it*. Some individuals achieve such unlearning by trial and error; most drug-dependent individuals are unable to do so and thus discover they need help to unlearn their drug-seeking habits (i.e., to successfully extinguish drug-seeking behavior).

Diagnosing Dependence and Abuse

Drug treatment is not designed for the low-intensity drug user who is readily able to control his or her level of consumption and for whom functional consequences have not yet accumulated. When progression to abuse occurs, the less intrusive ambulatory drug treatments are generally brought to bear. The most resource-intensive modalities, which involve extended pharmacological interventions or residential stays, are designed principally to treat drug dependence.

The importance of these distinctions has led clinicians and researchers to try to develop clear, standardized criteria for abuse and dependence. These criteria are most fully described in two authoritative, multiyear, multidisciplinary collaborative efforts built on extensive literature reviews and trials in research and clinical practice: the forthcoming 10th edition of the *International Statistical Classification of Diseases, Injuries, and Causes of Death* (ICD-10), a product of the World Health Organization, and the 3rd revised edition of the *Diagnostic and Statistical Manual of Mental Disorders* (DSM-III-R), published in 1987 by the American Psychiatric Association. In codifying diagnostic criteria for abuse and dependence, both classification systems have converged on formulations that emphasize two fundamental observations.

First, the criteria for dependence and abuse (the latter is called "harmful use" in ICD-10) apply uniformly to all psychoactive substances, which emphasizes the commonalities in drug-related behavior, physiology, and cognition or subjective awareness. The more specific pharmacological effects and sociolegal status of each substance are recognized but do not directly affect the diagnosis. Second, both schemes concede the irreducible complexity of drug phenomena. Rather than offering a single file of descriptors that every positive diagnosis must match (e.g., the classical signs of tolerance and withdrawal), the two systems lay out an array of functionally significant problems, diverse formations or combinations of which are accepted as equally significant for diagnostic purposes. Perhaps a small monument to this complexity is the fact that, despite cross-consultation between the two projects, and although each retains the same number of defining criteria (nine), there are various differences between them in shades of meaning (Table 3-2).

The convergence is most complete in defining the dependence syndrome: in the ICD-10, it is a cluster of physiological, behavioral, and cognitive symptoms or phenomena such that "the use of a drug or class of drugs takes on a much higher priority for a given individual than other behaviors that once had a higher value"; the DSM-III-R defines it as when "the person has impaired control of psychoactive substance use and continues use of the substance despite adverse consequences." A positive ICD-10 diagnosis is triggered when three or more criteria are present at some time in the previous year or continuously during the previous month. Similarly, any three DSM criteria precipitate the diagnosis of dependence. There are also degrees of dependence—mild, moderate, and severe—based on

TABLE 3-2   Correspondence Between the Criteria for Dependence[a] of the *International Statistical Classification of Diseases, Injuries, and Causes of Death* (10th rev. ed.; ICD-10) and the *Diagnostic and Statistical Manual of Mental Disorders* (3rd ed., rev.; DSM-III-R)

ICD-10	DSM-III-R
Progressive neglect of alternative pleasures or interests in favor of substance use.	Important social, occupational, or recreational activities given up because of substance use.
Persisting with drug use despite clear evidence of overtly harmful consequences.	Continued substance use despite knowledge of having a persistent or recurrent social, psychological, or physical problem that is caused or exacerbated by the use of the substance.
Evidence of tolerance such that increased doses of the substance are required in order to achieve effects originally produced by lower doses.	Marked tolerance: need for markedly increased amounts of the substance in order to achieve intoxication or desired effect, or markedly diminished effect with continued use of the same amount.
Substance use with the intention of relieving withdrawal symptoms and subjective awareness that this strategy is effective.	Substance often taken to relieve or avoid withdrawal symptoms.
A physiological withdrawal state.	Characteristic withdrawal symptoms.
Strong desire or sense of compulsion to take drugs.	Persistent desire or one or more unsuccessful efforts to cut down or control substance use.
Evidence of an impaired capacity to control drug taking behavior in terms of its onset, termination, or level of use.	Substance often taken in larger amounts or over a longer period than the person intended.
A narrowing of the personal repertoire of patterns of drug use, e.g., a tendency to drink alcoholic beverages in the same way on weekdays and weekends and whatever the social constraints regarding appropriate drinking behavior.	Frequent intoxication or withdrawal symptoms when expected to fulfill major role obligations at work, school, or at home or when substance use is physically hazardous.
Evidence that a return to substance use after a period of abstinence leads to a rapid reinstatement of other features of the syndrome than occurs with nondependent individuals.	
	A great deal of time spent in activities necessary to get the substance, taking the substance, or recovering from its effects.

[a]A dependence syndrome is present if three or more criteria are met persistently (DSM: continuously) in the previous month or some time (DSM: repeatedly) in the previous year.

the number of symptoms observed above the minimum criterion level and in particular the extent of social and occupational impairment. Diagnostic specifications for partial and full remission are also part of the classification schemes.

Abuse is a lesser category in both schemes. In DSM-III-R, psychoactive substance abuse is defined as follows: the persistence of psychoactive substance use for at least one month or repeatedly over a longer period of continuing use despite the recurrence or persistence of one or more known adverse consequences (social, occupational, psychological, or physical) or the taking of recurrent physical risks such as driving while intoxicated. The substance abuse diagnosis is triggered only if the person has never met the criteria for dependence for this substance. ICD-10 diagnoses "harmful use" when there is clear evidence that the consumption of a substance or substances is responsible for causing the user actual psychological or physical harm—negative social consequences (e.g., arrest, job loss, marital breakdown) are not considered psychological harm. (If, however, these negative consequences in turn cause psychological harm, it is unclear whether the pattern of use would then be deemed harmful.) The ICD-10 scheme puts less emphasis than DSM-III-R on the importance of earlier drug history; previous dependence does not preempt a current finding of the lesser diagnosis, as it does in the DSM system.

The critical commonality in these definitions and measures is that these criteria focus on impairment of control and undesirable functional consequences of excessive drug consumption. These consequences may range from health problems to lost social opportunities, but they are alike in that they are unwanted. Indeed, individuals who become dependent are dismayed by the negative effects of their drug consumption. When the doses and schedules of use become dense enough, they take on a life of their own, which can impair an individual's capacity to reduce or cease drug use in spite of accumulating harm. Helping to strengthen this capacity for choice or self-control over drug seeking—particularly when the individual lacks the protection of confinement (e.g., closed hospital wards or prisons) where there is limited opportunity to exercise choice—is the object of virtually all interventions (including mutual self-help groups) to rehabilitate drug-abusing and drug-dependent individuals. To achieve this goal, it is often necessary to help develop other capabilities (or to heal other disorders or damages) so that alternative ways of behaving become more accessible and their rewards easier to reap.

Recovery and Relapse

Dependence sometimes lasts indefinitely but slowly increases in severity. More typically, however, dependence is interrupted, followed (after several months to several years of drug use) by some period of recovery.[3] Although recovery is similar to abstinence in that drugs are not sought or used, the previous experience of dependence or extensive abuse leaves a variety of powerful residues. There may be craving and other strong drug-related emotions and sensations, which may take months to recede. There may also be permanently disabling physical illnesses and wounds. There will certainly be conditioned behavioral tendencies and responses closely associated with drug taking that are slow to extinguish fully and must be specifically countered if recovery is to last. A recovering individual may have to scrupulously avoid certain locations, situations, or people who were strongly associated with drug acquisition. The individual may carry indelible social stigmata, such as a record of criminal convictions. And there may be other losses created or aggravated by drug involvement: years without conventional employment, lack of formal education, irremediable family divisions, and deep emotional wounds.

Recovery is not an easy process, and first, second, or later episodes may be followed by relapse. Cycling one or more times from recovery back through relapse to dependence or abuse (more rarely, to low-level use) is so common that it must be seen as an intrinsic feature of the natural history of individual drug behavior.

Individuals may follow any one of a range of courses after an initial period of abuse or dependence. There is a cumulative literature on one such course that Winick (1962) called "maturing out" of drug dependence. Although that description of recovery is now viewed as too restrictive and therefore misleading, it does suggest the decades-long span across which the cycle of drug dependence/recovery/relapse can continue. The bulk of the literature on cycles of dependence and recovery concerns heroin, the major drug of dependence of the 1950s and 1960s; it is not yet known whether long-term patterns of dependence on the major drugs of the 1970s and 1980s, marijuana and cocaine, will be similar. There are strong reasons to think that the heroin literature is a good guide, including the fact that findings regarding recovery and relapse from alcoholism resemble findings in the heroin literature.

The classical study of recovery and relapse from heroin addiction prior to the availability of modern treatment modalities was carried out by Vaillant (1973), who followed 100 heroin addicts from New York City who were admitted to Lexington in the early 1950s. For most of the study period, the only form of drug treatment available was detoxification. Yet

---

[3] The term *recovery* is equivalent to the term *remission* generally used in clinical descriptions of other chronic relapsing disorders. *Recovery* is used more commonly in the alcohol and drug field and suggests the more active character of the recovery process, in contrast to the passivity implied by *remission*; that is, a disorder remits, but an individual recovers.

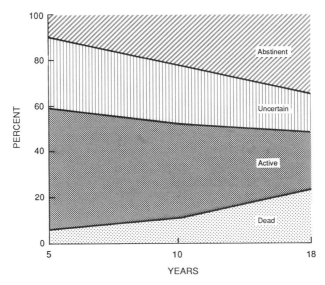

FIGURE 3-3 Status of 100 heroin addicts at three points in time after index hospital discharge. Source: Vaillant (1973).

the prevailing criminal approach to drugs, symbolized in New York by the Rockefeller "get tough" drug laws, guaranteed that there were powerful environmental incentives toward recovery. The results for this cohort are displayed in Figure 3-3. The number of actively heroin-dependent members declined as the cohort aged, but many remained until they died in a cycle of dependence, brief recovery (often while in prison only), and relapse. Deaths occurred at a sustained rate of approximately one per year—roughly the same as if this cohort of 100 men had been about 50 years old on average instead of less than 25 years old at the beginning of the period. Many became virtually permanent prison inmates as a result of unabated heroin use and other criminal behavior.

As these data and much subsequent research (e.g., McGlothlin et al., 1977; Nurco et al., 1981a,b,c) powerfully argue, dependent drug-seeking behavior and its subjective aspect, the strong desire or craving for drugs, are difficult to extinguish once they have been established in a familiar drug-supplying environment. Nevertheless, some proportion of individuals succeed in eliminating an established, chronic pattern of dependent behavior. Studies indicate that there is usually a complicated path to sustained recovery, more often than not involving one or more relapses. Individuals with severe problems (e.g., family disintegration, illiteracy and other educational failings, lack of legitimate job skills, psychiatric disorder) continue to have these difficulties (especially if they precede drug involvement) unless specific help is received to deal with them. Such problems disrupt the process of unlearning (that is, learning self-control over) drug-seeking habits and responses; consequently, these disadvantaged individuals are at intrinsically higher risk of relapse than persons with fewer or less severe problems.

The number of high-quality, long-term studies of recovery from dependence is relatively small, but the results have been consistent. Although many people do recover from dependence, recovery is seldom achieved, or even begun, before the individual recognizes that he or she has suffered and caused significant personal and social harm. Some proportion of individuals who are (or would be) diagnosed as drug abusing or dependent—a proportion that may vary somewhat with the specific drug and especially with the level of problem severity—recover without treatment. The evidence suggests that successful, nontreated recoveries are most likely to occur when the level of consumption and problem severity is low and the individual has (or gains) close friends and relatives—perhaps including coworkers, employers, or fellow members of mutual self-help groups—who provide daily support, encouragement, and disciplined help in avoiding relapse and engaging in non-drug-related activities. This kind of social support increases the chance of recovery whether or not formal treatment is received.

There is as yet, however, no way of discerning who will or will not recover without treatment or over what time frame recovery will proceed, and this discrimination deficit has two important implications. First, it is reasonable and ethically incumbent to presume that treatment is needed whenever abuse or dependence is present, even though this presumption means some individuals may undergo treatment who would otherwise recover even without it but perhaps at a slower rate. It is clinically sensible to titrate the intensity of the prescribed treatment to some degree according to the severity of the condition, the degree of preexisting social and personal support available to the individual, and the number of earlier attempts at untreated recovery. The need for treatment is clearest, and the indication for intensive treatment measures strongest, in cases of severe dependence and prior relapses.

The second implication of the inability to clearly discriminate those who may not need treatment in order to recover involves treatment evaluation. If a form of drug treatment contributes effectively to the recovery of various individuals who are so treated, it basically increases the overall group rate of recovery over what would have occurred in the absence of treatment. Evaluation of treatment effectiveness therefore depends not only on adequately describing the form of treatment and measuring the outcomes among those treated but also on being able to estimate the untreated recovery rate for that group. In practical terms, this means identifying the outcomes in an appropriate untreated comparison group. There are other ways to test treatment effectiveness—for instance, investigating whether larger doses of treatment have more effect than smaller doses, up to the prescribed limit or an optimum. Nevertheless, an untreated comparison group offers the ultimate test. This important methodological issue is discussed in Chapter 5.

ESTIMATING THE EXTENT OF THE NEED FOR TREATMENT

Diagnosing drug abuse or dependence in an individual based on history-taking, physical examination, and the information in previous records is a different matter from estimating how many individuals in the general population meet such diagnostic criteria. Individual histories have never been taken and physical test batteries for drug problems have never been performed on a fully representative sample of the whole U.S. population. A number of partial population studies have been conducted in the 1980s, however, and, taken together, these surveys provide a basis for estimating the extent of the need for treatment.

The most clinically sensitive population study was conducted using the DSM-III Clinical Research Diagnostic Criteria. Nationally adjusted prevalence estimates from household interviews in five metropolitan areas for 1981–1983 (Regier et al., 1988) indicated that, in a given month, 2.3 million adults—about 1 percent of the adult population—would have met the clinical criteria for a diagnosis of drug dependence or abuse. These authors further concluded that, over a 6-month period, a total of 3.4 million adults would have met these criteria because individual drug problems (and particularly patterns of abuse) undergo change across even this short a time span.

For the Presidential Commission on the Human Immunodeficiency Virus Epidemic (1988), the National Institute on Drug Abuse (NIDA) used 1985 household survey data (which were cruder than the Regier team's five-city instrument) to estimate that 6.5 million persons "used drugs in a manner which significantly impair[ed] their health and ability to function." More recently, for the September 1989 National Drug Control Strategy document (Office of National Drug Control Policy, 1989), NIDA used the 1988 household survey conducted by the Research Triangle Institute (NIDA, 1989) to estimate that 4 million persons (about 2 percent of the population aged 12 or older) had taken drugs 200 times in the past 12 months, thus defining the population most clearly in need of treatment.

These variations not only reflect divergent methods of estimating the need for treatment but also show that the extent of need is not static. One good indicator of this changing picture is provided by a data series collected since 1976 from local emergency rooms and medical examiners in cities around the country. The series consists of incidents in which specific drug involvement was noted in medical reports that specifically

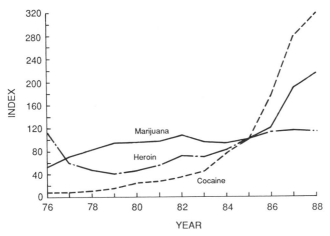

FIGURE 3-4 Trends in cocaine, heroin, and marijuana involvement in deaths and medical emergencies, 1976–1988. Index Year 1985 = 100. Sources: National Institute on Drug Abuse (1987); National Narcotics Intelligence Consumer Committee (1989).

called for this information. Figure 3-4 reports indices for cocaine, heroin, and marijuana from 1976 to 1988 in consistently reporting medical units, standardized to the 1985 value. The cocaine and heroin indices are an average of emergency room and medical examiner cases; marijuana is based on emergency room reports only. The paths of the three drugs have varied during the 12-year period, but all are clearly at higher levels in 1988 than in 1976—for cocaine, dramatically higher. These indices of severe drug problems project a very different picture from that seen in data tracking all current use (once or more in the past month). This type of threshold prevalence data, displayed in Figures 3-5a, 3-5b, and 3-5c for three age strata, shows quite a different set of trends for marijuana and cocaine across the 1980s, particularly among adolescents and young adults.

The committee has developed new estimates of the need for treatment by combining information from three data sources: the 1988 NIDA/RTI national household population survey; a number of surveys and longitudinal studies of criminal justice populations conducted or sponsored by the Bureau of Justice Statistics and the National Institute of Justice; and recent studies of the homeless population.

Household Survey Data

National drug use surveys to collect data from probability samples of U.S. household residents have been conducted at intervals of from one to three years since 1972. The 1988 survey of 5,719 adults and 3,095 adolescents, conducted by the Research Triangle Institute for NIDA, was the first to collect information on items that are part of the ICD-10 and DSM-III-R criteria for drug dependence and abuse. A thorough assessment of the reliability and validity of these survey items, including cross-validation with clinical workups or diagnostic interviews, has not been performed. Nevertheless, it is possible to use responses to relevant survey items on symptoms of dependence, negative consequences or problems attributed to

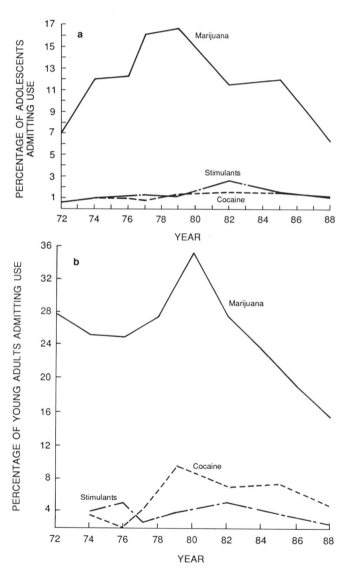

FIGURE 3-5 Continued on next page

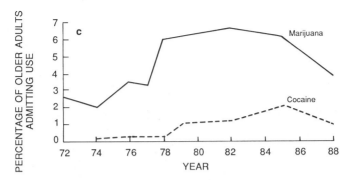

FIGURE 3-5 Trends in past-month drug use, 1972–1988, for (a) adolescents aged 12 to 17 years; (b) young adults aged 18 to 25 years; (c) adults aged 26 and older. Note: The stimulant line is missing in the figures where frequencies were too low for statistical reliability. Source: National Institute on Drug Abuse (1988b, 1989).

a drug, and levels of drug consumption to estimate more precisely than in previous efforts the need for treatment among household residents.

The data on each individual in the survey were classified to yield categories of clear, probable, possible, and unlikely need for treatment. Clear need was defined in terms of exceeding thresholds on three distinct criteria: illicit drug consumption at least three times weekly; at least one explicit symptom of dependence (usually two or more were present); and at least one other kind of functional problem attributed to drug use (usually two or more were evident). If an individual's level of consumption, number of symptoms, or number of problems fell below one threshold value but exceeded the other thresholds, a probable need for treatment was imputed. If there were at least monthly use and some indication of symptoms or problems, the individual's need was classified as possible. In all other cases, the need for treatment was deemed unlikely.

The committee believes that all of those individuals classified as having a clear need for treatment exceed the minimum diagnostic criteria for dependence. Those with a probable need for treatment exceed the criteria for abuse and, in some proportion of the cases, for dependence. Some of those with a possible need may meet the criteria for abuse—most will not. Appendix 3A details the procedures used to arrive at these estimates.

On this basis, out of an estimated 14.5 million individuals (about 7.3 percent of the household population 12 years of age or older) who consumed an illicit drug at least once in the month before the survey,[4] 1.5 million (0.7 percent of the population) can be categorized as having a clear

---

[4]The survey further revealed that an additional 13.5 million persons had used an illicit drug in the past year but not in the past month and 44.5 million individuals had used an illicit drug at least once but not in the past year.

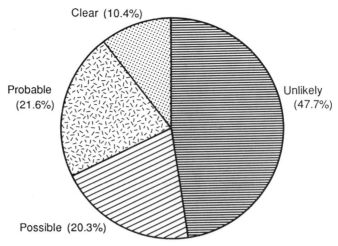

FIGURE 3-6   The estimated need for treatment among the 1988 household drug-consuming population (14.5 million individuals in the household population who had used drugs at least once in the past 30 days). Source: Institute of Medicine analysis of data from the 1988 National Household Survey on Drug Abuse, performed by Research Triangle Institute for the National Institute on Drug Abuse.

need for drug treatment at the time of the survey. Another 3.1 million individuals (1.6 percent) have a probable need; 2.9 million (1.5 percent) have a possible need. The other 6.9 million recent consumers are unlikely to need drug treatment (Figure 3-6).

The clear and probable need cases together comprise about 4.6 million individuals, which is one-third of the 14.5 million current-month drug consumers and about 2.3 percent of the total 1988 household population of 198 million individuals aged 12 and older. The clear and probable cases are two-thirds male and heavily concentrated among younger adults (aged 18 to 34); youths under the age of 18 make up 9 percent of the total (about 396,000 persons), and adults 34 years of age and older constitute another 16 percent (727,000 persons). Most of the adults participate in the labor force: 75 percent hold jobs, and 10 percent are unemployed. The 15 percent not in the labor force are primarily in school, retired, disabled, or have household responsibilities. The unemployment rate among clear and probable need cases is about double the 1988 national unemployment rate. Although a substantial majority of the household residents needing treatment maintain jobs in the legitimate economy, many have low incomes: 32 percent earn less than $9,000 per year, 38 percent earn $9,000 to $20,000, and 30 percent earn more than $20,000 per year.

Criminal Justice Populations

Among those groups that may not be well represented in the national household surveys are the nearly 2 percent of U.S. adults who are under the supervision (as inmates, probationers, or parolees) of judicial and correctional agencies of the federal government, the 50 states, the District of Columbia, and the nation's 3,000 counties. The sizable proportion of drug treatment clients who are also criminal justice clients—far exceeding the 2 percent share of the general population—indicates that the need for treatment among populations supervised by the criminal justice system merits a separate accounting. Moreover, the number of persons under such supervision has been growing at a steady rate (5 to 8 percent annually since 1973) that shows no sign of diminishing. Any future growth in the treatment sector, particularly on the public side, seems bound to involve an expanded interface with criminal justice populations.

On any given day in 1987, the last year for which complete counts are available, nearly 3.7 million adults were under criminal justice supervision or in custody (Allen-Hagen, 1988; Beck et al., 1988; Hester, 1988; Kline, 1988; Greenfeld, 1989). A minority of this group were serving sentences in state and federal prisons (580,000) or county jails (140,000) or were in jail awaiting prosecution (150,000); three out of four were under supervision in the community while on probation (2.24 million) or parole (360,000). About 50,000 minors were in juvenile justice or correctional institutions.

An even larger number of individuals were arrested during 1987 and thus came into contact with the criminal justice system for short periods. Of the 12.7 million arrests leading to 8.7 million jail admissions, 2.6 million arrests were for violent or property (income-generating) crimes and 937,000 were for drug law violations (Jamieson and Flanagan, 1989). A large proportion of other kinds of arrests (e.g., prostitution, gambling, weapons violations, simple assaults) involved drug consumers. At any one time, the bulk of these arrestees were in the community on bail or on recognizance while awaiting disposition of charges. The estimates presented in Appendix 3B suggest that more than a million of these 1987 arrestees clearly or probably needed drug treatment. However, there are better data available on individuals already under criminal justice supervision when arrested or those who come under that jurisdiction following arrest and disposition of charges. These data fall into two categories: those related to individuals in jails or prisons and those related to persons under community supervision (on probation or parole).

The prison and jail inmate population numbered 874,000 at the end of 1987. Inmates are not supposed to be consuming drugs while in custody (although there is clearly substantial leakage of drugs into correctional settings). Many have long prior histories of drug abuse or dependence, however, and enforced abstinence during incarceration hardly ensures continued abstinence after release.

Prior drug problems are quite common among state prison inmates.[5] A 1986 survey of inmates (Innes, 1988) found that 80 percent had used an illicit drug at least once, 63 percent had used such drugs regularly at some time in the past, 43 percent had used an illicit drug daily in the month prior to their offense, and 35 percent were under the influence of a drug at the time of the offense. State prison inmates typically began illicit drug use at age 15, were first arrested at age 17, and first began regular use of a "major" drug (heroin, cocaine, PCP, LSD [lysergic acid diethylamide], methadone) at age 18. The median age of the prison population was 28 years.

Confidential surveys conducted among prisoners demonstrate how drug involvement patterns have changed both in character and quantity over the past 15 years[6] (Table 3-3). In state prisons in 1974, one in four inmates reported having been under the influence of one or more drugs when he (or she, although 19 out of 20 inmates were male) committed the crime that prompted his incarceration. Heroin was the principal drug mentioned; marijuana was less common, and cocaine was rare. In 1979, with a third more prisoners in custody altogether, one in three prisoners had been under the influence of a drug. Heroin, however, was mentioned less frequently and thus was much lower in proportion and numbers. Marijuana had risen substantially on both counts, and cocaine prevalence had risen dramatically, although it was still less common than heroin.

In 1986, with two-and-a-half times as many prisoners in custody as in 1974, the number of heroin mentions had increased and was again

---

[5] Regarding prisons versus jails: generally, sentences that will involve a minimum of one year actually behind bars are served in prisons (state penitentiaries); those with shorter minimum confinements are served in county jails. (A few states have a single custodial system rather than separate county and state facilities.) There are also regular exceptions to this rule. The overall length of a sentence is almost always longer (generally by a factor of two to three [see Hester, 1988; State Statistical Programs Branch, 1989]) than the time to be served in custody; the actual amount of time served in prison depends on the state's mandatory release policies, the degree of prison overcrowding, the convict's behavior while in prison and on parole, and other considerations that affect correctional and parole policy.

[6] Prisoners serve sentences of varying lengths, and those with the longest sentences—generally for murder or rape—constitute a much larger share of a prison census than their entering numbers would suggest. Because of the length of sentences, a prison population, in reporting on pre-arrest drug patterns, is like a series of sedimentary layers that reflect criminal drug involvement in earlier periods. The pattern is complicated by the fact that many prison admissions are returned parole violators. At the end of 1988, about 43 percent of state prisoners had been newly admitted during the year, 18 percent had been returned during the year on parole revocations (about half of these with new sentences on top of the old ones), and 39 percent had been continuously in prison for a year or longer (Lawrence Greenfeld, Bureau of Justice Statistics, personal communication, July 1989).

TABLE 3-3   Trends in Numbers and Percentages of
Prison Inmates Who Reported Being Under the Influence
of One or More Drugs at the Time of the Convicted
Offense

Inmate Drug Status	1974		1979		1986	
	No.	%	No.	%	No.	%
No drug	163,000	74.7	204,000	67.7	338,000	64.6
Any drug	55,000	25.3	97,000	32.3	185,000	35.4
Heroin	35,000	16.2	26,000	8.7	36,000	7.0
Cocaine	2,000	1.0	14,000	4.6	56,000	10.7
Marijuana	22,000	10.3	53,000	17.6	97,000	18.6
Total	218,000	100.0	301,000	100.0	523,000	100.0

Sources: Innes (1988); Flanagan and Jamieson (1988).

comparable to 1974, although the proportion had not kept pace with the overall increase in the prison population. Cocaine prevalence now exceeded heroin by a large margin, and the marijuana figures continued to increase at a pace slightly ahead of the increase in all offenders imprisoned.

Based on questions about drug histories, it appears that most of those who were under the influence of a drug at the time of their offense also stated that they had histories of drug dependence and were using drugs on a daily basis when the offense occurred. *The great majority of those who were under the influence of drugs were not arrested for a drug offense per se* (possession, sales, etc.). Of all those who reported being under drug influence, 26 percent were in prison for robbery, 21 percent for burglary, 20 percent for a violent crime other than robbery, and only 14 percent for a drug offense. About the same percentage (42 to 43 percent) of all those incarcerated for robbery, burglary, or drug offenses indicated they were under the influence of a drug when the offense occurred; about 30 percent of all other imprisoned offenders reported drug influence as well.

Judged according to criteria similar to those applied to the household population, prisoners who were daily drug users at the time of their offense are considered to need treatment; in fact, all of them probably meet the diagnostic criteria for drug dependence. This group comprised 43 percent of all inmates responding to the 1986 state prison survey. Applying this finding to the 1987 state and federal[7] prison census of 584,000 (Greenfeld, 1989) results in about 250,000 inmates who need treatment. Taking a

---

[7] The federal prison population is around 50,000. These institutions were not surveyed with the state prisons, but at least the same proportion of these prisoners as of the state prison populations may be assumed to need treatment. (More than two-thirds of those confined in federal prisons are sentenced for property or violent crimes. In state prisons these offenders have the highest reported drug use, including one-quarter of the total who are serving time for drug offenses.)

similar proportion of convicted inmates serving time in county jails ($0.43 \times 140,000 \approx 60,000$) and juveniles in long-term custody institutions ($0.43 \times 25,000 \approx 10,000$) yields an overall daily estimate of 320,000 individuals in correctional institutions who need treatment.

At the end of 1987, probation and parole offices were supervising 2.6 million unincarcerated persons. The mix of offenses among parolees closely approximated that of the prison population from which they were drawn (and to which, in a large proportion of cases, they return following parole violations). An estimate that 43 percent of parolees (150,000) need drug treatment is therefore readily made.

The much larger probation population is the least well studied of all the criminal justice populations and consequently offers the most difficulty in accurately estimating treatment needs. For one thing, it includes a high proportion of less serious (nonfelony) offenses. But in general, one would expect there to be a significant number of probationers with drug problems. The prison- and parole-based figure of 43 percent would seem to be an upper bound; the estimate (see Appendix 3B) that 10 percent of all arrestees need drug treatment provides a lower bound. The midpoint of these two boundaries, 26 percent, represents about 580,000 probationers. Combining this figure with that for parolees (150,000) produces an estimate of approximately 730,000 individuals in the community under supervision of the criminal justice system who need treatment for drug problems.

The Homeless Population

Recent studies have estimated that from 200,000 to 700,000 people in the United States are homeless on any given night and as many as 2 million experience homelessness at some point during a year, staying temporarily in the intervals with family, friends, or acquaintances. About three-quarters of all homeless people are unattached adults; the balance are mostly women with children. There is evidence that the homeless suffer from a high prevalence of drug disorders; several recent studies have found prevalence rates of 10 to 33.5 percent, with a median value of 20 percent (Institute of Medicine, 1988b).

The homeless are by definition excluded from household population studies, as are individuals or families who are temporarily staying in someone else's household. The need for treatment in this otherwise unrepresented population could thus range from a minimum of 20,000 (10 percent of 200,000) to a maximum of 670,000 (33.5 percent of 2 million). For its estimate, the committee applied the median prevalence value of 20 percent of individuals having drug disorders to the midpoint one-night homelessness estimate of 450,000; however, it applied the lower prevalence estimate of 10 percent to an additional 775,000 "hidden homeless" or nonchronically transient (the midpoint of the difference between 2 million and 450,000). Adding the two prevalence figures yields a treatment-needing homeless population of about 170,000.

Pregnant Women

Pregnant women who are consuming illegal drugs, especially those with high rates of consumption, are of special epidemiological concern. Fetuses are vulnerable to maternal consumption of drugs during pregnancy, and there has been great concern about potentially serious consequences of maternal cocaine abuse and dependence for unborn babies in terms of premature delivery, small size at term birth, developmental somatic defects, and impacts on cognitive and behavioral development (Chavez et al., 1989; Zuckerman et al., 1989; Chasnoff et al., 1990). These risks from cocaine abuse or dependence appear comparable to the serious risks posed by tobacco or alcohol dependence. It is likely that the greater the severity of maternal abuse or dependence, the greater the risk of fetal damage from the pharmacological effects of the drug consumption itself and the greater the likelihood of maternal complications such as infection (most tragically, infection with the human immunodeficiency virus [HIV], which causes AIDS), malnutrition, and trauma.

The risks to children of drug-abusing or dependent mothers do not necessarily stop accumulating at birth. If maternal drug abuse or dependence continues, the future of these babies is further compromised or threatened on a day-to-day basis unless competent and loving care-giving by someone else can be arranged—often not an easy matter. The best alternative, therefore, is for the pregnant and postpartum mother to abstain from drug taking, and treatment may be an appropriate means toward this end.

The 1988 RTI/NIDA national household survey indicated that about 9.3 million women in high-fertility age brackets (15 to 35 years) used an illicit drug at least once in the previous year; 4.9 million did so within the past month. The overall expected birth rate for a group in this age bracket would be about 9 percent annually, with 7 percent pregnant in a given month. These numbers imply a probable range of 350,000 to 625,000 annual fetal exposures to one or more episodes of illicit maternal drug consumption. Of course, estimates of potential maternal drug exposure expressed as annual or monthly prevalence rates are not especially informative concerning the scope of risks of such fetal effects as low birth weight; more drug-specific, frequency-specific, and recency-specific analyses are needed for these determinations (cf. Zuckerman et al., 1989; Petitti and Coleman, 1990).

In terms of the classification methods used in this chapter, about 10 percent of all past-month users clearly need treatment (i.e., are dependent), and another 20 percent probably need treatment (most are classifiable as drug abusers). This implies that about 105,000 pregnant women annually are in need of drug treatment, based on the same diagnostic criteria applied to the general population. These statistical estimates assume that women who consume illicit drugs are on average just as likely as non-drug-taking age peers to give birth. No published studies shed direct light on this assumption, which may be too generous, considering that birth rates are much higher among married versus unmarried women and that married women are a much more abstemious group; on the other hand, it may not be generous enough, given that drug consumers, at least among teenagers, are more sexually active and more often pregnant than abstainers. At any rate, the estimate of 105,000 pregnant women needing drug treatment annually is a subset rather than an addition to the estimated numbers in need of treatment noted in previous sections.[8]

Summary

The committee's combined estimate of the point-in-time need for treatment on a typical day in 1987/1988 is approximately 5.5 million individuals (Table 3-4). This number includes about 1 in 50 household residents older than 12 years of age, more than one-third of all prison and jail inmates, and more than one-fourth of all parolees and probationers. The total estimate is about 2.7 percent of the U.S. population aged 12 years or older.

In finer grain, the survey data indicate that about 1.5 million persons in the household population *clearly* need treatment; the committee believes this to be a minimum estimate of the prevalence of drug dependence in that group. The survey questions used to estimate treatment needs in the criminal justice population are simpler and cruder than those used in the household survey. The criteria provided by these survey items are much more like the "clear" (that is, more severely impaired) than the "probable" householder treatment criteria; in other words, the individuals meeting these criteria (daily-user criminals) are likely to be drug dependent rather

---

[8] Working from a different base—studies among obstetrical patients—Chasnoff and associates have estimated that about 375,000 babies in the United States (more than 10 percent of live births) may be exposed annually to illicit drugs. This figure is within the committee's estimated range, although it is based on samples of uncertain representativeness that use a variety of methods. The major study (Chasnoff, 1989) involves 36 hospitals across the country. Nearly all of them are urban core medical centers serving large proportions of the innercity poor, who are likely to display illicit drug prevalence rates well in excess of the national average. In another study by Chasnoff and coworkers (1990), however, which covers a highly urbanized county in Florida, these investigators found rates of positive drug tests among prenatal clinic patients that approached those in some central cities, even among cases observed in private obstetrical practices.

TABLE 3-4 Estimated Need for Drug Treatment (in thousands) Among Surveyed Adult and Adolescent Populations, 1987–1988

Population	Total	Those Who Need Treatment
Household	198,000	
Clear need		1,500
Probable need		3,100
Homeless (sheltered, street, and transient)	1,225	170
Criminal justice clients		
Correctional custody	925	320
Probation and parole	2,600	730
Pregnancies (live births)	3,875	105
(Less overlaps)[a]		(−470)
Total needing treatment		5,455

[a]In theory, the need for treatment among parolees and probationers should be counted in the household surveys because it is generally a condition of parole and probation that certain signs of social stability, such as a fixed address in the community, be maintained. However, enforcement of such conditions is spotty. The efficiency of coverage of parolees and probationers in the national drug abuse household survey has not been examined. It would be simple to do so, however, by asking respondents whether they were currently on probation or parole. Such an item should be no more subject to nonresponse or validity problems than questions about illicit drugs. In the 1988 national survey on drug abuse, at least 70 of 5,800 adult respondents (including oversampled subgroups) would have been on probation or under parole supervision in the event of standard demographic likelihoods of participation.

There is some basis for estimating the efficiency of sampling probationers and parolees in the household survey. Criminal recidivism among parolees is very high; around two-thirds of all parolees are rearrested within a few years, and the figure is higher for those needing treatment. On this evidence, parolees have much reason to conceal themselves and are not likely to be residentially stable or accessible enough for complete enumeration and good representation in a household survey. The committee estimates that only 30 percent of those needing treatment, or 45,000 persons, are represented. About 20 percent of all probationers do not successfully complete probation. Those needing treatment clearly fail at a higher rate, probably 40 to 50 percent (see, e.g., Toborg and Kirby, 1984). This recidivism rate is not as high as for parolees, but it does suggest a reduced likelihood of being identified for participation in a household survey. The committee estimates that 50 percent, or 270,000 probationers needing treatment, may be represented there.

Overlap with the homeless estimate seems to require reasoning in the other direction. No data were located on rates of probation or parole status among the homeless. Yet the incidence of such status in this group seems likely to be higher than among the residentially stable. With the latter proportion placed at about 15 percent, doubling that yields 30 percent of the homeless drug-dependent or drug-abusing individuals on parole or probation—50,000 individuals.

The overlap of women who are pregnant (and give birth to live babies) with the household and other population figures is virtually total. The overlap of pregnancy, probation, and parole groups with homeless and household populations needing treatment is thus estimated at 470,000 persons.

Source: Institute of Medicine analysis of data from the National Household Survey on Drug Abuse conducted by the Research Triangle Institute; Innes (1988); Flanagan and Jamieson (1988); Greenfeld (1989); and Institute of Medicine (1988b).

than drug abusing. Considering the overlap in estimates, the committee therefore judges that at least 1.3 million household residents who are not currently under criminal justice supervision need treatment for drug dependence; 1.1 million individuals who are under justice supervision also need such treatment (one-third of these individuals are currently in jail or prison). About 3 million additional household residents probably need treatment; most of them would be diagnosed with the less severe condition of drug abuse. Another 100,000 homeless individuals who are not under criminal justice supervision also need treatment for dependence or abuse.

QUANTIFYING THE CONSEQUENCES

As a final component in considering the need for treatment, it is important to analyze the adverse effects—the burden—of drug abuse and dependence. In particular, to gauge the extent of this burden, it is important to use the same scale of measurement as that usually used to address the problem, namely, monetary cost. This approach, of course, is strictly economic and is not the ultimate measure of policy: in particular, the moral and emotional dimensions of the drug problem are virtually impossible to calibrate in monetary terms. But there is value in signaling the overall economic consequences of drug abuse and dependence, and this approach is a precursor to cost-effectiveness and cost/benefit studies that more closely assess the economic payoffs and merits of alternative responses and strategies (cf. Grant et al., 1983).

Most studies of the cost or burden of drug abuse (A. D. Little Co., 1975; Lemkau et al., 1974; Rufener et al., 1977b; Cruze et al., 1981; Harwood et al., 1984) have used a "human capital" approach, which has become fairly standard in estimating the costs of health problems (Rice, 1966; Cooper and Rice, 1976; Hodgson and Meiners, 1979). This method is conservative in that it measures only those dimensions of a problem that can be expressed as tangible losses from the stock of potentially productive labor and property in society. In so doing, it ignores the possibility that the actual or potential loss victims, as a group, might be willing to pay more to avoid these losses than the equivalent tangible costs alone. In other words, the pain, suffering, fear, and demoralization that accompany the tangible losses reflected in economic measures of drug problems are not fully accounted for by the human capital approach. There is also as yet no good analytical basis for quantifying the downstream costs of neurologic and other deficits of drug-dependent infants or the neglect and abuse of children by drug-impaired parents.

The last thorough estimate of the societal cost of drug problems, which covered 1983, was published several years ago (Harwood et al., 1984). Since then, a number of statistical updates and revisions have become available.

TABLE 3-5   Approximate Societal Costs (in billions of dollars) of the Drug Problem

Category	Cost
Victims of drug-related crime (1986)	
Lost work time	1.5
Stolen property	2.6
Lost lives/earnings	1.2
Cost of property repairs, medical services	0.2
Total	5.5
Crime control resources	
Federal anti-drug (1988)	2.5
State and local drug law enforcement (1986)	3.8
State and local drug offense adjudication, corrections (1986)	2.0
State and local crime control costs from drug-related crimes (1985)	4.5
Total	12.8
Criminal careers—lost productivity (1986)	17.6
Employee productivity losses (1983)	33.3
Drug-related AIDS (1985)	1.0
Drug treatment and prevention (1987)	1.7

Source: Institute of Medicine analysis of victimization costs using the methods described in Harwood and coworkers (1984; cf. Harwood et al., 1988). The figures for criminal victimization in 1986 are taken from Shim and DeBerry (1988). See Appendix 3C for additional description of sources.

The committee's more contemporary estimate, based on the most recently published data, is presented in Table 3-5.

The costs are of several types. The criminal aspect of drug use accounts for more than half of the amount estimated here: $5.5 billion worth of tangible losses to victims of property and violent crimes, $12.8 billion in enforcement costs, and $17.6 billion in productivity lost to legitimate economic enterprises because of time spent instead in prison or in criminal enterprises. Nearly equal in magnitude to the *sum* of these crime-related costs were the estimated reductions in the productivity of employees whose work performance was impaired by drug consumption. The health costs of drug problems in relation to AIDS and expenditures for drug treatment and prevention programs are other, not insubstantial costs, but they are much smaller than the costs incurred as a result of drug-related crime. Further details concerning the generation of estimates in Table 3-5 are provided in Appendix 3C. More elaborate new estimation analyses are currently being prepared by Dorothy Rice and colleagues for NIDA, referenced to index year 1985 (cf. Rice and Kelman, 1989), and by the Research Triangle Institute for the Bureau of Justice Statistics; neither set of results are yet available.

These cost estimates cannot be quantitatively disaggregated to show costs for drug use, abuse, and dependence, although it is certain that drug use as such is a small direct contributor to these costs. However, the roughly even division between crime-related losses and employment losses bears a rough correspondence to the estimate made above: those persons who are most clearly in need of treatment for dependence are almost evenly divided between the pool of several million criminal justice clients and the much larger base population, the source of the nation's regular labor force.

CONCLUSION

Few if any problems in American society are as complicated or as mutable as the issue of drug use, which has been one impetus for the proliferation of policy ideas and instruments. Because drug treatment is only one of several accepted policy instruments, the dominant question is how to calibrate its role—to determine how much treatment is needed, by whom, of what kinds, for how long, and at whose cost. In trying to make these kinds of policy decisions, particularly for the future, there are three important implications of the problem's complexity.

The first implication, which is elaborated in this chapter, is that careful methods and sophisticated knowledge are required to grasp the nature and quantify the extent of the need for treatment. A clear understanding of this aspect of the problem is particularly important when concepts such as "treatment on demand" or "required coverage" become the focus of debate. Those who are expected to underwrite the costs reflected by these concepts justifiably worry about stepping into a murky and bottomless pit of financial obligation. The need for treatment is great and probably still expanding, but the pit does have a bottom, and the murk can be cleared. Measures of the raw prevalence of drug taking—usually expressed in such terms as the 28 million Americans who took an illegal drug one or more times in the past year—are not good gauges of the extent of the need for treatment. Current prevalence statistics measure the pool of drug involvement for which some type of response—but not necessarily treatment—may be needed. The extent of the need for treatment becomes clearer if one focuses on two particular features that simultaneously have biological, psychological, and social significance: the level and pattern of consumption behavior, and the number and severity of functional problems an individual is experiencing or causing as a result of this behavior.

The overall prevalence of drug use is a poor absolute measure and an imperfect correlate of the extent and severity of problems, probably because different subgroups of the population have different trajectories of drug involvement. Although the number of users—that is, lighter consumers—may dip or soar over the short term, heavy consumers usually require some time to reach that level and are slower to change. Even good information about the distribution of drug consumption across the population leaves a margin of uncertainty about the need for treatment because a few individuals can consume heavily or regularly with seeming impunity while others have severe trouble at much lower doses and frequencies. These differences have much to do with the kind of social advantages and supports available to the individual.

This chapter outlines an analytical model to distinguish different types and stages of individual drug consumption and consequences: from abstinence through use, abuse, and dependence, and on to recovery and relapse. The two outstanding points about this model are the specific identification of a need for treatment with drug abuse and (especially) dependence, and the recognition that individuals continually move into and out of these conditions. The factors that propel individuals through the stages of this model are mainly learning and conditioning processes, which are strongly shaped by the economic, social, and cultural dimensions of a person's environment.

Drug abuse and dependence are distinguished from drug use through diagnostic criteria; in turn, these criteria, when applied to sample surveys of the population, permit moderately accurate estimates of the aggregate need for treatment. The committee analyzed a number of surveys of the general and special populations that contained questions similar to the diagnostic criteria and arrived at a new estimate of about 5.5 million people who need drug treatment (slightly more than 2.5 percent of the overall adolescent and adult U.S. population of more than 200 million people). It is estimated that about 1.1 million of these individuals are dependent on drugs and are clients of the criminal justice system; another 1.4 million are dependent but not under justice system supervision; and the other 3 million individuals are drug abusers in the household population who probably need less treatment both in terms of quantity and intensity.

The above breakdown leads directly to the second implication of the complex nature of the drug problem: different forms of treatment are needed. A wide variety of specific drug problems (some of which are in fact psychosocial or health problems) may precede drug abuse or dependence and exist apart from them; nevertheless, such problems contribute to drug-seeking behavior and affect opportunities for recovery and the chances of relapse. Many of these issues come to a head in selecting or negotiating the goals of treatment, which are the principal subject of Chapter 4.

The third implication of the complexity of the problem of drug consumption is that evaluating the costs and benefits of treatment is a very demanding task. The course of drug problems is diverse and full of branching probabilities, and it seems to be affected by many things about which scientific knowledge is still quite limited. Even though a single intervention may have little effect on an individual at the time it is delivered, the effects of serial interventions may accumulate significantly over a period of time. Determining how treatment affects the course of drug problems—what its incremental benefits may be—requires sophisticated analysis; considering current data limitations and analytical capabilities, such analyses cannot escape uncertainties.

These uncertainties might be greatly reduced in the event of a miracle cure for drug dependence. But none exists as yet, nor is such a cure a prospect for the immediate future. As with heart disease and cancer in the health domain, theft and assaultive behavior in the realm of crime, or homelessness and family dissolution in the area of social welfare, even the best interventions work only partially—some of the time and for some of the people. In none of these cases does the absence of a panacea excuse society from responding to the best of its ability or from working to find and improve the best ideas (even if they are only partially successful). The costs of drug problems are so high that reducing them even modestly is worthwhile. The complexity, uncertainty, and costs associated with drug abuse and dependence, as noted in this chapter, undergird the analysis of treatment effectiveness and costs and benefits in Chapter 5.

APPENDIX 3A
ESTIMATING THE NEED FOR
TREATMENT IN THE HOUSEHOLD POPULATION

Special analyses of the 1988 National Household Survey of Drug Abuse were conducted to Institute of Medicine specifications at the Research Triangle Institute to quantify the need for drug abuse treatment among the household population. Previous estimates using the national household surveys were based on the frequency of drug consumption only. Yet the diagnostic algorithms developed in DSM-III-R, ICD-10, and their predecessors refer to physiological and psychological symptoms of dependence and abuse and to psychosocial problems and consequences of consumption. These may be correlated with consumption frequency, but they are not simply isomorphic with frequency.

The household survey instrument does not directly employ all of the DSM or ICD criteria (see Table 3-2), but it includes numerous items that are very similar to them. The survey inquires about the current frequency of illicit drug consumption (days of use in the past month), symptoms of dependence in the past year, and problems and consequences of drug use in the past year. In this analysis, frequency of drug consumption was coded into eight ranges:

- no current illicit use of any drug;
- current use of unknown intensity;

[Most frequent use of any one drug in the past month:]

- once;
- 2 to 8 times;
- 5 to 8 times;
- 9 to 16 times;
- 17 to 24 times; and
- 25 to 30 times.

The symptoms of dependence were coded into three ranges: no reported symptoms from any drug; one reported symptom from any drug; and two or more symptoms from any drug. The survey questions used to elicit information on dependence were as follows:

In the past year:

Have you ever tried to cut down on your use of any of these drugs?

Circle the number next to each drug for which you have ever needed larger amounts to get the same effect or that you could no longer get high on the amount you used to use.

Circle the number next to each drug you have ever used each day or almost daily for two or more weeks in a row.

Circle the number of each drug you felt that you needed or were dependent on.

Circle the number next to each drug for which you've had withdrawal symptoms, that is, you felt sick because you stopped or cut down on your use of it.

Response categories for each of the above: cigarettes; alcohol; sedatives; tranquilizers; stimulants; analgesics; marijuana; inhalants; cocaine; hallucinogens; heroin; other opiates, morphine, codeine; never experienced this.

The problems and consequences of drug use were coded into three ranges: no reported problems from any drug; one reported consequence from any drug; and two or more consequences from any drug(s). The questions below were used to elicit information on drug problems; the drugs listed above (see the questions on dependence) were also used as response categories for these questions.

Have you had any of these problems in the past 12 months from your use of any of the substances on this card? If yes, write in which substances you think probably caused the problem.

TABLE 3A-1   Frequency of Illicit Drug Consumption
(for one month) and Estimated Prevalence by Level of
Consumption

Level of Consumption[a]	Sample Cases	Estimated Prevalence
Unknown	215	3,744,840
11	141	2,363,026
2–4	192	3,152,013
5–8	79	1,296,743
9–16	82	1,727,539
17–24	55	987,827
25+	63	1,206,790
Total	827	14,478,778

[a]Number of times drugs were used in previous month.

Source: Institute of Medicine analysis of data from the 1988 National Household
Survey on Drug Abuse, performed by Research Triangle Institute for the National
Institute on Drug Abuse.

Became depressed or lost interest in things.
Had arguments and fights with family or friends.
Had trouble at school or on the job.
Drove unsafely.
At times, I could not remember what happened to me.
Felt completely alone and isolated.
Felt very nervous and anxious.
Had health problems.
Found it difficult to think clearly.
Had serious money problems.
Felt irritable and upset.
Got less work done than usual at school or on the job.
Felt suspicious and distrustful of people.
Had trouble with the police.
Skipped four or more regular meals in a row.
Found it harder to handle my problems.
Had to get emergency medical help.

Tabulations of these three variables are reported in Table 3A-1 (levels
of consumption) and Table 3A-2 (cross-tabulations of the symptom and
problem indexes). Cigarettes and alcohol were excluded from the tabulations into categories. The symptom and consequence indexes (each with
values of 0, 1, or 2) were summed to yield a symptom/problem scale with
values of 0 through 4. Those individuals with a value of zero reported
neither symptoms nor problems in the past year; those with a value of 4

TABLE 3A-2 Estimated Number (in thousands) and Percentage of Current Drug Users Who Experienced Negative Consequences of Drug Use and Symptoms of Dependence During the Past Year (1988)

Symptoms of Dependence	Negative Consequences of Drug Use						Total		Sample Cases
	None		1		2+				
	No.	%	No.	%	No.	%	No.	%	
None	5,734	39.6	381	2.6	261	1.8	6,376	44.0	367
1	2,366	16.3	320	2.2	273	1.9	2,959	20.4	172
2+	2,669	18.4	489	3.4	1,986	13.7	5,144	35.5	288
Total	10,769	74.4	1,190	8.2	2,520	17.4	14,479	100.0	827
Sample cases	603		70		154		827		

Source: Institute of Medicine analysis of data from the 1988 National Household Survey on Drug Abuse, performed by Research Triangle Institute for the National Institute on Drug Abuse.

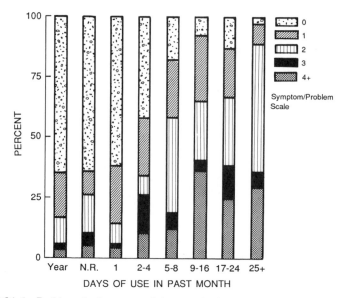

FIGURE 3A-1   Problems by frequency of drug use in the household population, 1988. Year
= no use in past month but at least once in past year; N.R. = no response on frequency
items. Source: Institute of Medicine analysis of data from the 1988 National Household
Survey on Drug Abuse, performed by Research Triangle Institute for the National Institute
on Drug Abuse.

experienced at least two symptoms and two problems. A value of 2 means
two or more symptoms with no problems, two or more problems with no
symptoms, or one of each. Similar interpretations apply to the indicator
values 1 and 3. The symptom/problem scale was then cross-tabulated with
the level of current use. The resulting matrix (Figure 3A-1) can be readily
transformed into relative need for treatment. In an ordinal sense, those
with the least need would be expected to be in the upper left of the
matrix (very low use, few or no symptoms/problems), whereas those with
the greatest need would be in the lower right corner (highest use, highest
symptoms/problems).

The categories of "clear," "probable," "possible," and "unlikely" need
for treatment are used to indicate the likelihood that the respondent
would require treatment (Figure 3A-2). "Clear" need is defined as a
consumption frequency exceeding twice weekly and a value of 3 or 4
on the problem/symptom scale. More-than-twice-weekly consumers with
two or fewer symptoms/problems are assigned to the "probable" category.
Also "probable" are those with a maximum use of any single drug of
from two to eight days per month and a scale value of 3 or 4. The
frequency index measures only the drug that is taken most frequently;

because many respondents take more than one substance, however, an individual may be taking other drugs less frequently and at different times. For relatively infrequent consumers, the major clinical sign is clearly the elevated symptom/problem count.

An individual who consumes an illicit drug five to eight times a month with a low problem/symptom count is classified as having a "possible" need for treatment. In the same class are consumption levels of two to four episodes per month and a scale value of 1 or 2, once-a-month consumption with scale values of 3 or 4, and unknown levels of use. All other individuals are considered relatively "unlikely" to need treatment.

Out of 14.5 million current-month drug consumers, the committee classified 1.5 million as *clear* candidates for treatment, 3.1 million as *probable*, 2.9 million as *possible*, and 6.9 million as *unlikely*. For purposes of estimating the need for treatment in the household population the clear and probable groups total 4.6 million. Sex, age, labor force participation, and earnings of this combined group are reported in Table 3A-3.

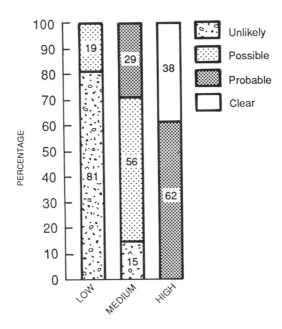

FIGURE 3A-2   Need for treatment by frequency of use in the household population, 1988. Source: Institute of Medicine analysis of data from the 1988 National Household Survey on Drug Abuse, performed by Research Triangle Institute for the National Institute on Drug Abuse.

98   *TREATING DRUG PROBLEMS*

The statistical properties of these estimates (standard errors) are complex and have not yet been computed. Research Triangle Institute staff consider estimates based on fewer than 15 to 20 case observations to have unacceptably high standard errors. Most of the estimated population characteristics presented here, however, have more than adequate sample cases. (For example, the estimate of 4.6 million persons with clear or probable need for treatment is based on 247 cases meeting the defined criteria.) To provide a sense of the likely statistical properties of these estimates, 95 percent confidence intervals for past-month drug use in subpopulations with estimated use by 5 million or fewer individuals are presented in Figure 3A-3. Larger population estimates have better statistical properties. (Note that the 95 percent confidence interval is generally smaller, relative to the

TABLE 3A-3   Estimated Need for Treatment (clear plus probable) in the Household Population by Gender, Age, Labor Force Status, and Earnings, 1988

Characteristic	Sample Cases	Estimated Prevalence	Percentage
Gender			
Male	154	3,169,412	68.4
Female	93	1,463,103	31.6
Subtotal	247	4,632,515	100.0
Age			
12–17 years	58	395,736	8.8
18–25	84	1,882,855	41.8
26–34	73	1,501,764	33.3
35 and over	19	726,788	16.1
Subtotal	234	4,507,143	100.0
Labor force status of adults (aged 18 and older)			
Employed	125	3,108,314	75.6
Unemployed	19	389,174	9.5
Not participating	32	613,919	14.9
Subtotal	176	4,111,407	100.0
Unemployment rate	144	3,497,488	11.1
Earnings of adults (those employed)			
Less than $9,000/year	38	1,000,047	32.2
$9,000–20,000/year	50	1,187,341	38.2
Over $20,000/year	37	920,926	29.6
Subtotal	125	3,108,314	100.0
Total	247	4,632,515	100.0

Source: Institute of Medicine analysis of data from the 1988 National Household Survey on Drug Abuse, performed by Research Triangle Institute for the National Institute on Drug Abuse.

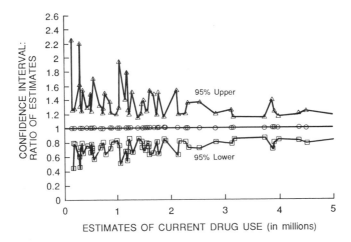

FIGURE 3A-3 Confidence interval of estimates of current illicit drug use by subpopulations. The estimates indicate the illicit use of drugs during any past month for subpopulations (combinations of age, sex, race, and region) with fewer than 5 million users. The reported 95 percent confidence intervals are divided by the estimates to produce ratios. Source: National Institute on Drug Abuse (1989).

value of the estimate, for larger estimates.) Smaller estimates have lower reliability.

The plot demonstrates scatter because various subpopulations were sampled at differential rates (e.g., youth and Hispanics were sampled at relatively higher rates, whereas adults aged 35 and older and whites were sampled at lower rates). Therefore, identical estimates for two different subpopulations can have very different statistical properties: an estimate of 500,000 youths needing treatment is much more reliable than an identical estimate for older adults because the estimate for youth is based on about 70 to 80 cases, whereas the estimate for adults aged 35 and older is based on only 10 to 15 cases.

APPENDIX 3B
ESTIMATING THE NEED FOR TREATMENT AMONG ARRESTEES

Information about drug use by arrestees is collected by the Drug Abuse Forecasting (DUF) system created by the National Institute of Justice. This program reports on a quarterly basis urinalysis results collected from arrestees in a dozen or more cities or urban areas ranging in size from Indianapolis to Chicago, Manhattan, and Los Angeles. Urinalysis can detect opiate or cocaine doses (for 48 to 72 hours), marijuana (for 1 to

4 weeks), and other drugs (for varying lengths of time; see Hawks and Chiang, 1986).

The DUF samples are not random but purposive, concentrating on drug charges and violent and property crimes according to individual stratified sampling schemes in each city. For this reason, the DUF results are not directly representative of all arrestees nationwide or even in the cities represented. For example, about 35 percent of DUF sample arrests in mid-1988 were for drug offenses, burglary, and robbery, exceeding the percentage of arrests for these charges in 53 U.S. cities of comparable size (more than 250,000 residents) by a factor of about 2.5 and exceeding their percentage of all U.S. arrests by about a factor of 3.

Drug use is pervasive among DUF arrestees. In the most recently reported summary statistics for the fall of 1989 (O'Neil et al., 1990), about two-thirds of male and female arrestees screened positive for at least one drug, ranging from 53 to 84 percent for men (in San Antonio and New York, respectively) and from 42 to 90 percent for women (in Indianapolis and Philadelphia). More specifically, cocaine traces were found in about one-half of the men (28 to 77 percent) and the women (22 to 79 percent), marijuana traces were found in about one-fourth of the men (13 to 48 percent) and one-fifth of the women (8 to 27 percent), and opiates were found in one-tenth of the men (2 to 23 percent) and the women (1 to 27 percent). About one-fourth of the sample were positive for more than one illegal drug.

Additional information is obtained from DUF interviews. Arrestees are asked whether they consider themselves dependent on drugs, whether they could benefit from treatment, or whether they are enrolled in treatment. A positive response to one of these items, in conjunction with a positive drug test, is interpreted as indicating a likely need for drug treatment. A positive test but negative verbal responses is interpreted as ambiguous evidence of need for treatment. Table 3B-1 indicates findings for early 1988. About 29 percent of DUF arrestees were classified as likely to need treatment, another 48 percent as possibly needing treatment (ambiguous results), and the final 24 percent as unlikely because they tested negative (some of these individuals may nonetheless have drug problems that require treatment, but they were not detected). Summary statistics on need for treatment in the DUF sample in early 1989 were published by Wish and O'Neil (1989).

There is some variation in these rates across different offense types, as reported in Table 3B-2. Probable need for treatment was higher for those committing income-generating crimes (robbery, 40 percent; burglary and larceny, 34 percent) and drug offenses (37 percent) than for those committing violent crimes (homicide, 16 percent; sex offenses, 21 percent; assaults, 25 percent).

TABLE 3B-1   Arrestees' Potential Need for Treatment (percentage of total cases) by City, Spring 1988, based on Drug Use Forecasting Data

City	Potential Need For Treatment			Cases
	Probable	Ambiguous	Unlikely	
Total	29.0	47.5	23.6	2,428
New York	51.0	39.7	9.3	257
Portland	26.6	51.3	22.1	263
Indianapolis	32.3	26.9	40.8	130
Houston	11.3	58.8	29.9	204
Detroit	29.9	41.9	28.1	167
New Orleans	15.2	60.7	24.1	191
Phoenix	21.9	46.2	31.9	251
Chicago	29.3	52.7	18.0	283
Los Angeles	41.0	39.0	20.0	446
Other	15.7	57.6	26.7	236

Source: Unpublished Drug Use Forecasting system statistics provided by Dr. Eric Wish, National Institute of Justice.

TABLE 3B-2   Arrestees' Potential Need for Treatment (percentage of total cases) by Charge at Arrest, Spring 1988, based on Drug Use Forecasting Data

Charge	Potential Need for Treatment			Cases
	Probable	Ambiguous	Unlikely	
Total	29.0	47.5	23.6	2,428
Assault	25.4	42.0	32.6	264
Burglary	33.6	52.2	14.2	247
Drug sale/possession	36.6	54.8	8.6	465
Weapons	18.6	50.0	31.4	70
Homicide/manslaughter	16.2	40.5	43.2	37
Robbery	40.0	41.8	18.2	165
Stolen property/vehicles	25.0	52.8	22.2	176
Sex offenses	20.9	38.4	40.7	86
Larceny/pickpocketing	34.1	41.1	24.7	287
Other	21.3	47.0	31.7	624

Source: Unpublished Drug Use Forecasting system statistics provided by Dr. Eric Wish, National Institute of Justice.

The proportion of arrestees needing drug treatment in the DUF cities can be roughly extrapolated to a national basis, adjusting for variations in the number of high-probable-need offenses (burglary, robbery, and drugs) reported in all large cities, smaller cities, suburbs, and rural areas. After this adjustment, about 700,000 arrestees nationwide would be likely to need treatment. If the ambiguous cases are added to this estimate, another 1.2 million arrestees might need drug abuse treatment. The number of individuals represented by arrests would likely be 10 to 20 percent lower owing to multiple arrests per year.

APPENDIX 3C
ESTIMATING THE COSTS OF DRUG PROBLEMS

Drug-related Crime—Victim Losses

There were 34.1 million personal and household victimizations in the United States in 1986 (Shim and DeBerry, 1988). These crimes cause injury, property damage and personal inconvenience worth billions of dollars per year, as well as forcibly transferring further billions of dollars from victims to perpetrators. It is conservatively estimated that more than 25 percent of property crime and about 15 percent of violent crime—a total of 9 million crimes—are related to drug abuse by the criminal. In other words, without the criminals' current and prior involvement with drugs, these crimes would not have been committed.

Using the methods of Harwood and coworkers (1984, 1988), victim losses from the drug-related crimes have been estimated at $1.7 billion, of which the largest proportions were for lost work time ($1.5 billion), property damage ($150 million) and medical care costs ($50 million). Further losses experienced by victims were attributable to the value of the property stolen, which for the 9 million drug-related crimes noted above was $2.6 billion.

Homicide is strongly linked to drug trafficking. Surveys of homicide arrestees have found that more than 50 percent are positive for drugs and 16 percent claim they are addicted to illicit drugs (Innes, 1988). Twenty-eight percent of inmates convicted of homicide or nonnegligent manslaughter claim to have been under the influence of illicit drugs at the time of the crime, and 12 percent admit to being daily users of heroin or cocaine (Innes, 1988). Conservatively, averaging the 12 percent who admit daily use and the 16 percent who claim addiction yields a causal involvement for drugs in homicide of 14 percent. This implies that 2,900 homicide deaths (out of the 20,600 total estimated by the Bureau of Justice Statistics) were drug related. The economic value of homicide victims' lost productivity was $1.2 billion.

Crime Control Resources

The federal government spent $2.5 billion on criminal justice activities specifically directed against the drug trade and drug traffickers in 1988, an increase from the $1.76 billion spent in 1986 (White House Office of Public Affairs, 1988). U.S. contributions to efforts to interrupt the international drug trade consumed $1.2 billion, whereas federal domestic investigations received $584 million. Federal prosecutions and corrections efforts cost $150 and $560 million, respectively.

Federal drug enforcement efforts have grown from $36 million in 1969 to $2.5 billion in 1988, with projected 1989 expenditures of $3.8 billion (Strategy Council on Drug Abuse, 1975; Office of National Drug Control Policy, 1989). State and local governments devote even more resources specifically to fighting the drug trade. A national survey of law enforcement agencies found that, in 1986, 18.2 percent of total expenditures were for this purpose (Godshaw et al., 1987), amounting to $3.8 billion out of nearly $21 billion in state and local law enforcement (police) efforts. Adjudication, legal, and correctional services dedicated specifically to fighting the drug trade cost a further $2 billion.

In addition, much violent and property crime is believed to be motivated by drug abuse (drug-related crime). Using conservative assumptions about the causal role of drug abuse in violent and property crime (about 15 percent and 25 percent, respectively, as discussed above), state and local criminal justice efforts against drug-related crime probably cost $4.5 billion in 1985.

Employee Productivity Losses

The largest economic impact of drug abusers derives from their abandoning the legitimate economy for the underground one and their potentially impaired performance in legitimate jobs. These impacts represent losses of potential legitimate productivity—services that are never delivered to the workplace because the drug abusers have entered criminal careers or been incarcerated or because they do not perform in jobs as well as their non-drug-abusing peers. Crime career and incarceration losses to the economy were $12.2 and $5.4 billion in 1986, which arise from significant commitments to crime career endeavors by 1.1 million persons and the incarceration of 200,000 persons on drug charges or drug-related offenses (updated estimates from Cruze et al., 1981, and Harwood et al., 1984).

Reduced productivity among those in the work force is the most complicated calculation; it may also be the largest burden resulting from drug abuse. Harwood and colleagues (1984) estimated that in 1983 nearly 8 million persons had severe prior histories of drug use (daily consumption of marijuana or other illicit drugs for a minimum of a month at some time in life) that were significantly related to their having a lower household income than their peers. The losses of legitimate potential productivity so estimated were $33.3 billion in 1983. The lost income represented by this cost directly affects the well-being of drug-involved individuals and their family members, who may be doubly afflicted (as may the drug abusers themselves) because of theft and partial or total reliance on social welfare.

Failure to earn a legitimate income affects public revenues through losses in tax contributions on earnings and expenditures. These costs are thus spread in various ways (that are difficult to quantify) from the individual to society.

Health Costs

Most drug treatment and prevention services are government supported, but there is also significant private payment for treatment. These services have received an enormous boost since the 1986 Anti-Drug Abuse Act, with the federal commitment escalating markedly in 1987, 1988, and 1989. Expenditures for drug treatment were at least $1.3 billion in 1987 (see Chapter 6); prevention activities (which target both drugs and alcohol) were $212 million in 1987 (Butynski and Canova, 1988). Drug abuse-related AIDS costs in 1985 were estimated to be $967 million (Rice et al., 1990). About 25 percent of all AIDS cases to date have a history of intravenous drug abuse (Institute of Medicine/National Academy of Sciences, 1988), a figure that represents a steady rise throughout the 1980s (Miller et al., 1990).

4

Defining the Goals of Treatment

A wide range of hopes have been fastened on drug treatment, in keeping with the diversity among those who take a strong interest in treatment programs: clients, their families, clinicians, outside payers, employers, and public agencies. How these different expectations can be reconciled and prioritized is a fundamental question—particularly for the development of measures to assess treatment outcome. Such assessments are in turn crucial at a time when competition for budgetary dollars is intense and health cost control measures are targeting substance abuse benefits for differential reductions—even though the public and the President rank the drug problem above national security and economic concerns as the country's most serious current issue (Gallup, 1989; Bush, 1990).

Every treatment program needs to have operational goals, which should be clearly understood and viewed as legitimate by all interested parties. These goals imply how program success is to be measured. Changes in the frequency of program clients' cocaine or heroin consumption and in their commission of (and subsequent apprehension for) violent crimes are typically the dominant themes of treatment outcome studies. With limited exceptions, changes in physical and psychological well-being, marijuana and alcohol consumption, general employment status, and the size of local drug markets are subsidiary issues. AIDS risk reduction as a measure of treatment outcome is only beginning to assume importance.

This chapter first reviews the diverse interests that have shaped treatment, the interplay between these interests, and their implications for setting realistic treatment goals. The committee focuses especially on client motives for entering treatment. What finally spurs most clients into treatment is the desire to relieve some kind of immediate drug-related pressure or to avoid an unpleasant drug-related consequence. Concerns about legal jeopardy loom large among these motives and have been analyzed more extensively than all other factors combined. In this chapter, therefore, the committee carefully examines how the criminal justice system affects the drug treatment system and particularly considers the implications for treatment of the large and growing pool of drug-involved individuals over whom the justice system exerts (or tries to exert) various kinds of authority.

Besides the criminal justice system, the workplace is the most significant formal institution potentially affecting referral to treatment, particularly through employee assistance and drug screening programs. Estimated productivity losses owing to drug problems add up to an impressive figure. There is limited evidence, however, about the connection between employee assistance or drug screening programs and drug treatment, and the data suggest that employer linkages are not a big part of the total treatment picture.

The various and complex motives displayed by clients in treatment, the differing severities and depths of their problems, and the differential involvement of the criminal justice system or employers yield a spectrum of potential with respect to recovery from drug problems. Programs in turn have developed strategies for selecting or recruiting across that spectrum, within the limits of their clinical resources, organizational commitments, and institutional environments. Partial recovery, particularly in terms of reduced drug consumption and other criminal activity, is a realistic expectation for most clients in treatment at any one time. Full recovery is an achievable goal only for a fractional group, whereas no recovery can be expected for another fraction.

In light of these observations, the most general conclusion of this chapter is that in setting and evaluating treatment goals, what comes out must be judged relative to what went in—and as a matter of more or less rather than all or none.

DIVERSE INTERESTS

The notion of successful drug treatment has many possible shadings. A number of drug treatment goals have been overtly or implicitly advanced in authoritative statements over the years (American Bar Association/American Medical Association, 1961; Office of Drug Abuse Policy, 1978; Office of National Drug Control Policy, 1989; Besteman, 1990; Courtwright, 1990). These goals are diverse enough that success in reaching one of them (although it may be related to other goals) is not necessarily a requirement for success in reaching the others. The following is a compendium of many of these treatment goals:

- substantially reduce the treated individual's use of illicit drugs—or, more stringently, end it altogether;
- substantially reduce—or end altogether—violent and acquisitive crimes by the treated individual against others;
- substantially reduce—or end altogether—the treated individual's consumption of legal psychoactive drugs, including alcohol and medical prescriptions such as methadone;
- reduce the treated individual's specific educational or vocational deficits;
- restore or initiate legitimate employment of the treated individual;
- change the treated individual's personal values to approximate more closely mainstream commitments regarding work, family, and the law;
- normalize or improve the treated individual's overall health, longevity, and psychological well-being;
- reduce specific drug injection practices and hazardous sexual behaviors, such as multiple unprotected sexual encounters, that readily transmit the AIDS virus between the treated individual and others;
- reduce the overall size, violence, seductiveness, and profitability of the market for illicit drugs; and
- reduce the number of infants born with drug dependence symptoms or other immediate or longer term impairments owing to intrauterine exposure to illicit drugs.

The length of this list of goals and the specific variations within it (reducing versus ending a certain behavior, individual versus more broadly sociological effects) have two distinct although related origins. First, different governing ideas about drugs have instilled different aspirations, theories, and philosophies into the treatment system. Second, drug treatment episodes involve multiple parties, and the ultimate results of any treatment episode are shaped by the differing objectives and behavior of those parties.

Analytically, the parties involved in drug treatment are *individual clients* entering treatment; *clinical programs* themselves, which offer different types of services; third-party *reimbursers* or payers of clinical expenses (e.g., insurers or public health bureaus); *regulatory agencies or other monitors* such as accreditors or utilization managers, who enforce or evaluate program compliance with specific legal or clinical standards; *family* members or others who are personally involved with individuals entering treatment; agencies that have legal or client relationships with these individuals, such as *criminal justice agencies* or *employers*; and the *public* through its appointed and elected representatives.[1]

The goals of clients, clinicians, program managers, payers, regulators, politicians, and other interested parties are often imperfectly matched. Conflicts and competition for control of clinical decision making are common. This pattern is visible not only in particular cases but also more broadly, as drug treatment policies, practices, and capabilities evolve with accumulating experience and vary with the changing balances between governing ideas.

For example, the moral censure of drugs and the desire to reduce the prevalence of drug-related crime were early and clear influences on the development of publicly supported treatment programs. It is impossible to understand the growth of the national treatment system apart from the national policy focus on cutting down street crime. But compassion for the suffering of the addict has also been a factor, together with a strong current of concern, especially in the 1960s, about improving economic opportunities in urban neighborhoods badly troubled by poverty, drugs, racial discrimination, and other problems. Concern has centered as well on protecting the civil rights and restoring the human dignity of drug-dependent individuals. In this context, community programs were viewed as a source not only of therapy for the treated individual and crime control for all of his or her neighbors but also of jobs, identity, community empowerment, and political achievements (Vocational Rehabilitation Administration, 1966; Brotman and Freedman, 1968; Martin and Isbell, 1978; Attewell and Gerstein, 1979; Besteman, 1990; Courtwright, 1990).

In contrast, most privately reimbursed drug treatment programs began with a much firmer adherence to the medical perspective associated with treating dependence on alcohol as a disease, a perspective with very different legal ramifications and in particular an orientation toward restoring employees to satisfactory job performance. Private treatment programs have also placed great emphasis on the dignity—or destigmatization—of the afflicted individual (Wiener, 1981; Institute of Medicine, 1990; Roman and Blum, 1990). More recently, the fear of harmful or criminal behavior—including drug transactions at the work site and negligence in job performance that might lead to injury or loss of life—has become a

---

[1] These categories of interest in treatment are not necessarily separate in practice. Family members may have legal relations with the individuals in treatment in the form of marital and parental responsibilities; the family or the individual may take full or partial financial responsibility for treatment charges; employers and criminal justice agencies are not only bound to some individuals in treatment by formal contracts or writs but may also be paying for the treatment; payers such as state agencies often double as program regulators; employers, agents of justice, and, of course, clinicians often develop strong personal concern for their clients within the professional framework of service or supervision. Furthermore, although some parties to treatment deal with each other only in a single episode, others do so across many episodes.

significant factor as well (Gust and Walsh, 1989). Most recently, high levels of concern about increasing expenditures on private treatment for drugs, alcohol, and mental illness (and every other health cost) are affecting the private treatment sector.

Plurality of interests is not a phenomenon unique to drug treatment, and it is not an insuperable obstacle to setting achievable goals. Even with clearly divergent intentions, different parties may be able to strike a bargain—that is, agree on a "social contract" for treatment—that everyone involved considers favorable, even though each party may get something less—or more—than it originally bargained for. The major result of complexity for present purposes is that it makes treatment processes highly contingent. If participants have differing goals, treatment processes are more susceptible to breakdown through client attrition or discharge, staff demoralization or mismanagement, program closing, or withdrawal of participation by a payer or other external agent.

In light of the diversity of treatment goals and the differing motives that underlie them, it is important to develop realistic expectations about what treatment can usefully accomplish. The principal issues reduce to a few central and relatively enduring questions: Why do individuals enter drug treatment? What are the implications of entry motivations for setting clinical goals? What are the actual and the optimal goals of drug treatment and the criminal justice system? What are the supporting relationships between them? Between drug treatment and employers? What should be the minimum acceptable results of treatment—partial or only full recovery?

REASONS FOR SEEKING TREATMENT

Individuals who seek admission to drug treatment offer a variety of reasons for doing so (Anglin et al., 1989b; Hubbard et al., 1989). The reasons they give are illuminating, although their logic proves to be unintelligible in some cases, and they may be evasive or deceptive in others. Three fundamentals are present in virtually every such instance. First, the applicant for admission to drug treatment has one or more uncomfortable and fairly urgent problems to resolve. Typically, the problems entail noxious physical or psychological stimuli (a serious infection, chronic depression), sharp social pressure (a felony case, an angry spouse), or the imminent threat of something quite unwelcome (e.g., imprisonment or assault). Second, the problems are related to drug use, although the client may or may not view them as issues separate from drug consumption. In fact, the relative severity of drug abuse or dependence may be only loosely coupled with the severity of the presenting problem. Third, the individual is ambivalent about seeking treatment.

Motives do not necessarily translate directly into outcomes. Reconfiguring client motivation is a fundamental clinical objective of many if not all good treatment programs. Moreover, there is reason to think that treatment processes affect individuals to some degree regardless of their initial motives. Nevertheless, the cardinal importance of the initial motivation to seek treatment is that these motives are likely to influence the probability that the client will stay in treatment long enough for the therapeutic process to take effect. For this reason, it is worthwhile to delineate treatment motivations in some detail.

The kinds of problems that lead applicants to seek treatment are well summarized in the scales of the Addiction Severity Index, a diagnostic screening interview and rating method designed to yield "a subjective estimate of the client's level of discomfort in seven problem areas commonly found in alcohol and drug dependent individuals" (McLellan et al., 1985:iii). The following categories are rated for severity:

• medical status (lifetime hospitalizations [excluding drug detoxification or treatment], chronic medical conditions, disabilities, severe symptoms in past 30 days [excluding drug withdrawal, intoxication, or overdose effects]);

• employment/support (level of formal education and training, occupational type, usual employment pattern, past 30 days' employment, income level and sources, dependents, recent job-finding efforts [if applicable]);

• drug use (use during past 30 days, recent dependence/abuse symptoms, lifetime use, length and date of last abstinence, lifetime overdoses and detoxifications, previous treatment episodes, recent daily cost of drugs);

• alcohol use (use during past 30 days, recent dependence/abuse symptoms, lifetime use, length and date of last abstinence, lifetime overdoses and detoxifications, previous treatment episodes, recent daily cost of alcohol);

• legal status (whether legal jeopardy prompted application, whether client has an active case pending or is on probation or parole, lifetime arrests by type, number of convictions and incarcerations, recent crimes committed);

• family/social relationships (marital status and satisfaction, living arrangements and satisfaction, relations with friends, recent and past conflicts with family or friends); and

• psychiatric status (treatment episodes, symptoms of depression, anxiety, confusion, or aggression during lifetime and in past 30 days, suicide attempts).

The literature on admission to treatment, much of which reports on the use of the Addiction Severity Index or similar instruments and reflects an abundance of clinical experience, indicates that treatment is sought primarily when there is a negative or threatening situation to be alleviated in any one—or more—of these areas (Brown et al., 1971; Ball et al., 1974; Gerstein et al., 1979; Hubbard et al., 1989).[2] Moreover, studies show that applicants often report either an unsuccessful attempt to deal with the admitting complaint without seeking treatment or an earlier successful resolution of this or a similar problem (at least temporarily) with the aid of treatment. Because some problems can be intermittent, yielding to quick solutions but returning again and again to trouble and frustrate the individual, initial brief flirtations with treatment are often followed by later, more extended episodes. In fact, half or more of a mature program's admissions can be expected to be repeat admissions to that program—without counting time spent in other programs. The prevalence of repeat admissions is generally highest in methadone programs, which require documentation of previous relapses and have the oldest clientele. In a typical long-standing methadone program, two-thirds of the clients are second or later admissions (Allison et al., 1985; Hubbard et al., 1989).

Controlling drug use is virtually always a part of treatment motivation, but the extent or proportion of that part varies. It may be the sole objective of treatment entry, or it may be no more than a base from which superordinate objectives are to be achieved. These objectives can be very specific: for example, to withdraw completely from a local drug market to avoid violent recriminations for a dishonest transaction (stealing someone's drugs, acting as a police informant, etc.); to influence a prosecutor or judge to reduce a heavy criminal charge or sentence, thus yielding probation rather than jail or a shorter rather than longer term of incarceration; to complete probation or parole successfully; to save a job threatened by drug-related absenteeism, ill temper, or errors; or to stave off a family rupture, such as expulsion from a conjugal or parental home or the loss of custody of a child.

---

[2] Because a large proportion of the available research literature on patterns of drug treatment motivation is drawn from studies of heroin addicts entering methadone and residential treatment in the 1970s, caution should be used in generalizing those findings to drug users of today. On the other hand, the street heroin addict of the 1970s was usually an experienced polydrug user, familiar with all manner of opiates (codeine, morphine, propoxyphene, dihydromorphinone), cocaine (always popular for intravenous or other use but not as widely accessible or as cheap as it is today), amphetamines, alcohol, marijuana, barbiturates, and other drugs. The heroin addict was distinguished largely by a strong preference for that drug, assuming its availability. Patients entering residential and methadone programs today are similar to those of earlier years but generally have higher levels of nonopiate use, especially cocaine. The durability over the years of drug experience patterns and other characteristics may also be true of outpatient counseling programs, whose clients have tended on the whole to be younger, less desperate economically, and more often oriented toward psychological interpretations of their problems (Sells et al., 1976; Hubbard et al., 1989). Seldom opiate users, these clients were and are heavy users of marijuana, alcohol, and now cocaine.

The motives can also be quite general: to restore generally run-down physical health; to put one's life back together; or to find or regain a sense of self-respect. Perhaps the most general of reported motives is a pervasive sense of weariness or melancholy, a cumulative and demoralizing realization that the increasing trouble that comes with sustained abuse and dependence is leading to a dead end. Depending on the modality, one-quarter to one-half of a national sample of treatment admissions reported depressive and suicidal thinking (Hubbard et al., 1989).

Recently (Kosten et al., 1988), as well as in previous years (Allison et al., 1985), health crises, problems involving serious jeopardy from the criminal justice system, and psychiatric/psychological problems are the most prominent motivations among those seeking relief from cocaine and opiate use in public programs.[3] In the case of women or married men, pressure precipitating admission to treatment often comes from family members; however, in general, these demographic types are a minority of those entering public programs.

Pressure from the criminal justice system is the strongest motivation reported for seeking public treatment. Those who entered outpatient and residential programs in a 1979–1981 national sample of public program admissions were directly referred by the criminal justice system about 40 percent of the time. Direct referral, however, is clearly a conservative measure of the broader influence of criminal justice pressure (Anglin et al., 1989b). Between one-half and two-thirds of admissions to these modalities had some form of legal supervision such as parole or probation. Very few methadone clients—less than 3 percent—were directly referred by justice agencies in the 1979–1981 sample (Allison et al., 1985; Hubbard et al., 1989), but probation or parole status was quite common. In other studies, large proportions of methadone clients have indicated subjectively perceived pressure involving their legal status (Anglin et al., 1989b).

Court orders or other criminal justice system referrals to treatment are not unknown in private programs, particularly in outpatient modalities (Harrison and Hoffmann, 1988; Hoffmann and Harrison, 1988). But it seems likely that these referrals are mostly drinking/driving rather than drug cases (the published statistics on private programs are dominated by alcohol admissions and do not differentiate motivations by primary substance problem). Threats from employers or family members as well as psychological anguish and personal health problems are prominent motivators in private-tier programs.

The implications of criminal justice involvement in an admission to drug treatment are important. Clinicians recognize that an applicant who

---

[3] Chapter 6 more thoroughly delineates how the public tier of programs differs from the private tier.

is on parole or probation or who has a case currently in court automatically brings a second (and perhaps a third or fourth) "client" along—that is, the parole officer, defense attorney, prosecutor, judge, and so forth. Sorting out the effects of program activities on the clinical client versus their effects on the criminal justice client is no easy matter. Is an individual to be counted a treatment success or a treatment failure if he or she complied perfectly with treatment rules but dropped out of treatment early when convicted and imprisoned on a preexisting felony charge and is still in prison at the 12-month follow-up? Is a client a treatment success or a treatment failure if he or she is on probation, refrains from drug-seeking behavior, but continues to live by larcenous activities—avoiding rearrest during the 12-month follow-up period? Should the client whose parole officer insists on almost daily contact be equated analytically with the client whose probation officer wants no more than a quarterly postcard? The client's progress during or after treatment may depend heavily on the detailed conditions of criminal justice supervision that applied when the client entered treatment. To understand this connection requires a closer look at the relationship between the criminal justice and treatment systems.

CRIMINAL JUSTICE AGENCIES AND TREATMENT

According to the estimates presented in Chapter 3, more than a million individuals now in custody or under criminal justice supervision in the community need drug treatment. Approximately 1 in 10 of these individuals is estimated to be currently in treatment; probably a similar number have had previous exposure to treatment. These figures indicate the significance of the criminal justice system as an environment for drug treatment—an important environment now as it has been in the past (see Besteman, 1990; Courtwright, 1990; Phillips, 1990). In the eyes of the public, criminal offenders constitute the most worrisome component of the drug problem and bulk large in estimates of the costs to society of drug use. It is difficult to envision any expansion of drug treatment without an expansion in its overlap with the criminal justice system (sharing of clients/supervisees/inmates).

Linkages between the justice and treatment systems occur at numerous points. Drug-involved offenders are sometimes sent to treatment rather than adjudication, a process known as pretrial diversion. Many courts and correctional systems use commitment or referral to community-based treatment programs as an adjunct to probation or conditional release (parole) from prison. There is also treatment within correctional facilities and correctionally operated or funded halfway houses.

Although the number of individuals in the criminal justice system as a result of drug-induced offenses has always been appreciable, it is much greater now than in the past—even as recently as 5 years ago. This increase is due to the 15-year trend of massive growth in the criminal justice system itself and in particular to the growth in volume of its correctional services—that is, time behind bars. Between 1973 and 1988, the number of arrests made annually by police increased an estimated 50 percent, from 8 million to nearly 13 million—much faster than the increase in the U.S. population. Overall, the police concentrated nearly all of this increased attention on adults: for example, from 1978 to 1987, the number of juvenile arrests declined by 13 percent whereas the number of adult arrests increased by 37 percent. (These shifts greatly exceeded changes in the age distribution of the population.) Adult arrests for drug crimes have increased disproportionately: an estimated 848,000 out of 937,000 total drug arrests in 1987 were adult offenders (Jamieson and Flanagan, 1989).

The consequences of arrest have also changed, and there is now a much greater likelihood than in the past that an individual convicted of a crime will spend time in custody and under subsequent community supervision. In 10 years, from 1978 to 1987, the average daily jail census nearly doubled, from 156,000 to 290,000; in 15 years, the prison census more than tripled, from 204,000 in 1973 to 625,000 in 1988 (Figures 4-1a and 4-1b). Periods of imprisonment for felons sentenced to state prisons now average 2 to 3 years; the average imprisonment is somewhat less for drug offenses and somewhat more for violent offenses (e.g., 3 to 5 years for robbery, 7 years for homicide). Total sentences extend much longer than the time served in prison. Under widespread mandatory release rules, about 45 percent of the sentence is usually spent in prison initially, with the remainder on parole, not counting reincarceration time as a result of parole violation. Altogether, about 3.3 million individuals were under criminal justice supervision of one sort or another on the designated census days in 1987 compared with 1.3 million in 1976. Three out of four of these individuals were in the community rather than behind bars.

Court Referral to Treatment

The largest effort to bring adjudicated populations into contact with treatment is court-ordered screening to assess suitability for placement in community-based treatment programs under pretrial or posttrial probation. A series of these types of court-related programs were organized beginning in 1972 under the Treatment Alternatives to Street Crime (TASC) program (Cook et al., 1988). Originally created mainly to serve opiate addicts, the program soon became a common mechanism for diverting lesser drug cases, such as marijuana possession in small amounts, to avoid "clogging the justice system" with offenders who were nonviolent criminals.

In a model program, TASC clinicians used pretrial screening to assess

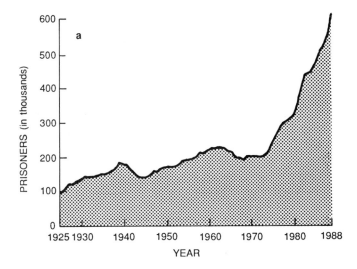

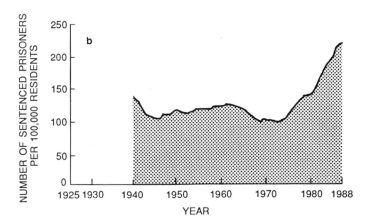

FIGURE 4-1   (a) Sentenced prisoners in state and federal institutions in the United States on December 31 of the years 1925–1988. Prison population data were compiled by a year-end census of prisoners held in custody in state and federal institutions. The 1988 figures are advance estimates subject to revision. Data for 1925 through 1939 include sentenced prisoners in state and federal prisons and reformatories, whether committed for felonies or misdemeanors. Data for 1940 through 1970 include all adult felons serving sentences in state and federal institutions. Since 1971, the census has included all adults or youthful offenders sentenced to a state or federal correctional institution with maximum sentences of more than one year. Sources: Flanagan and Jamieson (1988:484); Greenfeld (1989). (b) Rate (per 100,000 resident population) of sentenced prisoners in state and federal institutions in the United States on December 31 of the years 1940–1988. The rates for the period before 1980 are based on the civilian population, which is the resident population less the armed forces stationed in the United States. Since 1980, the rates are based on the total resident population provided by the Bureau of the Census. Sources: Flanagan and Jamieson (1988:485); Greenfeld (1989).

the treatment suitability and needs of drug-involved arrestees identified either by urine tests, a previous record of drug-related arrests, or interviews. These assessments were then used to ensure that treatment would be offered to those who both needed it and met qualifying criteria (see Phillips, 1990). Under such a program, when an accused individual was deemed suitable for treatment and the prosecutor and court agreed, he or she could accept referral to a community-based treatment program and the pending case would be suspended or a summary probation issued. If the individual completed the program successfully, the pending charges were dismissed or the probation discharged.

The federal "seed money" funding base for 130 TASC programs in 39 states was withdrawn in 1981, but 133 program sites in 25 states are now operating with support from state or local court systems or treatment agencies (Bureau of Justice Assistance, 1989). In addition, renewed federal support has recently become available as a result of the Justice Assistance Act of 1984 and the Anti-Drug Abuse Acts of 1986 and 1988. Some TASC programs have diversified, expanding from assessment and referral functions to counseling or testing; some currently contract with parole departments to assess and supervise prison releasees as well as probationers.

Early formative evaluations indicated that some TASC programs were efficiently managed and successful in introducing many of their contacts to treatment for the first time. They also seemed to yield promising results in terms of lower recidivism. Nevertheless, it is impossible to draw conclusions about the effectiveness of the TASC diversion approach. As the coordinators of a national TASC network point out, "TASC had no solid data base or data collection mechanism in place that would allow for long-term evaluation and comparison of the program's impact on drug-related crime or on the processing burdens of the criminal justice system" (Cook et al., 1988:102).

There are some data available, however, on the effects of TASC referral compared with other referral sources. Analysts of the national 1979–1981 Treatment Outcome Prospective Study (TOPS) developed a multivariate regression model of the effects of TASC referral compared with other client admission characteristics in residential and outpatient counseling programs (Collins and Allison, 1983; Hubbard et al., 1989). Criminal justice referrals to methadone programs in the sample were rare—too rare to permit reliable statistical results—but a substantial percentage (31 percent) of those admitted to outpatient nonmethadone and residential therapeutic community programs in the TOPS project were referred by criminal justice agencies, largely TASC programs.

After controlling for various preadmission characteristics (including criminal activity), TASC referral had a positive effect on the length of stay in treatment: retention increased for referred individuals by seven weeks on average in residential programs and six weeks for outpatient stays over the retention of nonreferred individuals. As Chapter 5 notes, longer retention is statistically associated with better response to treatment. These incremental differences, however, were not large enough to produce statistically significant differences in the outcome of treatment. At a minimum, this result showing increased retention means that legal pressure in the form of direct referral was clearly not detrimental to TOPS treatment outcomes, confirming the earlier results of 1969–1973 admissions to a national sample of programs (Simpson and Friend, 1988) and contrary to the reservations expressed by many clinicians before the implementation of TASC.

There is growing interest in TASC-type programs and "coerced treatment" as a mode of relationship between the treatment and criminal justice systems. The experience with community-based treatment during the 1970s was certainly favorable. When neither the treatment programs nor the criminal justice system was overwhelmed by cases, the deals struck between defendants, the courts, and the programs appear to have had clinically benign or positive effects; clients so acquired did at least as well in treatment as clients entering as a result of other forms of pressure. Whether this finding will hold up under the current circumstances of vastly increased criminal justice case-processing burdens is not yet known.

Prison and Parole Referral to Treatment

The large numbers of drug-involved prison inmates (see Chapter 3) and their propensity over the course of many years to commit a high volume of violent crimes in the community (Nurco et al., 1981a,b,c; Johnson et al., 1985) make the idea of treating the drug abusers and drug-dependent persons in this captive population an attractive one. Two objectives of prison—to isolate the criminal from doing harm in and to the community and to mete out punishment as promised by the law—do not require drug treatment. But a third purpose of prison, to deter the commission of future crimes by the convict after his or her release from confinement, could well be served by treating inmates—that is, if evidence supported the presumption that treatment would reduce drug use after prison and that this would in turn reduce recidivism. If one could efficiently and effectively deploy drug treatment in prisons, where so many drug-involved criminals are located, the potential reduction in community crime costs would be a large social benefit. A close look at the data on prisoners, drugs, and recidivism, however, leads to guarded expectations about whether and how much drug treatment might cut prison recidivism, notwithstanding its effectiveness in cutting drug use.

The reason for caution is that prisons are currently functioning much like revolving doors for clients, whether or not they are heavily involved with drugs. Another way to express this notion is that individuals in prison are generally in the middle of an extended career in crime. Despite the massive expansion in numbers of prisoners, there is not much room in prisons for younger first offenders because of the large (and increasing) number of more senior, returning parole violators and multiple offenders. In 1978, a study of young adults on parole found that, within six years after release, 69 percent had been arrested and 49 percent had been reincarcerated (Flanagan and Jamieson, 1988). Among a sample of 16,000 prisoners released to parole in 11 states in 1983, the average parolee had 8.6 prior arrests on 12.5 offenses, and 67 percent were on their second or later incarceration (Beck and Shipley, 1989). Sixty-two percent had been rearrested and 41 percent reincarcerated by the end of the third year after release. In the 1986 survey, three-fourths (74 percent) of all state prison inmates had been incarcerated before, and half had been incarcerated at least twice before (Innes, 1988).

Recidivism statistics also strongly suggest that longer (rather than shorter) incarceration—at least within the range generally incurred in today's prisons—does not necessarily reduce the probability of rearrest after release, although longer imprisonment by definition keeps criminals isolated from the community for longer periods. Beck and Shipley (1989) found that the rate of rearrest within three years of release was virtually the same for individuals serving as little as six months as it was for those serving as much as five years. Only the 4 percent of prison releasees who had served terms longer than five years—almost all of whom were convicted murderers, rapists, and armed robbers with multiple convictions—had a lower rate of rearrest (by about 14 percentage points) than the others. The lack of correlation of length of imprisonment (up to five years) with the probability of rearrest held steady after controlling for a variety of separate factors that predicted rearrest.

Drug involvement as such was not a principal feature differentiating recidivists from nonrecidivists in this population. In a multivariate logit analysis, five categorical attributes were found to *increase* the probability of recidivism: age when released (<25, 25–34, 35+), number of prior convictions (7+, 4–6, 1–3), prior probation or parole revocations (*yes*/no), prior incarceration (*yes*/no), and whether the current offense was for an acquisitive crime, namely, robbery, burglary, or theft (*yes*/no). More than 90 percent of prisoners with positive criteria on all five of these risk factors were recidivists (rearrested), as opposed to only 17 percent of prisoners with five negative criteria. With these five major factors (which are dominated quantitatively by age and number of convictions) taken into account, considering whether the individual had ever had a drug arrest (and 38 percent of the sample had) spreads these probabilities out by only about two more percentage points.

Although the prison-based studies show rather limited differences in recidivism between heavily drug-involved prisoners and other prisoners, there is ample evidence that, for those who use opiates and cocaine heavily, the relation of illicit drug consumption to current other criminality when in the community is a close one. When heavy drug consumers cut out or cut back on their drug use, their criminality of other kinds is also dramatically lower (Ball et al., 1981; Johnson et al., 1985; Speckart and Anglin, 1986); however, the causal direction here is not clear. The relationship between illicit drug use and other criminality tends to be reciprocal and "synergistic," each independently increasing the likelihood of the other. If drug treatment involves close surveillance in the community and a therapeutic focus on factors related directly to criminal occupation as well as to recovery from drug seeking, treatment may be able to affect the recidivist tendencies of prisoners and parolees to a greater degree than the modest leverage indicated by today's discouraging statistics on recidivism generally.

Preliminary Conclusions About "Mandatory Treatment"

The drug treatment and crime control systems share important goals—in particular, their clients' pursuit of less criminal and drug-involved lives. There are probably 40,000 individuals in drug treatment programs in jail or prison, out of nearly 1 million persons in custody on any given day. More broadly, many courts and correctional systems use commitment or referral to community-based treatment programs—usually programs involving close supervision, such as residential facilities—as alternatives or adjuncts to probation or parole. Half or more of the several hundred thousand admissions to community-based residential and outpatient drug treatment programs are on probation or parole at admission. These statistics are a direct manifestation of the criminal-medical policy idea (see Chapter 2).

There is frequent favorable reference today to "mandatory," "compulsory," or "required" treatment. The most important reason to consider these or related schemes to force more criminal justice clients into drug treatment is not that coercion may improve the results of treatment but that treatment may improve the rather dismal record of plain coercion—particularly imprisonment—in reducing the level of intensively criminal, antisocial, and drug-dependent behavior that ensues when the coercive grip is relaxed. In fact, getting more criminal justice clients into treatment could improve the results of criminal justice sanctions even if it actually diminished the average effectiveness of treatment. As it turns out, however, contrary to earlier fears among clinicians, criminal justice pressure does not seem to vitiate treatment effectiveness, and it probably improves retention to some extent.

The relevant evidence on criminal recidivism during and after "mandatory" treatment is reviewed in Chapter 5. It concerns mainly the effects of therapeutic prison programs paired with intensive parole supervision and postrelease continuity in community treatment. Some of these programs are at the discretion of the sentencing authority only, but more of those on which evidence is available involve initiative on the part of the inmate.

Most criminal justice pressure on community program clients does not involve forcing them into treatment. The pressure is more often indirect or involves some voluntary interest by the client. In the indirect case, the court (or other justice agency) simply insists that the client stay free of drugs or else be remanded into custody. The individual may then choose to seek treatment under the assumption that avoiding drug use (or at least avoiding abuse or dependence, which are far more troublesome and difficult to conceal) will be facilitated. In other cases, the court or other agency may offer the client a choice (through plea bargaining or negotiation): generally, a term in prison versus a period of probation or parole with treatment.

Criminal justice referral to treatment occurs for several reasons, including the belief that treatment may help reduce drug use and other criminal behavior. Increasingly, there is strong motivation to relieve court and prison overcrowding. Utilizing the treatment option takes responsibility for the case somewhat out of the criminal justice system, reduces the high cost of continuing incarceration, fends off the hanging sword of court-ordered population ceilings, and promises to deliver a degree of supervision beyond what probation or parole offices may typically be able to provide.

When referral occurs to relieve overcrowding, however, the stipulation "go to treatment and comply with the program, or *risk being returned to custody*" loses its credibility. The more overcrowded and strained the criminal justice system, the less pressure it can muster to help push people into seeking and complying with treatment. In view of the unrelenting growth of criminal justice populations, which threatens to swamp prison capacity and adjudication processes alike, any increase in these systems' ability to pressure people to enter or comply with treatment seems unlikely. Rather, increasing treatment capacity and improving the quality of treatment programs may be a way to keep the justice system situation from becoming even worse.

EMPLOYERS AND TREATMENT

Two-thirds to three-quarters of clients in the private drug treatment sector are drawn from the employed population (Comprehensive Care Corporation, 1988; Harrison and Hoffmann, 1988; Hoffmann and Harrison, 1988; Smith and Frawley, 1988). Just as the criminal justice system has been a locus of pressure toward treatment admission, employers have been seen as a similar lever for drug-abusing and drug-dependent employees. As a result of management concerns, union interest, and governmental actions, the role of employers in relation to drug treatment has become more extensive in the 1970s and 1980s than in previous years. Developments in the past two decades have been institutionalized in two kinds of drug-related workplace activities: employee assistance programs (EAPs) and drug screening programs (DSPs). Although they have some common qualities, there is a clear disjunction in the purpose and operation of these two kinds of programs.

Employee Assistance Programs

Employee assistance programs, or EAPs, began in the 1960s and were originally associated with the alcohol treatment field, resulting from the growth of concern about "hidden" alcoholics in all social classes. Indeed, it is only in the past 20 years that experts and activists have driven home the idea that the great majority of alcohol-dependent and alcohol-abusing individuals are not impoverished skid row inebriates but are spread throughout the working, middle, and upper classes, including the ranks of corporate executives (Beauchamp, 1980; Moore and Gerstein, 1981; Roman and Blum, 1987, 1990; Institute of Medicine, 1990). Today, EAPs serve a variety of management and employee benefit purposes, including the therapeutic management of drug problems.

The original role of the EAP was to enable supervisors (through an aggressive policy of supervisory training) to identify suspicious job deterioration before the situation was hopeless and to engage in "constructive confrontation"—originally called "constructive coercion" (Trice, 1966)—of the employee regarding his or her alcohol problem. This confrontation would then be followed by referral to treatment and follow-up as appropriate. Clearly, the goal of the EAP in this process was to return the deteriorating employee to satisfactory job performance; in pursuit of that goal, it provided training, assisted in confrontations, and made referrals. It was generally based in a central office and had its own credentialed specialists affiliated with the personnel or health department of a firm or union.

EAPs are common in larger, unionized firms and agencies.[4] About 26 million workers in private industry (31 percent of such workers; Bureau of Labor Statistics, 1989b) and 10 million public employees now have access

---

[4] A Bureau of Labor Statistics (1989b) survey indicated that EAPs are available to 4 percent of workers in establishments with less than 10 employees and 87 percent of workers in establishments with more than 5,000 employees. The same variation applies to drug screening programs, which are available to 1 percent of workers in sites with less than 10 employees and 68 percent of workers in establishments with more than 5,000 employees.

to an EAP. There has been steady growth: about 25 percent of Fortune 500 firms had EAPs in 1972, 57 percent had them in 1979, and virtually all such firms operate programs today. But EAPs have changed over time. Functions have been added (e.g., benefit management, brief counseling), and an industry of external EAP contractors has arisen. More significantly, the programs' original focus on alcoholism has broadened and now constitutes a larger social problem or "industrial social work" orientation: only one-third of a typical EAP's cases now involve alcohol or drug abuse, and the majority of cases are informal (and therefore confidential) "self-referrals" rather than formal supervisory referrals (Backer and O'Hara, 1988; Roman and Blum, 1990). All of these trends have made EAPs more and more like an employee benefit—one component of a total compensation package—and less and less like a management tool for maintaining desired levels of employee productivity on a day-to-day basis.

Along with the reduced role of alcohol in EAP goals and activities, there has been increasing attention to drugs; this trend is in part the result of a generational change, as those entering the work force after 1970 increasingly were found to be consuming illicit drugs as well as alcohol. The rapid emergence of marijuana and cocaine use in the work force of the 1980s met the expansionary crest of spreading EAP services and explicit substance abuse insurance coverage for employees and their families, generating a rapid increase (but from a very low base) in drug treatment referrals. In particular, the attention of EAPs to mixed alcohol and cocaine problems coincided with the addition of drugs to the scope of the private tier of alcohol treatment providers, with widespread and often highly publicized offerings of combined treatment (chemical dependency) protocols.

Typically, according to the corporate respondents surveyed by Roman and Blum (1990), about 4 percent of the employees in a firm providing an EAP consult the EAP in a given year. About 1.5 percent of employees specifically present a substance abuse problem, and in two-thirds of these cases, only alcohol, and not drugs, is clinically significant. These results correspond with a variety of data from individual firms reviewed by this committee during site visits. The bottom line is that about 0.5 percent of employees in an average EAP firm can be expected to consult the EAP (usually on a self-referred basis) for serious drug problems in a 12-month period. Applied to a work force of about 36 million individuals with access to an EAP, this suggests that about 180,000 candidates for referral to drug treatment may currently be seen by EAP counselors.

Yet, as the changing role of EAPs suggests, the actual linkage of employers to treatment has been much less substantial than the above figure suggests. Employer referrals or pressures play only a small role, based on the few data sets available on referral to private programs. According to counselor discharge evaluations supplied by programs subscribing to the Chemical Abuse/Addiction Treatment Outcome Registry follow-up system (Harrison and Hoffmann, 1988; Hoffmann and Harrison, 1988; these data mainly pertain to alcohol clients), the employer is mentioned as a primary motivator for treatment admission by only one-sixteenth of inpatients and one-tenth of outpatients. In these private-tier, midwestern, largely insurance-paid chemical dependency programs, greater numbers of both inpatients (one in seven) and outpatients (one in three) were reportedly motivated to seek treatment primarily by the courts—most presumably as drinking/driving cases—rather than by their employers.

Drug Screening Programs

The growth of drug screening programs (DSPs) has been a significant development of the 1980s, encouraged strongly by the federal government and most recently required of federal contractors by the Drug-Free Workplace Act of 1988 (P.L. 100-090, Title V, implemented by Executive Order 12564, 1989). The growth of DSPs has been led by large companies, and there is increasing regulation by the states (Intergovernmental Health Policy Project, 1989). These programs are drug specific and rarely, if ever, test for alcohol.

There are two fundamental kinds of DSPs: for employees and for job applicants. Most of the employee testing takes place at scheduled intervals (e.g., annual physical exams, prospective promotions to sensitive positions) or for probable cause rather than on a random basis, although random testing has attracted the most attention and controversy. In 1988, about 16.6 million or one-fifth of private-industry employees worked in organizations with some kind of DSP. Two-thirds or 11 million of these employees were in establishments that have programs to test current employees, and 14.7 million were in workplaces that test applicants (Bureau of Labor Statistics, 1989b). Applicant testing is the lion's share of DSP activity: about 953,000 employees and 3.9 million job applicants were tested in the 12 months prior to the mid-1988 Bureau of Labor Statistics survey. About 84,000 employees (8.8 percent of those screened) and 466,000 applicants (11.9 percent of those screened) tested positive. Most of the positive tests yielded evidence of cocaine or marijuana use.[5]

---

[5] These DSP results are not necessarily representative of overall employee or applicant drug consumption patterns. Most employee testing is based either on a strong suspicion of drug use (which greatly raises the likelihood of positive results) or the necessity to maintain a drug-free status in positions with particular safety hazards (which probably lowers that likelihood). In addition, these results most likely underreport casual use (false negatives) because of conservative cut-off levels, limited test sensitivity, and intervals between periods of use; however, they may also include a number of false positives (American Medical Association Council of Scientific

How Employers View Drug Treatment

Of the half-million positive DSP tests of job applicants, it is unknown how many—if any—lead to treatment. The overwhelming rule, however, is that employers simply deny the job application when the test is positive. Drug screening programs thus are used far more frequently to keep people from working than to make them fit for it. As for employee testing, about 60,000 of the estimated 84,000 positive results occurred in firms with EAPs, which are more likely than employers without EAPs to consider treatment an appropriate response. Nevertheless, in one survey of 1,238 EAPs (Backer and O'Hara, 1988), virtually none reported that more than "0–5 percent" of their clients entered treatment as a result of DSP activities, even though more than a third (35 percent) of the reporting EAPs were in firms or agencies with drug testing.[6]

The evidence, although thin, thus suggests that there are sharply fewer annual employer-related referrals to treatment than the combined figure from EAPs and DSPs of up to 264,000 potential cases. In the committee's judgment, a figure of around 50,000 annual employer referrals to treatment, which is to say, direct employer pressure to seek treatment, seems plausible. This number is roughly equal to the daily census of drug treatment clients inside jails and prisons; it is a fraction of the annual criminal justice referrals to treatment through TASC and related programs. Most of the employer referrals are to private-tier programs, about which research knowledge is especially sparse (see Chapter 5). Until that base of knowledge is improved, no better estimate is possible.

Despite the large productivity implications of drug abuse and dependency, employers appear to use their potential leverage very gingerly with regard to treatment. They do voice great concern about the cost implications of covering drug treatment under employer-sponsored health plans. This seeming disparity derives from two factors. One is the tendency to lose sight of drug treatment as such within the much larger pool of alcohol and psychiatric ("nervous and mental") benefit claims. The second factor is

---

Affairs, 1987). The errors are thus in different directions and of different magnitudes, and it is impossible to estimate the net resulting bias.

[6] The comparable figure in the Bureau of Labor Statistics sample was that 45 percent of EAPs were in DSP firms. This comparison is noted because the Backer and O'Hara survey needs to be viewed cautiously; the survey response rate was 16.2 percent, and the sample of EAPs was not selected from an enumerated list or sampling framework. The U.S. General Accounting Office (1988) reviewed 10 other surveys of employers from 1985 to 1989. None of them were representative samples, and most had low return rates similar to the Backer and O'Hara survey. Most companies indicated a willingness to refer current employees with positive drug screening results to a rehabilitation program on a case-by-case basis, but there was no indication how often referral took place in practice. In 439 EAPs surveyed by Blum and Roman in 1984–1985, those with DSPs reported the same rate of drug-related referrals as those without screening programs.

the high growth rate in payouts for inpatient care for drug abuse diagnoses that are attributable not to employees but to their covered dependents, particularly adolescent girls. These issues are assessed further in Chapter 8, but their prominence strongly reinforces the impression that employers view drug treatment more as part of the problem of high employee benefit costs than as part of the solution to a pervasive productivity problem.

AMBIVALENCE AND THE SPECTRUM OF RECOVERY

Even drug consumers who are badly impaired or severely pressed by legal or other problems are often ambivalent about seeking treatment. They may yield in the end only because pressure from family members, the law, deteriorated health, psychological stress, or a combination of such factors becomes too intense to deny. They may also find themselves impelled to seek treatment finally because attempts to relieve the pressure through other means, such as unassisted self-control, have proven futile.

Ambivalence toward treatment has several sources. First, it is always necessary to remember that the population involved *like the drugs they consume.* Drugs "work" for them, providing psychological and physical effects they have learned to value. Beyond the drug effects as such lie personal satisfactions for drug consumers in their ability to acquire and use drugs, both of which require a certain amount of practical and ritual competence (Preble and Casey, 1972; Johnson et al., 1985). It is easy, moreover, for the heavy consumer to mistake the satisfaction of drug wants and needs for the satisfaction of most (if not all) other wants and needs. This mistake is readily compounded because sustained drug experience may make an individual quite adept at meeting drug-specific requirements (e.g., knowing which drugs to buy and from whom, how to get the most effect from a drug) and less capable of satisfying other requirements, such as holding down a job. In addition, there is moral and logistical support for drug behavior to be found among other drug consumers, who may be close friends and family members. Their moral support for drugs may well extend to active disapproval of treatment (Eldred and Washington, 1976).

Finally, most forms of drug treatment, if implemented according to best clinical practice, are rigorous. These programs impose environmental schedules and controls and require a substantial amount of emotional work and behavioral change on the part of the client. Their requirements range from such logistical conditions as restrictions on mobility, keeping appointments for psychotherapy, and urine testing to more deep-seated issues such as clinical frankness and movement toward behavioral and emotional maturity. Unfortunately, clinical rigor has probably diminished in recent years as declining resources cut deeply into program operating capabilities. For example, programs that formerly used once-a-week urine testing have cut back in many cases to monthly tests, in compliance with minimum federal regulations. Psychotherapy and other service hours have typically been reduced by half or more from earlier levels (Hubbard et al., 1989).

Nevertheless, even at reduced levels of program rigor, drug consumers' ambivalence about participating in clinical procedures or program activities may lead to their breaking off the admission process before it is completed. Ambivalence generally continues during the first days and weeks of treatment exposure, presenting a stubborn challenge to clinicians. Where admission pressures such as threats to personal safety, legal jeopardy, health problems, or other motivational sources are not especially durable and the individual's goal of immediate relief is not accompanied by the need to protect positive assets or by a strong desire for longer term relief from drug seeking and its associated life circumstances, it is often difficult to overcome a person's reluctance to comply with demanding clinical requirements. Remitting pressures and continuing ambivalence undoubtedly contribute appreciably to the rapid early attrition curves seen in many drug treatment programs.

These judgments about the relation of motivation and attrition are difficult to prove or quantify with available research evidence. All measurements that correlate with early treatment dropout do so rather weakly (Hubbard et al., 1989). This weakness may be the result of imprecision in measuring the motives for seeking treatment and imprecision inherent in the dichotomies typically employed in client surveys, such as self-referral versus other-referral, on probation or parole versus not on probation or parole, and no versus any "perceived legal pressure." It may also be the case that a more general quotient or index of treatment motivation needs to be developed, taking into account the balance between severity of problems, attractiveness of assets in jeopardy, and features of the client's extended individual history of drug experience. Measurement problems aside, it is clear that initial motivation is but one element in a constellation of factors affecting the duration of treatment. Some of the other elements that have been studied, including qualities of program staff and specific treatment procedures, are reviewed in Chapter 5.

Full, Partial, and Nonrecovery from Drug Problems

An individual's initial motivation with respect to changes in his or her drug consumption varies from a desire for full recovery—aiming to achieve a lifetime of continuous abstinence—through more modest intentions, which can be called partial recovery, to not seeking recovery at all. The desire for lifelong abstinence is straightforward and easy to understand, but it is far from universal among clients in treatment. It is most likely to be found among those for whom the retention of valuable personal assets hinges on abstinence, forming a powerful counterweight to the attractions of drugs. More affluent and socially conventional clients often have a comfortable home, a good job, respectability, and an intact non-drug-using family at the time of admission, and these assets serve as incentives that support abstinent motivation. Less advantaged clients, those who are without most or all of these attributes or without evident prospects for securing them (even though they may greatly desire such things), have few preadmission assets. Indeed, it may be that the only resources these individuals possess, the threat of whose loss acts as an incentive, are their lives and their rights as citizens— even as second-class citizens from whom certain fundamental rights have already been withheld, as in the case of parolees. In other words, for socially disadvantaged individuals who are heavily involved in drug use and whose positive personal assets are limited, avoiding a long stretch in prison may be the only motivational counterweight strong enough, at the outset, to balance the lure of easily available drugs. The ethical and civil rights implications of this inequality between the well-off and the disadvantaged are troubling; nevertheless, this description accurately depicts the current state of affairs.

Clients may formulate exterior motives for entering treatment as "to get [someone] off my case." External pushes are usually allied to some degree with positive pulls or motivations to change. The positive motives are often not strong enough in themselves to initiate or sustain compliance with treatment, but reinforcement through external pushes into treatment and therapeutic pressure within treatment may be effective in doing so.

Clients often enter treatment as a self-conscious strategy to achieve partial recovery. That is, their purpose is to use treatment to help them gain control over their drug behavior—not to extinguish it entirely but to enable them subsequently to moderate it, perhaps for the first time in many years (e.g., to reduce their use to the manageable level they may have attained during an earlier, happier period of their drug-using careers). The purpose of these clients may be, for example, to keep daily drug use down to a clinical prescription (perhaps methadone, a tranquilizer, or a mood elevator) plus some drinks and an occasional "hit" of marijuana, methamphetamine, or some other "treat." Most important to this kind of applicant or client is to avoid taking the major drug of dependence (usually cocaine or heroin) or, if a "slip" happens in a moment of weakness, to have some protection and instantly available help against falling back into a full-blown, full-time habit (Wesson and Smith, 1985). These are users for whom treatment is a crutch, but one that produces both individual and social benefits. The challenge they offer to the quality of counseling and clinical acumen in a program is to make the crutch perform well, to satisfy and at the same time try to upgrade their recovery aims.

In contrast to the motive toward partial recovery, some clients have no wish at all to modify their drug consumption but seek program admission only to falsely certify such intentions in the eyes of family members or criminal justice agents (or both). How programs respond to these "bad attitudes" varies. Some programs work hard to discover and stop any deception on the part of clients and to confront them early on with the choice either of working to reform these attitudes and their accompanying behavior or of leaving treatment. Other programs subscribe to the philosophy that drug use and related attitudes such as deception (including self-deception or denial) are the fundamental clinical problems for which the person was admitted and that, for such cases, staying in treatment represents an improvement in health status, even if the improvement is small. Therefore, it would be impermissible to deny these individuals further treatment. It is a truism among clinicians, however, that such persons are probably heading for even deeper trouble, and later many of them seek treatment again with a different attitude.

Setting Realistic Goals

Drug problems that are serious enough to need treatment are usually chronic and relapsing in nature—generally, they are embedded in several ways in the client's life, they built up over time, and they have often inscribed permanent social, emotional, and physical scars. Recovery from chronic, relapsing conditions takes time and requires much effort from an individual; how much the client wants to work toward recovery undoubtedly makes a difference in treatment. But people who seek drug treatment vary in what they want to gain and in who else is involved. For clients seeking admission, treatment is the solution to a problem or problems too serious to ignore and too large to handle without help. Full recovery from dependence, including complete abstinence from drug use, may not be necessary to solve the problem that led them to treatment, although it may be the answer, or part of the answer, to even larger problems that an individual seeking treatment does not acknowledge or yet want to solve. All of these elements affect how much effort the prospective client is willing to put into the recovery process.

Drug treatment clinicians have devised ways to respond to these varying client features and have incorporated these methods into program policies and goals. Program policies are not all dry abstractions and pious sentiments; rather, they are rules of thumb for selecting clients for admission, dispensing discipline or extra attention, or deciding on discharge. Every program admits applicants to some degree according to its reading of an applicant's motives and situation, including the role of third parties such as the law and third-party payers. Programs vary in how eager they are to accept or avoid the harder cases, how intensively they are willing (or able) to work to treat the most difficult problem clients, and how heavily or swiftly or carefully they impose sanctions for noncompliance with the treatment plan.

Abstinence from illicit drug consumption is the central clinical goal of every kind of drug treatment, but it is not the complete goal. Clinicians also want their clients to stay out of jail and away from criminal activities, to be physically healthy, to adopt productive roles in family or occupational settings, to feel comfortable and happy with themselves, to avoid abuse of or dependence on alcohol. Full recovery in all of these senses can be realistically envisioned in some fraction of cases—a fraction that depends in part on the kind of population from which the program recruits its clients. But full recovery is not a realistic goal for other individuals, and those others make up the majority of admissions to most drug programs. For another fraction of applicants, even partial recovery as a result of the particular treatment episode is unlikely, although a period in treatment may plant or nurture the seeds of more serious efforts toward treatment and recovery in the future.

In summary, the pragmatic objectives of treatment in most cases are modest: to reduce illicit drug consumption, especially of the primary drug of abuse, by a large percentage—perhaps to nothing for an extended period—*relative to the consumption one could expect in the absence of treatment*; to reduce the intensity of other criminal activity if present; to permit the responsible fulfillment of family roles; to help raise employment or educational levels if the client so desires and the program has the resources available for such an effort; and to make the client less miserable and more comfortable physically and mentally. These goals are incremental: instead of absolute success and failure, there are degrees of improvement.

In light of the substantial losses to society resulting from active drug abuse and dependence, the committee considers a quantitative reduction in illicit drug consumption and the problems that accompany it for an individual client to be a socially and personally valuable result. An extended abstinence, even if punctuated by slips and short relapses, is beneficial in itself and may serve as a critical intermediate step toward lifetime abstinence and recovery. A useful shorthand for this pragmatic goal is that *drug treatment strives to initiate, accelerate, and help sustain the recovery process.*

Treatment goals may be influenced or guided by theoretical contemplation or rigorous induction, but they are typically selected and ordered by a complex process of social trial, error, and negotiation. Goals also vary because individual problems vary from client to client. Some clients' drug abuse or dependence is entangled in a chaotic life of violent criminal acts, ruptured family relationships, illiteracy, and psychological disturbance. For other individuals, drug abuse or dependence is a deviation from a pattern of conventional social successes and advantages. Treatment goals also vary because social concerns with different elements of drug problems differ over time and across institutional settings.

Programs have different orientations that affect the kinds of clients they recruit and the depth of their commitment to the "total client." A program may be oriented primarily toward an intensive short-term (e.g., four- to six-week) treatment protocol, viewing its task only as ensuring that the first steps toward recovery are taken, leaving the client, family, and other interested parties to complete the recovery process. A program that for the most part recruits socially advantaged individuals will not need to provide or help the client find vocational, educational, housing, welfare, or primary medical services.

A program with a longer term treatment protocol may view its primary responsibilities more comprehensively—to deal not only with the initial steps toward recovery but also with any other aspects of the client's circumstances that may increase his or her vulnerability to relapse. If these negative circumstantial aspects are prominent, then that program sets itself a much more challenging task than the program whose clients have few problems other than drug-seeking behavior with which to contend. Often, a program must develop channels to vocational, educational, housing, welfare, psychiatric, or primary medical services or else gain the resources needed to offer the necessary services itself, particularly for clients who are so disorganized that they have to have everything packaged together in one place. Such programs are prepared to view joblessness, psychological depression, or homelessness as part of the diagnosis they need to treat. That kind of perspective does not mean that these clinicians believe that joblessness, psychological depression, or homelessness are universal causes of drug problems or that the country must deal with unemployment, melancholy, and housing problems nationwide in order to help any individual client. It does, however, make these programs intrinsically more expensive to administer. The justification for the higher level of resources expended per client hinges on the prevailing norms surrounding assistance to the disadvantaged and the effectiveness with which programs are able to employ these resources to produce better recovery outcomes.

CONCLUSION

The picture of drug treatment goals that results from this chapter's analysis is not simple, but it has a certain coherence. That coherence resides in the principle that what should be expected from treatment is relative—relative to who is being treated and to how severe his or her problems are, and relative in that success should be viewed as a matter of more or less rather than all or none.

To define a reasonable set of treatment goals, it is necessary to consider certain characteristics of those being treated: depth of drug dependence, extensiveness of criminal activity, state of physical health, history of employment, status of family support, what specific problem(s) precipitated treatment, who besides the individual client has become concerned with what he or she is doing, and the seriousness of the client's intentions. The goals of treatment are to address and significantly improve these characteristics; the effectiveness of treatment is gauged by how much it improves them compared with what would probably occur without treatment.

In general, the primary goals of treatment have centered on reducing heroin or cocaine intake, predatory crime, and client death rates; at a secondary level, they involve marijuana or alcohol intake, unemployment or poor job performance, and lack of education. Improving family conditions and psychological well-being are sometimes viewed as ends in themselves, at other times as side effects of reaching primary goals, and at still other times as important prerequisites to reaching primary goals.

More is known about the primary than about the secondary issues. For example, predatory criminal behavior persists even in the teeth of extensive arrest and imprisonment. For this reason, criminal justice agencies have frequently turned to drug treatment programs for help in dealing with the drug-dependent criminals under their supervision in hopes of slowing down the increasing burden of recidivism and overcrowding. Employers, on the other hand, are much more committed to the use of drug testing, the most recent and rapidly growing employer program in this connection, to keep individuals with drug problems from entering the work force rather than to push toward recovery those who are already in it. This agenda may explain the fact that increasing drug treatment costs seem to them far more a threat to be eliminated than a productivity opportunity to be seized, an issue to which the committee turns in Chapter 8.

Because recovery clearly is possible and because most people enter treatment in search of it, albeit under pressure and with very mixed and confused motives, the committee believes that any worthwhile treatment program or method should be able to demonstrate that it has accelerated recovery among most of its clientele. However, rapid and full recovery is sufficiently unusual outside of treatment that it should not be viewed as the sole measure of treatment success. Partial recovery is better than no recovery. There is a real difference between hundreds or thousands of illegal and unhealthy acts over a period of time and a handful or even scores of such acts, and that difference should not be ignored when programs are called on to account for their clients' behavior.

5

The Effectiveness of Treatment

The question that people ask drug treatment experts most often and most insistently is a simple one: Does treatment really work? In the committee's judgment, and that of most experts, the available clinical experience and research data add up to a similarly short and pointed answer: It varies. This answer should be no surprise, as the question is naive. Virtually everything in Chapters 2, 3, and 4 of this report leads one to expect the effectiveness of treatment to be a complicated matter to understand and assess. Drug treatment is not a single entity but a variety of different approaches to different populations and goals. Response to treatment is not a matter of all or nothing, complete success versus total failure, but of degrees of improvement. Moreover, the setting for evaluation is not the quiet purity of a controlled laboratory experiment but the tangled complexity of real lives and programs under pressure from many directions.

The committee's strategy under the circumstances has been to put forward a line of questioning that is straightforward but somewhat more elaborate and revealing than "Does treatment really work?" These questions, which are listed below, cannot all be fully and confidently answered at present. Consequently, they must continue to be asked about each kind of treatment.

• *What are the basic concepts or modalities of treatment*? That is, what are the underlying designs or theories of treatment, what specific types of drug problems or population groups are being addressed by each design, and what are the best results that have been obtained under ideal conditions?

- *How well does each modality work in practice?* How adequate in terms of methodology are the evaluations of real programs, and what do the best of these evaluations reveal?

- *If a modality is not working as well as might be expected, what are the reasons?* For example, is the implementation or replication of the modality flawed or incomplete? Are the wrong kinds of clients being treated? Are there unexpected side effects? Does the environment interfere with the effectiveness of the treatment?

- *Do the benefits of the treatment justify its costs?* In other words, is treatment a sound investment of scarce public and/or private resources?

- In addition to these questions about treatment as it presently exists: *How might further research help to improve treatment?*

In responding to the first of these questions, this chapter considers serially the four major types or modalities of drug treatment: outpatient methadone maintenance, residential therapeutic communities (TCs), outpatient nonmethadone (OPNM) treatment, and inpatient/outpatient chemical dependency (CD) treatment. As indicated in the brief description of these modalities in Chapter 2, each type of drug treatment has developed since the 1950s. TCs derived largely from Synanon, which began in California in 1958. Methadone maintenance developed from studies on a hospital ward in New York in 1964; CD programs grew out of hospital-based approaches to treating alcoholism in Minnesota in the 1960s. Outpatient nonmethadone treatment[1] goes back at least to psychoanalytic treatment of "toxicomania" in the 1930s, but the community mental health movement, youth crisis counseling, "drop-in centers," and "free clinics" of the 1960s adopted quite different orientations that have substantially shaped the OPNM programs seen today. Although every modality has specific roots, all have continued to evolve since their introduction.

The most extensive usable results of research on the effectiveness of

---

[1] Because methadone maintenance programs are virtually always conducted on an outpatient basis but are set apart by the specific reference to methadone, all other outpatient programs are conventionally lumped together as outpatient nonmethadone or outpatient drug free. In light of the frequent use of other psychotropic medications during outpatient treatment, the committee views the term "nonmethadone" as more accurate than "drug free." The lumping together of all outpatient nonmethadone treatment is testimony to the prominence and distinctive nature of methadone maintenance and the fact that the population it serves is sufficiently homogeneous and different from the populations served by other outpatient programs. It should also be noted that methadone may be used in modalities other than maintenance, which technically refers to a planned treatment duration of 180 days or longer. (Shorter periods—usually 3 weeks to 2 months—are considered methadone detoxification.) Planned methadone-to-abstinence tapers of longer than 180 days are also incorporated into some program plans.

drug treatment are from several moderately sized clinical experiments and natural or quasi-experiments and from prospective longitudinal studies involving thousands of clients. There have been two large-scale, multisite, federally sponsored studies of publicly supported programs: the 12-year follow-up of a 1969–1971 Drug Abuse Reporting Program (DARP) national admission sample cohort and the Treatment Outcome Prospective Study, or TOPS, which involved a 10,000-person national sample of 1979–1981 admissions to 41 drug treatment programs in 10 cities. The Drug Abuse Treatment Outcome Study (DATOS), a third large-scale national prospective study, is scheduled to begin in 1990.

The committee addresses the paradigmatic questions separately within each modality. Although many treatment seekers try more than one treatment modality over the course of their drug careers (they build up a "treatment career" as well), the average profiles of clients admitted to the major modalities are quite different. Both treatment seekers and treatment programs engage in a great deal of individual selection into which many factors enter. For example, programs are geographically and economically differentiated in their accessibility to various types of potential clients; methadone clinics are relatively low in cost and typically located in inner-city areas; chemical dependency units are generally expensive and found in affluent suburbs. The typical demographic and drug-taking patterns of the different modalities' populations (a reflection of who *stays* in treatment from among those who are admitted) are quite distinctive. As a result, one cannot simply compare the performance or results of each modality with the others as if their client populations were interchangeable. Moreover, because some clients move between programs and there is evidence that treatment effects may, in part, be delayed and cumulative, it is hazardous to ascribe all the effects of a treatment episode to that episode alone; adjustments must be made to take prior treatments into account.

The most extensive and scientifically best developed evidence concerns methadone maintenance. A lower although still suggestive level of evidence is available concerning therapeutic communities and outpatient nonmethadone treatment. The lowest level of evidence is available for chemical dependency. Where the evidence on treatment effectiveness approaches adequacy, its overall tendencies are clear.

• Treatment reduces the drug consumption and other criminal behavior of a substantial number of people. Clients exhibit their best behavior while actively enrolled in treatment; their behavior is often poorer following treatment than during it, although still better than before admission.

• There are large variations in effectiveness across programs, which seem to be related to the varying quality of clinical management and competence. Practices in methadone maintenance dosing are a clear instance of this variation; there is also variance owing to differences in the characteristics of the populations being treated, such as the severity of their problems at admission.

• The length of time in treatment is a very important correlate of outcome; that is, longer treatment episodes yield better outcomes than shorter ones. Retention is presumably related to general program quality and specific client motivation to remain in treatment; however, no predictive treatment motivation test is available, and the role of treatment in facilitating motivation or averting impulsive decisions to "split" from treatment is not yet well understood.

• The benefits of treatment programs on the whole outweigh their costs, but variations in cost-benefit methodologies and results are great.

It should be noted that, except to describe the model, there are virtually no data to answer critical questions regarding independent self-help fellowship groups such as Narcotics Anonymous and Cocaine Anonymous or the Oxford Houses. Although the ideas underlying the Anonymous fellowships were incorporated at the outset into the clinical approaches[2] of TCs and CD programs and clients in these modalities are encouraged to participate in Anonymous meetings, the fellowships have shied away from involvement in formal evaluation protocols. Because drug-related Anonymous groups have been meeting in most cities longer than drug treatment programs have been present, and because they generally welcome individuals who are in treatment as well as those who are not (except that many Anonymous groups are antipathetic to individuals in methadone maintenance), they are in essence a part of the environmental baseline over which the incremental effects of the more formal treatments must be measured.

Two special topics are set slightly apart from the main lines of the chapter: the role of detoxification, which is often carried out in hospital settings, and the effects of treatment that occurs within correctional institutions. In the committee's view, it is not tenable to consider detoxification a treatment modality for the rehabilitation of drug abuse and dependence. Rather, it is a way of moderating some of the effects of overdose or withdrawal, and it may serve as a gateway to treatment. Correctional programs seem to fall largely into one of three types: they are either therapeutic communities, outpatient-type programs whose clients happen to live in prison, or drug law education programs carrying the name of treatment.

---

[2]Although CD programs incorporate numerous therapeutic components in addition to Alcoholics Anonymous-type meetings, the 12 steps of the Anonymous creed are so fundamental to the CD modality that the latter has been referred to as the "professionalization of Alcoholics Anonymous." There is no scientific literature on the Oxford House approach, which combines residential proximity with the fellowship principles.

The committee considers the need and opportunity for research relevant to treatment effectiveness to be so important that this chapter presents several recommendations for research on treatment methods and services. With recent budget increases for research, there is no overall lack of resources that could be devoted to such studies. Rather, the challenges of treatment-oriented research are arduous and demand certain kinds of commitments that are altogether too easy to slight in the rush to distribute cascades of research funding to more glamorous (e.g., high-technology) research ventures.

METHADONE MAINTENANCE

What Is Methadone Maintenance?

Methadone maintenance is a treatment specifically designed for dependence on narcotic analgesics, particularly the narcotic of greatest concern in the United States, heroin.[3] The controversies surrounding methadone maintenance[4] have made it the subject of literally hundreds of studies. From these studies, including a few vitally important clinical trials, strong evidence has accumulated about the safety and effectiveness of methadone.

---

[3] There are three main types of narcotic analgesics: those derived from opium, such as morphine, heroin (diacetylmorphine), and codeine, and the two major synthetics, meperidine (best known as Demerol) and methadone. There are numerous congeners of each major narcotic type that have varying degrees of activity. The natural and synthetic compounds have dissimilar chemical bases but share certain critical structural properties that result in their penetrating and affecting the "endogenous opioid" neurotransmitter system in similar ways. There are significant differences, however, in how the major narcotic types are absorbed and metabolized outside the brain; these difference affect the duration and rate of their central nervous system effects.

[4] There continue to be widespread negative beliefs among the general public and some policymakers about methadone (see, for example, the results of focus group discussions reported by the Technical Assistance & Training Corporation [1989]). The drug is suspected, for example, of being unsafe even in clinically controlled usage; it is said to "rot" the bones (or the brain, or the liver) and to create lassitude or stupefaction among individuals who take it for any length of time or at any dose except a minimal one. It is also said that indefinite maintenance is "just substituting one addiction for another," so the most important clinical goal should be to "get off methadone" as soon as possible. It is thought that most of the people enrolled in methadone maintenance programs sell some or all of their daily methadone dose and use the proceeds to buy heroin and other drugs. Putting all of these beliefs together, methadone can be portrayed as an assault on the well-being of communities in which methadone maintenance clinics are located, rather than a therapeutic response to local drug problems.

This set of beliefs about methadone is based partly on shards of experience (often reported by journalists), partly on philosophical or ideological premises that may be impervious to evidence, and partly on frank skepticism about the existence of a therapeutic rationale or base of evidence underpinning methadone maintenance treatment. This section should at least be useful in addressing the last of these sources of belief.

The idea is not unfamiliar that a treatment for a chronic health disorder could involve long-term, even permanent pharmacological maintenance using a powerful drug that is nevertheless safe if properly administered. Perhaps the most obvious examples are treatments for endocrine problems: insulin for diabetes, thyroxine for thyroid deficiency. A treatment for chronic mood disorders (manic-depressive cyclothymia) using lithium chloride for long-term maintenance is a psychiatric example. Although methadone maintenance was viewed as revolutionary when it was first developed in the United States, the historical sketches in Chapter 2 and in Courtwright (1990) point toward early twentieth century instances in U.S. cities of morphine maintenance as a treatment for opiate dependence. In Great Britain, heroin maintenance was also practiced, although it has largely been replaced there by methadone maintenance. The application of maintenance concepts to the treatment of drug dependence therefore is not medically unusual. But to understand how methadone maintenance operates as a treatment for heroin dependence, three aspects must be stressed: the significance of clinically defined goals, the pharmacological basis of drug substitution, and the embedding of substitution in a broader clinical behavioral strategy.

Goals

Methadone maintenance cannot be understood apart from the correct stipulation of the major goals of treatment, primarily to reduce illicit drug consumption and other criminal behavior and secondarily to improve productive social behavior and psychological well-being. It is critical that methadone is a legally prescribed drug for the purpose of treating dependence.[5] Yet even more critical is that individuals who receive methadone maintenance treatment should reduce their use of illicit drugs and their commission of other crimes (e.g., selling drugs, stealing money, using weapons to obtain funds to support their drug consumption) ideally to zero but at least by an appreciable amount. Improved social productivity and well-being would be important further measures of the effectiveness of methadone maintenance. The goal of ending the licit dependence on methadone itself is well down the list—so that the risk of increased crime or illicit drug use weighs heavily against arbitrary limitation on the duration of methadone maintenance. Nevertheless, this goal has been given much higher priority in many programs, as discussed later in the chapter.

---

[5] The argument has been made that even illegally marketed methadone represents a significant public health improvement over street heroin. Although this result is theoretically plausible, an opposite result is equally plausible, and there is little evidence to support either theory. Therefore, in policy terms, street methadone sales are a negative effect.

Substitution

At the base of methadone maintenance is an empirical observation that was made before the biological reasons for it were well understood: all of the effective narcotic analgesics may be substituted for one another with adjustments in dose and route of administration. Substitution is possible because there are basic similarities in their objective and subjective effects; in particular, in dependent individuals there is parallel or cross-tolerance to elevated doses and cross-suppression of respective withdrawal effects. Key differences involve how quick, how strong, and how long-lasting these actions are; they are also apparent in the precise mixture of effects for each drug.

Cross-dependence is particularly important in detoxification. Most drugs of widespread abuse and dependence (heroin, cocaine, alcohol) act quickly and dramatically and wear off in a matter of hours. By the same token, the associated primary withdrawal syndromes tend to be striking but short; there is usually, however, a somewhat more protracted but less dramatic phase of sustained withdrawal symptoms such as sleep disturbance, agitation, or mild depression. The general approach to detoxification is to moderate the more severe symptoms, often by substituting a long-acting drug, which can then be tapered down to zero, leaving only the lesser symptoms.

Methadone may be prescribed not for maintenance purposes but for a shorter period—three weeks was once standard, although the period may legally extend up to six months—to moderate withdrawal symptoms. Detoxification generally begins with an escalating dosage to reach a point such that the patient stops using other opiates and withdrawal symptoms are not evident. Then the methadone dose is tapered down to zero. Individual responses vary, but usually this method does not completely suppress withdrawal symptoms during and after the tapering period; rather, it keeps them mild for a time—until the tapering procedure does not provide enough methadone to prevent the more discomfiting withdrawal symptoms. It is common for individuals to drop out of methadone detoxification some time during the second week of a typical three-week planned detoxification period. Sometimes other medications are given during methadone detoxification to manage particular symptoms.

As shown by the long record of experience with detoxification of heroin dependence, those detoxified were universally found to have a very high susceptibility to relapse—usually well in excess of 90 percent of followed cases (see Vaillant, 1973). After detoxification, and often before its procedures had been completed, there was a resumption of craving for opiates. Dole (1988) and others have theorized that the extensive use of opiates may bring on alterations in the brain neurotransmitter/receptor systems affected by opiates, leaving many individuals with a virtually permanent craving that can only be assuaged by drugs of the opiate family.

Methadone has several unusual pharmacological properties that have made it especially suited to a maintenance approach. Unlike many opiates, it is effective orally, a significant advantage in that oral dosing is more hygienic than the needle and more easily titrated than smoke. Because of methadone's particular pattern of absorption, metabolism, and elimination, a single dose within a train of level doses, in the typical maintenance range of 30 to 100 milligrams per day (mg/day), takes effect gradually and wears off slowly, yielding a fairly even effect across a period of 24 hours or longer. Methadone is thus conducive to a regime of single daily maintenance doses, eliminating dramatic subjective or behavioral changes and making it easy for clinician and client to fit into a routinized clinic schedule.[6] This pattern is very different from the shorter action and more dramatic highs and lows of heroin, morphine, and most other opiates. The long-term toxic side effects of methadone, as of other opiates if taken in hygienic conditions in controlled doses, are notably benign.

The short-term clinical effects of methadone were first studied at the Lexington addiction research center in the 1950s, and research continued there and elsewhere into the 1960s. Since the mid-1960s, about 1.5 million person-years of methadone maintenance have accumulated in the United States. Not all clients have been closely observed for medical side effects, but the thousands of research cases that have been carefully observed yield a well-documented conclusion:

[P]hysiological and biochemical alterations occur, but there are minimal side effects that are clinically detectable in patients during chronic methadone maintenance treatment. Toxicity related to methadone during chronic treatment is extraordinarily rare. The most important

---

[6] There was extensive research from the late 1960s to the late 1970s on a longer acting methadone congener, levo-alpha-acetylmethadyl (LAAM), that requires less frequent doses—every two or three days instead of daily. LAAM has been studied in a series of phased clinical trials but has not yet been approved for nonexperimental use, although its safety and freedom from toxic side effects appear comparable to those of methadone (Savage et al., 1976; Ling et al., 1978; Blaine et al., 1981). Overall, during the trials, methadone was more successful than LAAM in retaining clients in treatment (by 20 percentage points), largely because more LAAM recipients felt that the medication was not "holding," that is, not keeping opiate withdrawal symptoms from beginning to emerge between doses, a result that Goldstein and Judson (1974), after a double-blind study, judged to be more psychological than physiological in origin. LAAM recipients who stayed in treatment used less heroin and performed better on other clinical measures than methadone clients, particularly those on lower methadone doses. Some clinicians reported a substantially improved therapeutic climate in LAAM clinics owing to the more relaxed three-days-per-week visiting schedule (Goldstein, 1976). There are probably clients who would do better on LAAM than on methadone, and vice versa, with results for both likely to improve with better dose optimization and counseling about differences between the two drugs. A revival of interest in LAAM and an attempt to restore the initiative toward approval by the Food and Drug Administration for nonexperimental use are under way.

medical consequence of methadone during chronic treatment, in fact, is the marked
improvement in general health and nutritional status observed in patients as compared with
their status at the time of admission to treatment. (Kreek, 1983:474)

The most common physical complaints during methadone maintenance
are insomnia and weight gain, but these are clinically related both to the
consumption of other drugs and alcohol (consumption that continues and
sometimes increases among a fraction of clients, the size of which varies
from program to program) and to preexisting or coexisting abnormalities
common in this population and in the general population.

Clinical Behavioral Strategy

In terms of the social history and individual model of drug-seeking
behavior reviewed in Chapters 2 and 3, a program of controlled methadone
maintenance at an appropriate dose level could have recovery-inducing
effects on heroin dependence. These effects may be felt through two paths
corresponding to the two most common motivational processes that operate
during heroin dependence: pleasure seeking and withdrawal avoidance.

With regard to pleasure seeking, methadone is an effective analgesic.
Yet the effect of an accustomed (tolerated) dose is merely a dim echo
or reminder of heroin's most intense effects, not so much a "rush" as a
reassurance—which may wear better in the long run and is certainly less
disruptive in the short run than the euphoric heroin high with its associated
itchiness and dreamy nods. There is also a more subtle and perhaps equally
valuable effect: if heroin and methadone are both in the body, their active
metabolites compete with each other for access to sites of action in the
brain. If the methadone dose is high relative to the heroin dose, the latter
will not have a very distinctive effect, and the individual taking methadone
will find heroin less rewarding. As a result, the shooting of heroin "over"
the methadone may become self-extinguishing.

On the other side of the pharmacological fence, methadone maintenance prevents symptoms of heroin withdrawal, which, although not
life-threatening or excruciating, are immiserating (a good parallel is a head
cold or a bout of influenza). The critical condition is that the dependent
person feeling withdrawal symptoms knows that all of these unwelcome sensations can be banished within minutes with a dose of an opiate. Recurrent
withdrawal symptoms stimulate drug seeking during heroin dependence,
and the ability of methadone maintenance to keep them at bay is a major
attraction and benefit.

In its initial clinical trials, which began in inpatient settings and then
were extended to outpatient sites, methadone maintenance proved capable of stabilizing the psychological functioning of the heroin-dependent

individual at a near normal state. Methadone in effect eliminated the alternating phases of euphoria, somnolence, and agitated concern characteristic of the incipient stage of withdrawal from heroin dependence. The clinicians conducting the trials observed that clients on methadone were not obsessed with acquiring the next dose, became interested in the prospects for improving the conventional strands of their lives, and were generally functioning without notable drug impairment or side effects. An individual on methadone was capable of participating in counseling, psychotherapy, and remedial education and training (most of the same rehabilitative services delivered in therapeutic communities and outpatient treatment). This capability was partly the result of the intrinsic pharmacological effects of methadone and partly because, unlike street heroin, it was provided reliably, in legitimate clinical settings, and in reliable doses.

Methadone maintenance was originally defined as the administration of methadone together with rehabilitative and counseling services, and this definition, along with many detailed specifications about facilities and staffing, was built into federal regulations as a required protocol for a licensed methadone maintenance program. These regulations permit methadone to be dispensed only by licensed maintenance or detoxification programs or by hospital pharmacies. (In hospitals, methadone is prescribed mainly for severe postoperative or cancer pain and occasionally for short-term inpatient detoxification.)

Methadone programs are nearly always ambulatory, with daily visits to swallow the methadone dose (usually provided in a 3- to 4-ounce plastic bottle of sweetened, orange-flavored water) in the clinic, except for the traditional Sunday take-home dose. After several months in the program with a "clean" drug-testing record and good compliance with other program requirements such as counseling appointments, clients may regularly take home one or more days' doses between every-other-day, twice-weekly, or even weekly visits—a revocable range of privileges. Some methadone clients voluntarily reduce their doses to abstinence and conclude treatment after some time; others remain on methadone indefinitely.

The role of counseling is multifold. In the first instance, the design of methadone maintenance programs includes numerous monitoring and adjustment features that stress the need for clients to wean themselves away from street drug seeking. Program clinics have specific hours for dispensing, counseling, and medical appointments; there are codes of proscribed behavior (e.g., no violence or threats of violence), and monitored drug tests are conducted at random intervals—at least monthly and as often as weekly, although the cost of the tests have led financially strained programs to cut them back to the minimum. Counseling includes the assessment of client attitudes and appearance (important in themselves and as clues to drug behavior) and the gathering of information about employment, family, and criminal activities; counselors offer psychotherapy and individualized social assistance and recognition, depending on their caseloads and their training for such tasks.

In most clinics, counselors participate in staff decisions with regard to changing dose levels, requirements for therapeutic contacts, award and revocation of take-home privileges, and decisions regarding termination from the program. Clinical experiments have studied methadone dosage and behavioral techniques (contingent rewards and sanctions for "dirty" urines and missed and late counseling appointments) as part of the modality's repertoire. The clinical trial literature has demonstrated important success in the use of methadone dosage supplements or decrements and take-home privileges to punish or reward clients for noncompliance with such clinical rules as the proscription on continued drug use and the requirement of cooperation by timely attendance for dispersing, participating in counseling, and paying required fees (Stitzer et al., 1983).

The drawbacks to methadone maintenance have been well recognized since its inception: the client is still at least mildly dependent; the drug reduces heroin craving and stabilizes the individual psychologically but does not necessarily modify or rehabilitate other behavior; clients often still use or abuse and sometimes become dependent on other drugs including alcohol; and it is possible for take-home methadone to be diverted from therapeutic uses and sold to permit the client to buy heroin or other drugs. Moreover, methadone has no direct pharmacological bearing on abuse or dependence on alcohol or other drugs, especially cocaine, which has become such a serious and widespread problem in the 1980s. The important question is this: Does the modality reach its primary goals in enough cases to outweigh these limitations and drawbacks?

How Well Does Methadone Work?

The goals of methadone maintenance—to reduce illicit consumption of heroin and other opiates, to reduce other criminal activity, and to help clients become more socially productive and psychologically stable— constitute a continuum that can be cut at various points to designate "success" versus "failure." At the outset of its use, the modality was specifically targeted toward those who were most severely dependent, as judged by substantial histories of relapse from earlier detoxification episodes (frequently in jail); this commitment was built into the early regulations requiring documentation of at least two years of heroin use and two prior relapses.

Early trials of methadone maintenance in New York (Dole and Nyswander, 1965, 1967; Dole et al., 1966, 1968, 1969) noted two striking findings: the majority of clients would remain in treatment for as long as it was available to them, in substantial contrast to the usual experience in out-patient psychotherapy; and methadone maintenance significantly improved the condition of clients as revealed by studies that considered behavior in the community for periods of several months to several years. Although there was some use of other drugs, including heroin, especially in the first few weeks after admission, such use generally fell off over time, contrasting sharply with the increasing return over time to heroin dependence that was the norm after detoxification or other typical medical or psychiatric treatments. The steadiness of employment increased somewhat, but a much more dramatic change was the sustained reduction in criminal behavior, especially drug trafficking crimes.[7]

The most convincing results about the efficacy of methadone mainte-nance—the capacity of the treatment to induce client changes independent of initial selection or motivational effects—come from a handful of clinical experiments that are widely separated in time and place but that consistently yield very distinctive findings. In these studies, heroin-dependent, heavily criminally involved populations who were randomly assigned to methadone maintenance or a control condition (an outpatient nonmethadone modality) demonstrated clinically important and statistically significant differences in favor of methadone on the gauges of drug use, criminal activity, and engagement in socially productive roles such as employment, education, or responsible child rearing.

In the landmark experiment, Dole and colleagues (1969) randomly assigned 32 well-motivated criminal addicts to either a methadone treatment group ($N = 16$, of whom 4 declined treatment before program initiation) or a year-long control/waiting list group ($N = 16$). Out of the combined control and refuser group ($N = 16 + 4 = 20$), every individual became re-addicted to heroin soon after release, with 18 individuals returning to jail and the other 2 being lost to the study. At 7 to 10 months after initiation of the study, only 3 of the 12 addicts in the experimental group had been reincarcerated. Furthermore, although 10 of these 12 individuals had used heroin since the program was initiated, for 6 of the 10 this use was limited to the first 3 months of the program.

Gunne and Gronbladh (1984) have also reported a small but persuasive study (Figure 5-1). Thirty-four heroin-dependent individuals applied for admission to the only methadone clinic in a Swedish community; 17 were

---

[7] Observational studies of the original Dole-Nyswander program cohorts, which probably en-gaged the most highly motivated clients and had relatively high-quality staff and resources, yielded good data over time confirming the long-term efficacy of methadone maintenance (Dole et al., 1968; Gearing, 1970, 1974; Dole and Joseph, 1978). Studies in these and later programs also indicated the close relation of retention in treatment and good outcomes; attrition after a short period in treatment was associated with higher rates of relapse (Simpson et al., 1979; Hubbard et al., 1989).

randomly assigned to methadone maintenance, and 17 were assigned to outpatient nonmethadone treatment (these individuals could not apply for admission to the methadone clinic again for 24 months). Two years later, 12 of the 17 clients on methadone were no longer using illicit drugs; 10 were employed, and 2 were in school. Five still had drug problems, and of these, 2 had been discharged from treatment for severe abuse of sedative-hypnotic drugs. Of the 17 individuals who went into the outpatient nonmethadone program, only 1 was doing well; 2 were dead, 2 were in prison, and the rest had returned to taking heroin. After two years, then, 71 percent of methadone clients were doing well, compared with 6 percent of controls. Five years after the study began, 13 of the methadone clients remained in treatment and were still not using heroin, and 4 had been excluded from treatment because of unremitting drug problems. Among the controls, 9 had applied for and entered methadone maintenance; of these, 8 individuals were not using drugs and were socially productive. Of the 8 controls who did not apply for methadone when eligible, "five are dead (allegedly from overdose), two in prison and one is still drug free" (Gunne and Gronbladh, 1984:211).[8]

Another perspective on the effectiveness of methadone treatment is offered by the results of several "natural experiments." In one such study, Anglin and McGlothlin (1984) examined the introduction of the methadone maintenance modality to California in 1971, viewing it as a quasi-experimental intervention. They had previously begun a long-term observational study of heroin-dependent individuals who had been apprehended by law enforcement agencies in 1961–1963 (McGlothlin et al.,

---

[8] One other significant experimental study was reported by Newman and Whitehill (1978) from Hong Kong. This study demonstrated both the attractiveness or retentive power of methadone as such and the difficulties of conducting randomized clinical trials with drug-dependent populations when they are able to act on their own strong preferences about treatment assignment. (Another illustration of that difficulty in the United States was reported by Bale and coworkers [1980].) Newman and Whitehill studied 100 male heroin addicts who were seeking methadone maintenance. The men were hospitalized for one week and stabilized on 60 mg/day of methadone. They were then randomly assigned to ambulatory methadone maintenance or to slow detoxification. The maintenance group started out at 60 mg/day and ended by averaging 97 mg/day. The detoxification group was taken down 1 mg/day over 60 days, after which they were given placebos. The medication was given on a double-blind basis: neither patients nor clinicians had certain knowledge of which group they were in.

About 60 percent of maintenance patients were retained in treatment for the entire 2.5-year trial period, a rate commensurate with retention studies in the United States. In contrast, the patients who were detoxified dropped out of treatment rapidly. By the time they reached the placebo state, only 20 percent remained in treatment; nearly all had dropped out by the end of a year. Dropouts from the control group were subsequently recruited into methadone maintenance and had the same retention rates from that point on as the original maintenance group. Most of the control group sensed that they were being detoxified rather than maintained, and many quit the study to reenroll in methadone maintenance.

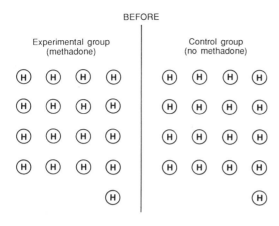

BEFORE

Situation before the randomization study: each circle represents an individual 20 to 24 years old. "H" indicates regular intravenous heroin abuse. The left half represents the experimental group, which will be accepted for methadone maintenance treatment; the right half represents the controls who will not be given methadone maintenance.

AFTER 2 YEARS

Two years after acceptance or decline: white circles = no drug abuse; H = abuse of heroin or (in the experimental group) hypnotic depressants; P = subject in prison; black circle = subject deceased; crossed circle = patient has been expelled from treatment.

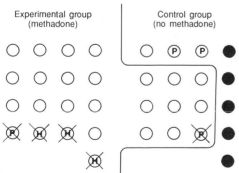

Five years after admission: nine persons from the original control group have been accepted in the methadone maintenance program.

FIGURE 5-1 Clinical trial of methadone maintenance versus outpatient nonmethadone for heroin addiction conducted through the Swedish Methadone Maintenance Program. Source: Gunne and Gronbladh (1984).

1977). Drug consumption and criminal involvement in this study population were high just prior to the introduction of methadone, despite the fact that all members of the population had been incarcerated and supervised for several years in the 1960s by the state's Civil Addict Program (CAP). Some of the study population had already stopped using heroin before the introduction of methadone; this group was termed the inactive user sample. Some of the remainder entered methadone treatment when it became available (the methadone sample), and the rest did not (the active user sample; Figures 5-2a, 5-2b, and 5-2c). McGlothlin and colleagues (1977) had found during their earlier study that the active user and methadone samples had reduced drug and crime activity while under CAP supervision but had quickly resumed their prior high activity levels once CAP supervision ended. After the advent of methadone programs in California, a major difference was observed between those in the active user group and the methadone clients, a difference that persisted for at least three years after the introduction of methadone.

Overall, the findings of this natural experiment indicate that a certain proportion of addicts (i.e., the inactive sample) had responded favorably and permanently to a particular form of criminal justice supervision involving specialized prison treatment and intensive parole. Of those who did not, a significant proportion entered methadone maintenance when it became available and responded very well to it (compared with otherwise very similar individuals who did not enter a methadone program): those pursuing methadone maintenance substantially reduced their drug use and criminal activity and (to a lesser degree) increased their employment.

Similar results have been reported in natural experiments involving the limited introduction of publicly supported methadone maintenance programs in a number of California cities and towns in the early 1970s and the subsequent closure of some of these programs for fiscal and political reasons. In cities where methadone maintenance became much less accessible as a result of such closures, former clients as a whole did appreciably less well at the two-year follow-up (in terms of heroin use, other criminal behavior, and, to a lesser degree, employment) than comparison groups in locations where there was continued access to treatment. In cities where public programs closed but private ones opened, those who transferred to the alternative methadone maintenance programs did much better (in terms of staying free of drugs and out of crime) than those who did not or could not continue treatment (McGlothlin and Anglin, 1981; Anglin et al., 1989a). In these as in all other studies, longer retention in methadone as opposed to early attrition from the program was associated with much better results measured by reduced heroin use and other criminal activity.

Why Do the Results of Methadone Treatment Vary?

A significant proportion of methadone maintenance clients do not respond well to treatment, for a variety of reasons relating to the clients themselves and to the programs. This proportion averages about one in four, although there is wide variation from program to program (U.S. General Accounting Office, 1990; Ball et al., 1988). It is clear that some clients who are admitted enter methadone maintenance for purposes other than to receive counseling and other services or to pursue recovery. These clients are not compliant with clinical rules and are less likely than others to be (or become) motivated; most leave treatment after short periods. It is much easier to identify these clients after the fact than before; programs screen out some but not all such clients through pretreatment intake reviews. There are also probably some clients who would recover just as quickly without methadone maintenance, but they choose methadone treatment because it is helpful or attractive in some ways that other treatments (or no treatment) are not. The proportion of such clients is variable—it may be as low as 1 in 20 or as high as 1 in 10. These clients are beneficial in terms of positive program statistics but somewhat exaggerate the degree to which the program is actually generating worthwhile effects.

The largest group of clients is clearly at some point in the middle. The evidence from experimental and quasi-experimental studies clearly points toward the existence of a substantial number of heroin-dependent individuals who perform at least moderately well in response to methadone maintenance and who would do poorly without it, even when other kinds of treatment are available.

There is compelling evidence that program factors such as methadone dosing policies and counselor characteristics affect the behavior of such relatively malleable clients above and beyond any initial differences in motivation. The strongest treatment retention and outcomes (measured as improved social functioning) were seen in the initial methadone clinical trials (Dole and Nyswander, 1965, 1967) and in cohorts admitted to methadone treatment in New York during the pilot stage of developing the treatment (Gearing, 1970, 1974). This phase of history was characterized by careful screening of clients, self-selection by addicts—as a result of admission waiting lists of up to a year—and extensive adjunctive services provided by highly skilled and motivated clinical staff (Lukoff and Kleinman, 1977).

Later evaluations found that retention rates and outcomes were somewhat poorer when the New York programs had reached large-scale operation, were no longer highly selective in admissions, and had reduced their waiting time for admission to a few weeks (Dole, 1971; Dole and Nyswander, 1976; Dole and Joseph, 1978). Some observers attributed this decline to strains on system capacity and the onset of rigid and antipathetic

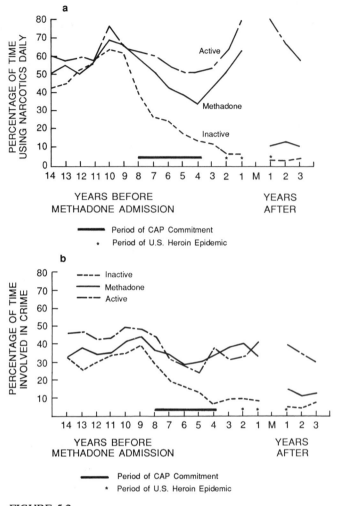

FIGURE 5-2

federal regulations in contravention of good clinical practices (Dole and Nyswander, 1976). Kleber (1977:268) has contended that the programs' primary problems were greatly reduced selectiveness in admissions and the shortage of skilled and motivated staff: "it is not surprising that retention rates dropped and the number of urines containing heroin rose. What is surprising is that the figures were not worse than they were."

Program performance (in terms of client retention and continued use of drugs) has also been observed to vary across programs at the same point in time. The Treatment Outcome Prospective Study, for example, showed a large degree of variation in clinically important client outcomes across nine

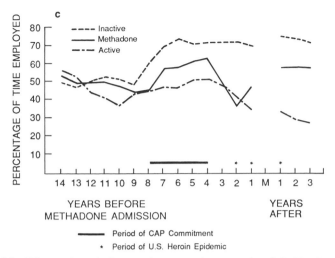

FIGURE 5-2 Effects of methadone maintenance in a sample of California ex-parolees who participated in the Civil Addict Program (CAP) measured on three parameters: (a) percentage of time reported as daily narcotic use; (b) percentage of nonincarcerated time spent in criminal activity; and (c) percentage of nonincarcerated time the individual was employed. CAP clients were divided into three groups: inactive users, active users, and methadone recipients. Source: Anglin and McGlothlin (1984).

methadone maintenance programs. Twelve-month retention rates averaged 34 percent of admissions, but five programs had low rates of 7 to 25 percent, whereas two programs had rates greater than 50 percent. Regular heroin use by clients at follow-up (approximately three years later) was reported by 21 percent of the entire follow-up sample, but two programs had rates greater than 30 percent, and three had rates of 11 to 14 percent (Hubbard et al., 1989).

Variation in performance has been linked most strongly to variations in methadone dosage policies. Programs that are committed to maintaining low average doses (30–50 mg/day) as a virtual goal of treatment—because of therapeutic philosophy or because state regulators strongly discourage higher doses—are less tolerant of occasional client drug use, missed counseling appointments, and other such treatment lapses, and have markedly lower client retention rates than more tolerant higher dosage programs. This lower tolerance does not, however, act as a stimulant to better client behavior or as a conveyor to move poorly responding clients out and bring in or keep better ones. There is solid, experimentally grounded evidence (see the major review by Hargreaves, 1983, and the associated conclusions of the expert consensus conference; reported in Cooper et al., 1983) that higher dose levels are fundamentally more successful in controlling a client's illicit drug consumption while he or she is in treatment. Although dose levels must necessarily be adjusted according to individual variations in metabolism and size, programs that maintain an overall average dose of 60–100 mg/day yield consistently better results than those averaging less. Doses in excess of 120 mg/day are seldom needed.

The most recent illustration of the importance of dose levels—and the fact that many programs continue to be committed to low-dose regimes in spite of strong evidence against their relative effectiveness—comes from a study reported by Ball and coworkers (Ball et al., 1988; Ball, 1989; see also Dole, 1989). Dramatic differences in client use of opiates and retention in treatment were found among six methadone clinics in three eastern cities studied in 1985–1986 and selected to begin with as well-regarded programs. In the best clinic, urinalysis revealed that 10 percent of enrolled clients in the sample had used drugs intravenously in the month prior to the one-year follow-up. In the two worst clinics, more than 55 percent of clients had used intravenous drugs in the previous month.

Discriminant function analysis found that the most important factor in predicting intravenous drug use was the methadone dose level (Table 5-1). Among clients in treatment from 6 months to 4.5 years the odds of recent heroin consumption decreased at each higher level of methadone. There was also a dose-related decrease in the chances of cocaine use, although the gradient was less steep. (This trend probably has little direct pharmacological cause but instead arises from the generalized behaviors of drug marketing and drug seeking: those who are actively seeking heroin are more likely to seek out or at least happen upon cocaine while doing so, and vice versa.) The programs with the highest illicit drug consumption among clients not only had low methadone doses but also had high rates of staff turnover and poor relationships between staff and clients. Knowledge of and sensitivity to the clinical significance of appropriate dose levels is probably one sizable element in a constellation of clinical competencies and strategies that contribute to the greater or lesser effectiveness of methadone maintenance programs. There are only rudiments of standards for training, credentialing, continuing education, evaluation, and clinical performance of counselors and other treatment program staff. It is remarkable how few research efforts have focused on this larger area of competence, appropriate training, and different service arrangements in the clinical management of methadone clients. A serendipitous experimental study by McLellan and colleagues (1988), which demonstrated striking differences in counselor effectiveness within the framework of a large, stable, well-regarded methadone maintenance program,[9] is a lonely beacon in the literature.

---

[9] Only four counselors participated in the McLellan study, however.

TABLE 5-1   Heroin or Cocaine Consumption of 338 Methadone Clients (in treatment from 6 months to 4.5 years) in Past 30 Days by Methadone Dose

| | | | Percentage Who Used Drug Within Past 30 Days | | | |
Dose (mg/day)	N	%	No Heroin	No Heroin or Cocaine	Any Heroin	Any Cocaine
0–39	105	100	69	57	31	29
40–59	99	100	86	68	14	28
60–79	89	100	94	80	6	18
80–100	45	100	98	89	2	9
Total	338					

Source: Unpublished data from Dr. John C. Ball, Addiction Research Center, National Institute on Drug Abuse. See also Ball and colleagues (1988).

Costs and Benefits of Methadone Treatment

Analyses of the economic costs and benefits of methadone maintenance have been derived from a handful of treatment effectiveness studies, and their results are rather sensitive to how these effectiveness studies are interpreted. An early simulation by Maidlow and Berman (1972), for example, concluded that methadone maintenance could yield lifetime benefits to society of $348,000 compared with average treatment costs of $13,200, a benefit/cost ratio of 26 to 1. However, their assumptions about the effectiveness of methadone were overly optimistic. A simulation by Rufener and colleagues (1977a) was more firmly grounded, yielding a smaller but still quite healthy benefit/cost ratio of 4.4 to 1 for a short period of time. Extended over lifetimes this result would not be too disparate with that of Maidlow and Berman; however, the Rufener team's assumptions about effectiveness also appear to be too optimistic.[10]

Using more realistic effectiveness data—but from only low-dose programs—McGlothlin and Anglin (1981) compared clients who left methadone maintenance when a community clinic was closed in Bakersfield, California, with clients in another community's program, which remained open. For men, the ratio of crime-related economic benefits to treatment costs was 1.7 to 1, over a short, two-year period. Additionally, the continuous

---

[10]Rufener and coworkers (1977a) examined the cost-effectiveness of three major treatment modalities (methadone maintenance, TCs, and outpatient nonmethadone) based on an analysis of the DARP data base (Sells, 1974a,b). Methadone maintenance was decidedly the most cost-effective treatment in terms of lowest cost per opiate-free days, non-opiate-free days, days not spent in criminal activity, and legitimately employed days. Goldschmidt (1976) similarly compared methadone maintenance and therapeutic communities, but his effort identified the benefits of both the in-treatment and posttreatment periods. He concluded that methadone and therapeutic communities produced similar "effectiveness units" (percentage of addicts meeting success criteria). The cost advantage of methadone, however, made its cost-effectiveness about twice that of therapeutic communities.

treatment group reported significantly higher rates of employment than those who had been closed out of treatment, although this factor was not formally valued in the study. The results for women were contrary but can be considered little more than a preliminary indication because the sample size was too small for statistical stability. A study of a public clinic methadone program closure in San Diego (Anglin et al., 1989a) showed virtually no net economic loss but also no net gain. In this instance, a private methadone program picked up a large proportion of the clients on a self-pay basis.

The most comprehensive examination of economic benefits and costs of drug treatment was performed with data from the TOPS (Harwood et al., 1988). The data included the average cost of a treatment day in methadone programs in 1979 and detailed interview measures of rates of criminal activities in the TOPS sample in the year before treatment, the period in treatment, and the year after discharge (where applicable). The study also factored in estimates of the average cost to society of particular crimes, based on surveys conducted in 1979 by the Bureau of Justice Statistics. The benefits of methadone maintenance treatment in terms of reduced crime-related costs to law-abiding citizens (including the value of stolen goods) were $13 per day compared with the $6 per day average cost of the program. Moreover, multivariate regression analysis found significant benefits in the year following discharge, such that retention for an additional day in treatment was worth $11 per day in delayed benefits. The final benefit/cost ratio was therefore 4 to 1. An alternative and much more conservative cost/benefit model in which only increases in employment (which were limited) rather than reductions in goods stolen (which were much larger) were valued found a cost/benefit ratio of about 1 to 1. Using either model, methadone maintenance pays for itself on the day it is delivered, and posttreatment effects are an economic bonus.

Conclusions

Methadone maintenance is a treatment that is designed for severe dependence on heroin. Prior to admission to a methadone program, the great majority of clients are consuming large amounts of heroin and other illicit drugs and committing predatory crimes (including drug selling) on a daily basis, a behavior pattern usually extending back several years or more. Although methadone is a relatively long-acting narcotic analgesic and produces dependence symptoms, the consumption of a clinically adjusted oral dose yields a steady metabolic level of the drug, produces little if any behavioral or subjective intoxication, and does not impair functioning or generate appreciably morbid side effects. Once such a solid, comfortable level is reached, suppressing the psychophysiological cues that precipitate and reinforce opiate craving, the client is amenable to counseling and related services that can help shift his or her orientation and lifestyle away from drug seeking and related crime and toward more socially acceptable behaviors.

Methadone maintenance has been the most rigorously studied of all the drug treatment modalities, and the studies have yielded positive results (although some programs have good and others poor client compliance with rules against illicit drug use and criminal activity). Nevertheless, methadone maintenance is a controversial treatment: its critics contend that methadone clients have "merely" switched their dependence to a legally prescribed narcotic and that many clients continue to use heroin and other drugs intermittently and to commit crimes, including the sale of their take-home methadone. In the committee's judgment, these controversies and reservations are neither trivial nor in themselves compelling. The issues are to what extent undesirable behaviors are reduced and positive behaviors increased as a result of methadone maintenance (in comparison with no treatment or with alternative treatment measures) and whether poorly performing programs can be improved. The extensive evaluation literature on methadone maintenance yields the following conclusions:

• There is strong evidence from clinical trials and similar study designs that heroin-dependent individuals have better outcomes on average (in terms of illicit drug consumption and other criminal behavior) when they are maintained on methadone than when they are not treated at all or are simply detoxified and released, or when methadone is tapered down and terminated as a result of unilateral client request, expulsion from treatment, or program closure.

• Methadone dosages need to be clinically monitored and individually optimized, but in general most clients have substantially better responses when maintained at the higher rather than lower end of the dose ranges currently being prescribed (up to 100 mg/day).

• During and after methadone maintenance treatment, criminal behavior declines and employment increases relative to untreated comparison groups, and the utility of these results substantially exceeds the cost of the treatment, especially when both the crime and employment dimensions are considered over an extended time period.

Methadone maintenance is not the answer for every heroin-dependent individual. At any one time, perhaps one-eighth to one-fifth of all individuals who were recently dependent on heroin can be found in a methadone maintenance program.[11] This figure could undoubtedly be increased if program quality were optimized, hostile stereotypes of methadone treatment

---

[11] This estimate derives from experiments such as that of Bale and colleagues (1980), which is described in the following section, and from national surveys of the treatment system, described in Chapter 6, combined with estimates of the prevalence of heroin dependence.

eliminated, and availability extended. When viewed in terms of lifetime prevalence, the number of current heroin-dependent individuals who will at some time enter the portals of methadone is higher, probably 30 to 40 percent. This range, like the preceding figure, is necessarily only an approximation because the research data that could give more precision to these estimates are inadequate, particularly in light of such recent developments as the AIDS epidemic. Nevertheless, in the committee's judgment, an improved network of methadone maintenance clinics might realistically be capable of reaching and dramatically accelerating the recovery of one-third of all those who become dependent on heroin.

THERAPEUTIC COMMUNITIES

What Is a Therapeutic Community?

The residential therapeutic community, or TC, is a way of defining the nature of individual drug problems as much as a therapeutic approach to the rehabilitation or, more frequently, the habilitation of drug-dependent persons. It is from this understanding that the TC derives its encompassing and intensive approach.

TCs were originally developed to treat the same problem as methadone maintenance programs: the "hard-core" heroin-dependent criminal. The residential TC has a broader perspective, however; it treats individuals who are severely dependent on any illicitly obtained drug or combination of drugs and whose social adjustment to conventional family and occupational responsibilities is severely compromised as a result of drug seeking—but who were compromised before drug seeking entered the picture. In this context, the specific drug (or more accurately, combination of drugs) represents a sociological fact more than a pharmacological foundation for treatment. In the 1980s, cocaine dependence has overtaken heroin dependence in the TC population. The profile of TC clients is also more demographically diverse than that of the heroin-dependent population. Generally, on average, TC clients in the early 1970s, when there was a national counting system, were several years younger and predominantly white by a modest margin, a pattern that has continued in later, more partial statistics (e.g., the 1979–1981 Treatment Outcome Prospective Study sample; Hubbard et al., 1989).[12]

The TC's group-centered methods encompass the following, all of which are grounded in an interdependent social environment with a direct link to a specific historical foundation:

---

[12]TC clients were 57 percent white, 34 percent black, and 9 percent Hispanic. Methadone clients were 16 percent white, 58 percent black, and 26 percent Hispanic (Sells, 1974a).

- firm behavioral norms across a wide range of proscriptions and specifications;
- reality-oriented group and individual psychotherapy, which extends to lengthy encounter sessions focusing on current living issues or more deep-seated emotional problems;
- a system of clearly specified rewards and punishments within a communal economy of housework and other roles;
- a series of hierarchical responsibilities, privileges, and esteem achieved by working up a "ladder" of tasks from admission to graduation; and
- some degree of potential mobility from client to staff statuses.

Because the therapeutic regimen of TCs has not been uniformly codified—and even if it had, would necessarily still involve substantial clinical discretion and creativity—there are great differences across programs in their recommended lengths of stay, staff-to-client ratios, and types of staff. These differences, which may be determined more by financial realities than by therapeutic philosophies, may have a great deal of influence over the differential clinical effectiveness of TCs.

De Leon (1986:5,7–8) has summarized the approach as follows:

The TC views drug abuse as a deviant behavior, reflecting impeded personality development and/or chronic deficits in social, educational and economic skills. Its antecedents lie in socio-economic disadvantage, poor family effectiveness and in psychological factors . . . affecting some or all areas of functioning. . . . Thinking may be unrealistic or disorganized; values are confused, nonexistent or antisocial.

Physiological dependency is secondary to the wide range of influences which control the individual's drug use behavior. Invariably, problems and situations associated with discomfort become regular signals for resorting to drug use.

Thus, the problem is the person, not the drug. . . . In the TC's view of recovery, the aim of rehabilitation is global. . . . The primary psychological goal is to change the negative patterns of behavior, thinking, and feeling that predispose drug use; the main social goal is to develop a responsible drug free lifestyle. Stable recovery, however, depends upon a successful integration of these social and psychological goals.

Sugarman (1986:66,69) elaborates further:

All models of the TC involve a set of explicit behavior norms which members support and a set of contingent sanctions, positive and negative. . . . [H]ierarchical programs have extensive and demanding limits, strictly enforced, on the grounds that addicts need to learn self-control, and to experience the security of a firm framework of order. . . . Behavioral limits and sanctions plus positive peer pressure engender a short-term process of behavior modification. Even though this changed behavior is dependent upon the external controls of the social setting, still it has a real significance. . . . The message is: you can change in ways that you would not have thought possible.

The self-sufficient group is a particularly important setting for learning the nature of social responsibility and the interdependence of individual interests. Ideally, the ordinary family and the ordinary peer groups that a child experiences in growing up convey this kind of learning; in practice, the lesson is often missed.

To a significant extent the TC simulates and enforces a model family environment that the client, so to speak, should have had during critically formative preadolescent and adolescent years. The TC tries to make up for lost years of formation in an intensive, relatively short period of time—approximately 6 to 12 months of residential envelopment and an additional 6 to 12 months of gradual reentry to the outside community prior to "graduation." There is encouragement as well of continued alumni involvement for the benefit of role modeling for new residents, recognition and reinforcement for the graduate, and psychological and financial support for the program.

How Well Do Therapeutic Communities Work?

Conclusions about the effectiveness of TCs are limited by the difficulties of applying standard clinical trial methodologies to a complex, dynamic treatment milieu and a population resistant to following instructions. Randomized trials or natural experiments in the community, which would permit a well-controlled comparison of clients admitted to TC treatment versus an equivalent group (e.g., persons seeking treatment but denied admission, individuals admitted to other treatment modalities or arbitrarily excluded from TC treatment as a result of program closure) are not feasible or appropriate; when attempted, such experimental protocols have failed (see Bale et al., 1980). Currently, the strongest conclusions on the effectiveness of TCs are based on nonrandomized or nonexperimental but rigorously conducted studies of clients seeking admission to therapeutic communities. It is therefore worthwhile to look more closely at the nature, strengths, and weaknesses of such evidence.

The Character of Nonexperimental Evaluations

In nonrandomized or nonexperimental studies of treatment effects, conclusions generally depend on two kinds of comparisons. One is the contrast of observed TC outcomes with the record of similarly troubled individuals from the pretreatment era (e.g., those seen at Lexington or other prisons or hospitals). The problem with such comparisons is that one cannot be certain that the people of one historical period are totally similar to those of another. Likewise, there may or may not be similarities between a group seeking TC (or any other specific) treatment and a group seeking detoxification, or between a self-selected group from the community and a group culled from the drug-dependent population by the criminal justice system. Those seeking admission to TCs might (although they just as easily might not) represent a different kind of drug population or a very specialized slice of the population, or at least a different enough slice to honestly confound any comparisons of this sort. Because the same data are not collected on the different groups being compared, one cannot really reduce this uncertainty very much.

The second comparisons are internal ones, between those who enter TC treatment and those who apply for it but break off the process before entry, and between clients staying for longer versus shorter periods of treatment (receiving, in effect, larger and smaller "doses" of TC). In this case, the groups at least are being compared within the same time and data collection frame. Still, there may be selection effects that threaten the validity of the comparison, that is, its capacity to determine treatment effects. Those who stayed may have been different to begin with from those who left earlier. For example, they may have been intrinsically more or less likely to do well, treatment or no treatment (because of lesser or greater initial criminality, shorter or longer drug histories, better or worse family support). These differences may bias the comparison one way or another—either in favor of or against treatment effectiveness.

To guard against such biases, researchers rely on baseline measurements and statistical adjustments to control for preadmission client characteristics that might account for differential retention or outcome.[13] These procedures increase one's assurance that the results are not confounded by selection effects; however, because some pretreatment characteristics that might conceivably affect retention and outcome may not have been measured well or even measured at all, they do not offer as much assurance as a successfully implemented, randomized clinical trial with minimal attrition.

The lack of randomized trials involving TCs is in some ways not surprising; most medical and criminal procedures became widely used without the benefit of such trials. The early success stories from the therapeutic communities Synanon and Daytop Village, in contrast to most treatment modalities' gloomy prior experience with heroin addiction, were positive and convincing enough that many clinicians and policymakers backed the establishment of TCs in the late 1960s and early 1970s. The scientific community paid them relatively little attention (a notable exception was Yablonsky, 1965), and many researchers viewed randomized trials as impossible to perform because heroin cases are so prone to noncompliance.[14]

---

[13]The causal model here attributes the client's status at a later point in time to three kinds of factors: predisposing conditions, which are controlled for by the baseline measurement procedures (e.g., why the client sought treatment, how much recovery the client wants to achieve); exterior factors during treatment, which are assumed to affect clients more or less at random; that is, they are not correlated with being admitted to treatment (changes in the price of drugs, for example, or police attitudes toward an individual, or the likelihood of being caught in a job layoff); and the units of treatment received, the element whose effects the researcher really wants to measure. There are three corresponding sources of error: unmeasured predisposing conditions, exterior factors that are correlated with being in treatment, and variations in the consistency of treatment units.

[14]The problem of heroin-dependent individuals' noncompliance with experimental and control

The Bale Study

The one notable attempt to undertake an experimental evaluation of the effectiveness of TCs compared with groups who were not treated or who were treated in other ways was conducted in California by Bale and coworkers (1980). This study, which examined methadone maintenance as well as TCs, did not work well as a random-assignment trial; in addition, the subject population was skewed from national norms. Nevertheless, its results are unique, important, and deserving of detailed attention for they underwrite much of the confidence that can be attached to results from studies that had no untreated control groups.

The subjects were 585 heroin-addicted male veterans who sought and gained entry to the Veterans Administration (VA) Medical Center in Palo Alto, California, for a 5-day opiate detoxification program during an 18-month intake period in the mid-1970s—who also met the study's requirements.[15] When asked, about one-fifth of the subjects denied any interest in transferring to a VA drug treatment program after detoxification (some later changed their minds). The balance (plus the changers) were randomly assigned to either of two methadone maintenance clinics or one of three residential programs, each a different kind of 6-month TC.

The clinical staff invested significant time in trying to enlist every subject in his assigned program, and the overall rate of transfers from detox to VA programs doubled as a result. Nevertheless, the random-assignment design was thoroughly compromised (Tables 5-2a and 5-2b). Less than half of the randomly assigned subjects entered and spent as long as a week in any of the VA treatment programs, and only half of those entered the specific programs they had been assigned to (the others waited out at least a 30-day exclusion period to enter their own preferred program). Altogether, 42 percent of the total study cohort did not enter

protocols is not specific to experiments involving TCs. Noncompliance has compromised attempts to compare alternative pharmacologically based modalities, as vividly demonstrated in several large-scale studies, including the attempted comparison of the effectiveness of methadone maintenance versus maintenance with the narcotic antagonist naltrexone (National Research Council, 1978) or methadone versus the longer acting methadone congener LAAM (Savage et al., 1976; Ling et al., 1978).

[15] There were 710 total drug detox admissions; exclusions from the study sample were for pending felony charges (51), major psychiatric problems (41), falsified eligibility for VA treatment (13), and miscellaneous reasons (19). The study population differed from the opiate-dependent DARP sample in several important particulars: they were all honorably discharged veterans (100 percent versus 25 percent in the DARP), all male (100 percent versus 77 percent), and mostly high school graduates (71 percent versus 39 percent) and ex-convicts (80 percent versus 60 percent) who used other drugs in addition to heroin (72 percent versus 52 percent). They were also less often black (41 percent versus 54 percent) or Hispanic (13 percent versus 22 percent) and more often employed (76 percent versus 57 percent) in white-collar jobs (36 percent versus 11 percent).

TABLE 5-2A   Subject Compliance (percentage) with Assignment to a
Therapeutic Program

Program Entered	Program Assigned				Detox (self-selected)	Total
	TC I[a]	TC II	TC III	Methadone		
	(79)[b]	(147)	(137)	(94)	(128)	(585)
None	44	40	36	28	59	42
Non-VA	9	16	20	20	28	19
TC I	18[c]	1	2	5	0	4
TC II	13	24[c]	9	9	6	13
TC III	13	10	22[c]	8	2	11
Methadone	4	10	12	31[c]	4	12
Total[d]	100	100	100	100	100	100

[a]TC = therapeutic community.
[b]Numbers in parentheses are subjects assigned to the program.
[c]Percentage entering program to which assigned.
[d]Totals may not add to 100% due to rounding.

Source: Bale et al. (1980).

TABLE 5-2B   Subject Compliance (number and percentage) with
Assignment, Combining Therapeutic Communities (TCs)

Program Entered	Program Assigned							
	TCs		Methadone (eligibility requirement)		Detox (self-selected)		Total	
	No.	%	No.	%	No.	%	No.	%
None	143	39	26	28	76	59	245	42
Non-VA	58	16	19	20	36	28	113	19
TCs	129[a]	36[a]	20	22	11	8	160	28
Methadone	33	9	29[a]	31[a]	5	4	67	12
Total[b]	363	100	94	100	128	100	585	100

[a]Number or percentage entering program to which assigned.
[b]Totals may not add to 100% due to rounding.

Source: Bale et al. (1980).

any kind of treatment during the follow-up year, about 28 percent entered
one of the VA TCs, 12 percent entered a VA methadone clinic, and 19
percent entered a non-VA program.

The lack of compliance affected the study so profoundly that research
analysts (who were independent of the clinical staff) were obliged to switch
from the simplicity of randomizing assumptions to the use of multivariate
statistical procedures to control for initial differences in age, ethnicity, prior

treatment, drug use patterns, and criminal history among treatment and nontreatment groups.

At the one-year follow-up, those who had been successfully recontacted (the follow-up contact rate was 93 percent) were divided among the no-treatment (41 percent), non-VA (21 percent), short-term TC (14 percent), long-term TC (14 percent), and methadone (11 percent) options.[16] Controlling for pretreatment characteristics, the no-treatment, non-VA treatment, and short-term TC groups were statistically indistinguishable from each other at the follow-up. Compared with these groups, however, the long-term TC and methadone client groups (comprising one-fourth of the total sample originally contacted during the detox program) were clearly different. The long-term TC and methadone clients were:

- two-thirds as likely to have used heroin in the past month (41 percent versus 64 percent);
- three-fifths as likely to have been convicted during the year (22 percent versus 37 percent);
- one-third as likely to be incarcerated at year's end (7 percent versus 19 percent); and
- one-and-a-half times as likely to be at work or in school at year's end (59 percent versus 40 percent).

The long-term TC group ranked somewhat better than the total methadone group on each measure, but the differences were not large enough to be statistically distinguishable in a sample of this size.

Other Significant Follow-up Studies

Beyond the efforts of Bale and colleagues, there is a significant controlled observational literature on therapeutic communities. The bulk of these studies have focused on clients admitted to particular programs such as Phoenix House and Daytop Village in New York; in addition, the DARP (Simpson et al., 1979) and the TOPS (Hubbard et al., 1989) separately examined clients who were admitted to about 10 TCs across the country (not the same programs and 10 years apart).

---

[16]Retention in treatment was not high for the 6-month residential programs. About 13 percent of the clients stayed less than 1 week (these were considered "no treatment"), 57 percent dropped out within 7 weeks, and 85 percent left treatment before 6 months. In contrast, about 65 percent of clients entering methadone maintenance were continuously in treatment for the follow-up year.

The TC group was therefore divided at the median length of stay (for all admissions who had remained longer than a week), which was 50 days. The short-term group stayed in treatment about 3 weeks on average; the long-term group stayed about 20 weeks on average. The methadone group on average stayed in treatment about 40 weeks.

The most extensive outcome evaluations from a single program come from Phoenix House in New York. De Leon and coworkers (1982) studied a sample of 230 graduates and dropouts and found that before admission the two groups were very similar with respect to criminal activity and drug use but that dropouts had somewhat greater employment. After treatment, the status of both groups was much better than before, but graduates had dramatically superior posttreatment outcomes compared with dropouts (Table 5-3).[17]

The Drug Abuse Reporting Program provided further important controlled observational findings about the effectiveness of therapeutic communities (Sells, 1974a,b). The mean and median lengths of stay in the traditional TCs involved in the DARP were close to 7 months, which was well below the average 16-month treatment plan. At 12 months after admission, 71 percent of those admitted had left the TC voluntarily or by expulsion, although only 5 percent had completed their treatment plan by then; the ultimate graduation rate was 23 percent (Simpson et al., 1979).

Most of the DARP's outcome measures at one year after discharge (daily opiates, daily nonopiates, arrests, incarceration) were significantly better for TC clients compared with the outcomes of detoxification-only and intake-only cases (Simpson et al., 1979). As in the Bale study, the multivariate-adjusted outcomes for TCs and methadone maintenance clients (matched for time since admission) on daily opiate use, nonopiate use, employment, and a composite index were quite similar. The length of stay in treatment was a positive, robust, significant predictor of posttreatment outcomes (drugs, jobs, and crime). Among clients staying more than 90

---

[17] One smaller study that is notable for its careful execution followed a random sample of graduates and dropouts from a Connecticut TC (Romond et al., 1975) with an 18- to 24-month treatment plan. The authors found few pretreatment differences between the graduate and dropout groups except that women were much less likely than men to graduate. All 20 graduates in the sample were successfully contacted; 10 of 31 dropouts in the sample were not located, and 1 refused an interview, yielding 20 successful contacts. Graduates had spent on average 21 months in treatment, compared with 5.7 months for dropouts (range: 10 days to 16 months). Interview data were corroborated through formal and informal community networks.

Graduates had consistently better outcomes. Only 1 of 20 graduates relapsed to dependence for some part of the follow-up period, another 5 sometimes used nonopiate drugs, and 14 remained drug free throughout the interval; altogether, graduates spent 0.5 percent of the follow-up period dependent. Of the 20 dropouts interviewed, 14 relapsed to dependence for some of the follow-up period, 2 more used nonopiates occasionally, 1 was incarcerated for the entire period, and 3 had used no drugs; 35 percent of the dropouts' posttreatment time was spent as drug dependent. Ninety-four percent of the graduates' posttreatment time had been in school or employed, and at the time of the interview, none were institutionalized and 2 had some criminal justice involvement (probation, parole, pending case). Forty percent of the dropouts' posttreatment time had been in school or employed; at the time of the interview, 4 were in other drug programs, 1 was in a psychiatric hospital, 4 were in jail, and 7 others had a pending court case or were on probation or parole.

days in treatment, there was a positive and linear relationship between outcome and retention. The outcomes among clients staying less than 90 days were indistinguishable from detox-only and intake-only cases, and there was no discernible relation between outcome and short lengths of stay.

The final results of the TOPS, which were derived using multivariate logistical regression to control for pretreatment demographics, drug use, and criminality, yielded the familiar positive relationship between length of stay and outcome but with no clear threshold (Hubbard et al., 1989; see Figure 5-3). One year or more in a TC was significantly related to reduced heroin use, lower crime involvement, and increased employment at a 12-month follow-up. The odds of having problems with heroin or crime were about two-fifths as great for the long-term residential clients as for early dropouts, and their odds of having a job were nearly 1.7 times higher. Cocaine use followed a similar pattern, but the effect was not statistically significant. Alcohol problems were not related to treatment retention.

In summary, multisite evaluations of the DARP (Simpson et al., 1979; Simpson, 1981) and the TOPS (Hubbard et al., 1989) both produced strong results supporting those of Bale and coworkers and the one or two useful

TABLE 5-3   Follow-up Results of Treatment at Phoenix House (New York City) Measured on Crime, Drug Use, and Employment Indices (percentage)

Index	N	Pretreatment	Post-treatment	p
Crime				
Total	226	96.5	29.2	<.001
Dropouts	154	97.4	40.9	<.01
Graduates	72	94.4	4.2	<.001
Dropout/graduate				
differences (p)		Not signif.	<.001	
Drug use				
Total	229	94.3	32.3	<.001
Dropouts	156	96.8	43.6	<.05
Graduates	73	89.0	9.2	<.001
Dropout/graduate				
differences (p)		Not signif.	<.001	
Employment[a]				
Total	230	32.6	75.7	<.001
Dropouts	156	36.5	66.0	<.001
Graduates	74	24.3	95.9	<.001
Dropout/graduate				
differences (p)		<.10	<.001	

[a]Employed more than 50 percent of the time.

Source: De Leon et al. (1982:Table 5).

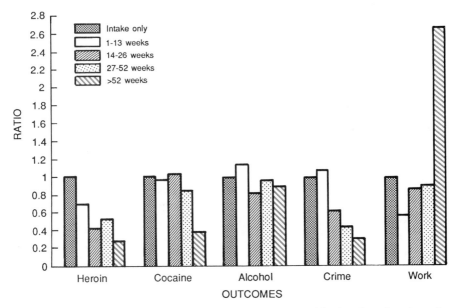

FIGURE 5-3 Outcomes and retention in therapeutic communities based on data from the Treatment Outcome Prospective Study and shown as odds ratios derived from multivariate analyses. The odds that members of the intake-only group will report a successful outcome at follow-up are compared with the odds for those who were in treatment for 1–13 weeks, 14–26 weeks, 27–52 weeks, and 53 or mor weeks. The intake-only odds are standardized or set equal to 1 for each criterion; the other group odds are expressed as ratios of 1. Source: Hubbard et al. (1989).

single-program studies. Even in the absence of clinical trials, it is difficult to credit any explanation of these results other than the following: TCs can strongly affect the behavior of many of the drug-dependent individuals who enter them, and retention in treatment after some minimum number of months—how many seems to vary with the program—is positively and significantly related to improved outcomes as measured by illicit drug consumption, other criminal activity, and economically productive behavior.

Why Do the Results of Therapeutic Communities Vary?

No one really knows why there is such variation in TC performance and client responses (although strong views are often expressed about the matter) because there has been virtually no systematic research about the determinants of client success and failure in TCs. It is highly plausible that the results of TC treatment depend on its primary elements: the client's motivations, the quality and quantity of staffing, and the psychosocial organization and therapeutic design of the program. The committee heard anecdotally that TC staffing has been problematic during the 1980s as a result of constant budget pressures (staff numbers or salaries can be cut or held down more readily than room-and-board expenses) and rising competition with private-tier outpatient and chemical dependency treatment providers for credentialed, experienced staff. Yet there are no studies that specifically investigate how TC staffing relates to the effectiveness of treatment.

There are clearly wide variations in outcome indicators across programs. Client-Oriented Data Acquisition Process (CODAP) reports published from 1976 through 1981 make it possible to examine variations across cities in client status at discharge. The crude city differences are not adjusted to account for differences in the characteristics of clients treated in the various cities, nor can they be broken down to the program level. Nevertheless, the 1976–1981 CODAP reports demonstrate graphically that effectiveness varied significantly from area to area and undoubtedly even more so from program to program.

The year 1980 was one of relative program stability: the treatment system had been in place from five to six years and had not yet been disrupted by the massive system changes that resulted from the institution of block grants with their devolution of management responsibility to the states. Yet very large variations were seen in the treatment "completion" rates reported for that year by residential programs (Figure 5-4), most of which were TCs. From the figure it is apparent that TCs in some cities diverged widely from the national average. Although the average residential completion rate across the nation was 10 percent, a sizable number of communities had averages well below and above this rate: 23 cities had rates between 5 and 15 percent, 9 cities were below 5 percent, 13 were between 15 and 24 percent, and 9 were above 25 percent. These variations have not been analyzed for possible attribution to differences in client characteristics, treatment process, quality of staff, or random processes. There is also currently no usable evidence of national scope showing whether client discharge statuses still exhibit such differences across geographic areas, or why.

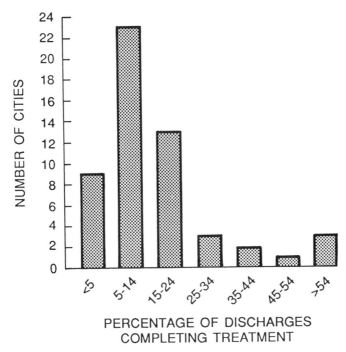

FIGURE 5-4 Variations in "completion" rates of opiate clients in residential programs in U.S. cities, 1980. Source: National Institute on Drug Abuse (1981).

Costs and Benefits of Therapeutic Community Treatment

Most evaluations of TCs indicate that they are cost-effective or cost-beneficial, or both. There have been fewer rigorous evaluations of costs and benefits than of cost-effectiveness, however. A simulation by Maidlow and Berman (1972) showed that a TC produces $213,000 of economic benefits to society per client at a cost of $14,700 (a benefit/cost ratio of 14.5 to 1). These authors concluded that TCs were highly cost-beneficial compared with prisons (which were much more expensive and had high recidivism rates). Rufener and coworkers (1977a) focused only on benefits after treatment (ignoring benefits during treatment) and tried to sort out the benefits that accrue variously to the client, the government account, and society as a whole. They estimated that the combined benefit/cost ratio of TCs after the treatment period was 1.9 to 1. As discussed earlier, however, both of these sets of benefit/cost ratios are biased upward because the assumptions used to produce them were overly optimistic compared with what is now known about treatment retention and effectiveness.

A more realistic cost-effectiveness study using the DARP data base

(Rufener et al., 1977a) found that TCs generally produced greater differentials than methadone or outpatient nonmethadone treatment in terms of legitimate income and employment status after treatment versus before. But methadone was decidedly more cost-effective—measured as the cost per added day of desirable outcome—because it was cheaper. Of course, these comparisons work only to the degree that those entering one treatment would as readily have entered the other.

A cost/benefit study of the Gaudenzia House TC (Griffin, 1983) compared the expense of operations over a five-year period with the benefits from reduced criminal activity and increased social productivity. The analysis distinguished the benefits to be derived from treatment "successes" and "failures," finding positive ratios of benefits to costs for both groups (9 to 1 for "successes" and 3.4 to 1 for "failures"). Benefits accrued even for "failures" because while in residence for treatment they were unable to commit as many street crimes (analogous to the incapacitation effect of incarceration) as they would have if not in residence.

Most recently, Harwood and colleagues (1988) analyzed the TOPS data base, examining the reduced crime-related impacts on society that result from drug treatment. A particularly important finding was that TC treatment, as with methadone treatment (see the section above entitled "Costs and Benefits of Methadone Treatment"), virtually pays for itself during the time it is delivered, owing to the reduced criminal activity of clients in treatment relative to either the pre- or posttreatment periods. Further benefits accrue after leaving treatment. The final benefit/cost ratio for TCs was 3.8 to 1 using the primary measure (the costs of crime) and 2.1 to 1 using a more conservative employment-oriented measure.

Conclusions

TCs are for the most part designed to treat individuals who are badly impaired by drug problems and other deficits, and client decisions about whether to seek TC treatment reflect an awareness of that design. Even those who do seek treatment often drop out of TCs in short order, in contrast to the much higher retention rates of those who enter methadone maintenance. There is, nevertheless, a sizable population who not only find TC treatment initially attractive but also will remain in this modality for a substantial fraction (up to the whole course) of planned treatment. This segment is distinct from the typical methadone maintenance population: it is appreciably younger, more heavily white, and more likely to use multiple drugs.

The committee considers the evidence about the following to be fairly persuasive (although not ironclad): those clients who stay in TCs for at least a third or half of the planned course of treatment, a threshold that seems to vary greatly from program to program—that is, those who stay in treatment for at least 2 to 12 months, varying from program to program for reasons that are not yet clear—are much closer to achieving the treatment's goals at follow-up than those who drop out earlier. The outcomes of the earlier dropouts basically cannot be distinguished from those of individuals who did not enter any treatment modality.

These improvements over nontreatment, which are estimated to be in the neighborhood of one- to two-thirds reductions in the rates of primary drug consumption and other criminal activity and half-again increases in the rates of employment or schooling, vary with the amount of time spent in treatment. TC graduates have outcomes that are even better than these rates, but they are a small percentage (usually 15 to 25 percent) of total TC admissions. What is most important here is that graduates are not the only ones who benefit themselves and society as a result of spending time in a TC. Even for those individuals who "split" early, even for those who show no later effects, the TC may be a good social investment considering that a day in a TC is a day away from street crime.

OUTPATIENT NONMETHADONE TREATMENT

What Is Outpatient Nonmethadone Treatment?

Outpatient nonmethadone (OPNM) programs range in duration from the one-time assessments and referrals of drop-in and "rap" centers to virtual outpatient therapeutic communities with daily psychotherapy and counseling intended to continue for a year or longer (Kleber and Slobetz, 1979). In between are the vast majority of programs, which see clients once or possibly twice weekly and deliver services based on theoretical approaches from psychiatry, counseling psychology, social work, therapeutic communities, or the 12-step Anonymous creed. Some programs contract extensively with Treatment Alternatives to Street Crime agencies or probation departments (see Chapter 4), monitoring the shared clients' compliance with probation conditions—particularly through administration of drug tests—and offering no other therapeutic services.

Some OPNM programs utilize psychoactive medications prescribed by psychiatrists or other physicians on staff. These agents may be medications used initially in detoxification to ameliorate withdrawal symptoms, maintenance antagonists that prevent intoxication (e.g., naltrexone), medications to control drug cravings after withdrawal (especially innovative cocaine pharmacotherapies), or drugs that address psychiatric disorders (depression, mood disorders, schizophrenia, etc.). Programs with the requisite resources may deliver or link their clients to formal education, vocational training, health care (such as AIDS testing or treatment), housing assistance (especially for homeless clients), support for battered spouses and children, and other social services.

The diversity of OPNM treatment defies easy summary and is matched by the heterogeneity of its client populations. These populations generally are not abusing opiates, usually are not involved in the criminal justice system (at least, were not so during the DARP and TOPS periods), and include significant proportions of abusing rather than dependent individuals—differing in all these respects from typical methadone and TC clients.

How Well Does Outpatient Nonmethadone Treatment Work?

The major conclusion that can be offered about the effectiveness of outpatient treatment is a familiar one: clients who remain in treatment longer have better outcomes at follow-up than shorter term clients. These conclusions are based entirely on multivariate results of the two major multisite evaluations, the DARP and the TOPS. In the Drug Abuse Reporting Program study of clients entering treatment from 1969 to 1972 (Sells, 1974a,b; Simpson et al., 1979; Simpson, 1981), OPNM clients exhibited statistically significant follow-up improvements relative to pretreatment in terms of employment and consumption of opiates and nonopiates, but not in terms of arrest rates, which were much lower before treatment than they were in TC or methadone maintenance clients. The DARP comparison groups, those in detox programs and those who only made contact with treatment during intake, reported no significant pre- to posttreatment changes except in opiate consumption (Simpson et al., 1979).

Analyses of retention (Simpson, 1981) produced results identical to those for TC clients: clients staying in treatment less than 90 days showed no improvement relative to the detox and intake-only clients, whereas those staying longer had improved outcomes on a composite score that incorporated drug, criminality, and productivity scales. For the 90-days-plus group, outcome scores were strongly and significantly correlated with total length of stay.

The larger and more recent Treatment Outcome Prospective Study (Hubbard et al., 1989) collected data on 1,600 OPNM clients admitted to 10 programs. Clients again reported better performance during and after treatment than before admission, and multivariate analyses strongly related posttreatment outcomes to length of stay, using multivariate logistical regression to adjust for client drug use histories and sociodemographic characteristics at admission (Figure 5-5). The analysis suggested that the critical retention threshold may be six months, but only 17 percent of TOPS outpatient clients were retained this long. OPNM dropout rates were quite

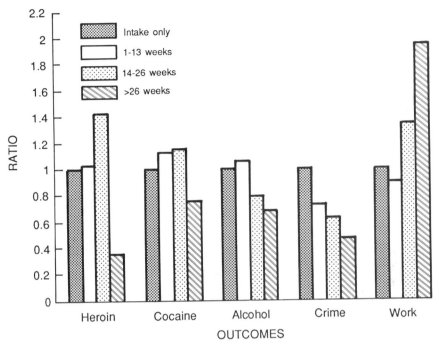

FIGURE 5-5 Outcomes and retention in outpatient nonmethadone programs based on data from the Treatment Outcome Prospective Study and shown as odds ratios derived from multivariate analyses. The odds that members of the intake-only group will report a successful outcome at follow-up are compared with the odds for those who were in treatment for 1–13 weeks, 14–26 weeks, and more than 26 weeks. The intake-only odds are standardized or set equal to 1 for each criterion; the other group odds are expressed as ratios of 1. Source: Hubbard et al. (1989).

high—significantly higher than for methadone or TCs. At four weeks the programs retained only 59 percent of clients; 18 percent eventually completed the course of treatment.

Why Do the Results of Outpatient Nonmethadone Treatment Vary?

There is no answer to this question for OPNM programs. Although there is evidence of variation in program retention rates, there is very little information about what the "active ingredients" in this treatment modality are that might lead to these variations. One can only speculate that the same factors that emerge from methadone and TC research, in particular, staff quality and program design, may be equally important here.

Benefits and Costs of Outpatient Nonmethadone Treatment

Both of the major multisite studies, the DARP and the TOPS, have been analyzed with respect to the costs and benefits of OPNM treatment. Rufener and colleagues (1977a) compared the cost-effectiveness of the major treatment modalities for the DARP subsample of opiate clients. For this population, OPNM generally had poorer cost-effectiveness than methadone and TCs, but no attempt was made to address whether OPNM was more cost-effective than no treatment or whether longer treatment was more cost-effective than brief episodes.

Harwood and coworkers (1988), using the methods described above for methadone and TCs, estimated a benefit/cost ratio of 1.3 to 1 for OPNM in the TOPS data base. Compared with a similar detox sample, increased treatment retention in OPNM programs had a modest but measurable impact on the amount of theft while in treatment, even though the OPNM treatment population was less criminally active than the populations in methadone treatment and TCs. An alternative measure, improvement in the amount of legitimate employment, produced a benefit/cost ratio of 4.3 to 1, indicating that the benefits of OPNM are more pronounced in terms of the secondary goal of employment rather than as reductions in already low levels of criminal activity. Unlike the results of TC treatment, crime-related benefits of OPNM after discharge were not discernible.

CHEMICAL DEPENDENCY TREATMENT

What Is Chemical Dependency Treatment?

Chemical dependency (CD) treatment (also called the Minnesota model, 28-day, 12-step, or Hazelden-type treatment) is the predominant therapeutic approach taken by the privately financed inpatient and residential programs identified in Chapter 6 as the "private tier" of providers. Virtually all of these programs were originally oriented toward alcohol problems but have increasingly served clients with illicit drug problems. The CD theory of the disorder and the modality's treatment approach have expanded from a focus on alcoholism that depended on the Alcoholics Anonymous principles (the 12 steps) to one more broadly addressing dependence on any chemical substance. Cook (1988a,b) has provided a concise historical review of the development of the Minnesota model. He notes the similarities between the underlying theories that shape CD and TC treatment but observes that they developed almost completely independently of each other.

Almost exclusively, the goal of CD treatment is abstinence from alcohol and drugs. The client is viewed as a victim of a disease process but also as the person with the primary responsibility for making behavioral changes that will promote abstinence, which will in turn eliminate problems resulting from alcohol or drugs.

In its most sophisticated formulation, the CD approach views drug problems as having multiple causes. There is a physiological phenomenon at work, but psychological and sociocultural dimensions are of equal importance. The physiological component often requires some pharmacological intervention as an integral aspect of treatment. The treatment's psychological dimension highlights the impact of emotional, motivational, and learning problems on dependence. Sociocultural models explore the relation of drinking and drug problems to socialization processes and environments. CD treatment practices represent a blending of the Alcoholics Anonymous model of recovery, certain insights and prescriptions of somatic medicine, and psychiatric and behavioral science principles.

Chemical dependency treatment is usually an intensive, highly structured three- to six-week inpatient regimen. Clients begin with an in-depth psychiatric and psychosocial evaluation and then follow a general education-oriented program track of daily lectures plus two to three meetings per week in small task-oriented groups. Group education teaches clients about the disease concept of dependence, focusing on the harmful medical and psychosocial effects of illicit drugs and excessive alcohol consumption. There is also an individual prescriptive track for each client, meetings about twice a week with a "focal counselor," and appointments with other professionals if medical, psychiatric, or family services are needed. Recently, there has been increasing emphasis on family (or "codependent") therapy and the concept that others may be acting as "enablers" of drug and alcohol consumption.

Clients actively engage in developing and implementing a recovery plan, which is patterned on the "step work" (working through the 12 steps that lead to recovery) of Alcoholics Anonymous. Self-help is a large part of therapy; clients work with each other and are generally required to attend Alcoholics/Cocaine/Narcotics Anonymous (AA/CA/NA) meetings.

Aftercare is considered quite important in CD treatment, but there are relatively few program resources devoted to it. It can last from three months to as long as two years and range in intensity from a simple monthly telephone follow-up to intensive weekly group therapy and individual counseling as needed. Clients are urged to continue an intensive schedule of AA/CA/NA attendance through the follow-up period, with continued contacts thereafter at a lower rate.

CD treatment has some elements in common with the TC approach: abstinence as a goal, striving for behavioral changes to achieve abstinence, the client taking primary responsibility for his or her problems, and recovery in the context of mutual support, including that of counselors. But there are noteworthy differences between the two modalities. The inpatient or residential phase of the CD treatment plan is short relative to TC treatment, and the extended follow-up or aftercare phase is seldom if ever a strong and integrated program element. Because the hospital-based services of CD treatment do not require clients to perform housekeeping duties, there is more time for psychotherapy and educational work; in the TC process, however, housekeeping and other program maintenance responsibilities are considered an integral component of therapeutic learning. CD program staff, like TC staff, are a mixture of stable, recovering (from alcohol or drug dependence) individuals and professional clinicians from traditional health care, mental health, and social service disciplines. However, CD staff tend to be more heavily credentialed.

CD treatment is full of educational work, including writing, reading, and lectures; there is little of the daily job routines or ladder of work responsibilities that are intrinsic to TC treatment and by which client progress is symbolized. (In CD programs, progress is made by ascending spiritual steps.) Most TCs depend heavily on advanced clients to direct the progress of new clients. Prior to admission, CD clients are usually enacting some stable social roles, whereas TC clients almost always have massive functional and social deficits. CD programs, with their residential treatment duration, are more attractive to clients with greater initial functional and social resources: indeed, the prototypical CD client used to be fortyish, middle class, employed, white, and dependent on alcohol. Today, although the clientele is more diversified (programs are now seeing more clients with combined cocaine/alcohol problems, as well as a segment of adolescents with both psychiatric and drug diagnoses), these origins continue to shape the CD approach.

How Well Does Chemical Dependency Treatment Work?

Although CD programs have come to play a major role in the drug treatment world, the research data on this type of treatment for illicit drug problems are weaker than for the other modalities. There are no relevant experimental or quasi-experimental studies; there were no CD programs in the DARP or TOPS samples. Only one of the available observational studies of CD programs employs an untreated comparison group (Rawson et al., 1986),[18] and none have collected data on admissions with short lengths of stay. There is also practically no use of multivariate statistics.

---

[18]This study reported on 83 individuals who responded to advertisements offering referral to cocaine treatment and who then self-selected a CD program, an outpatient program, or no treatment following an education/information session. The study found no significant differences between the CD and no-treatment groups eight months later.

The extent of reasonably certain knowledge about CD treatment is that clients who present drug problems at admission have poorer outcomes at the posttreatment follow-up than alcohol clients (with no illicit drug consumption) in the same programs. This finding is consistent across studies by the CareUnit system, the Chemical Abuse/Addiction Treatment Outcome Registry (CATOR) follow-up service, and the Hazelden center in Minnesota.

The CareUnit study (Comprehensive Care Corporation, 1988) sampled 1,002 adult clients who stayed at least five days in 1 of 50 different CareUnit programs in 1987. (CareUnits treated 46,000 adults and adolescents in more than 200 locations.) About 53 percent of the sample had used multiple substances before admission, and 29 percent reported polydrug consumption on a daily basis. Clinical program staff interviewed 723 clients from the sample at least one year after discharge. Sixty-one percent were classified as recovering at follow-up (fewer than four instances of use since discharge). Abstinence was poorer for preadmission consumers of illicit drugs (54 percent for those who had used cocaine and 48 percent for those using marijuana) and polydrugs (56 percent) than for consumers primarily of alcohol (63 percent). The strongest indicator of outcome was attendance at self-help groups after discharge: only 48 percent of nonattenders were recovering, compared with 79 percent of those attending the groups more than 29 times.

The CATOR study is a multisite comparison of independent programs. Hoffmann and Harrison (1988) found that at least 38 percent of clients in 22 adult inpatient programs in the Midwest had an admission history that included illicit drugs. However, the study excluded clients with fewer than 10 days in treatment, followed virtually no one who did not complete treatment, and reached only 37 percent of completers at the two-year follow-up interview. Few results were detailed specifically for individuals with drug problems, but the authors note that "[p]revious CATOR analyses have consistently found that polydrug users have the poorest prognosis for abstinence, followed by regular marijuana users. . . . The relationship of use pattern to recovery is confounded to some extent by age since the polydrug and marijuana groups contain a larger proportion of younger patients" (p. 31).[19]

Why Do the Results of Chemical Dependency Treatment Vary?

There are no useful studies that distinguish the reasons why some clients in CD programs recover and others do not. As with other treatments,

---

[19] Studies of Hazelden drug clients (Laundergan, 1982; Gilmore, 1985) are too limited methodologically to merit detailing, which is unfortunate, given the prominence of this program. The findings are consistent with CATOR and CareUnit results in indicating lower abstinence rates at follow-up for drug clients than for alcohol-only clients.

client motivation and program staff quality are suspected factors. But there is no readily available information on variations in drug client outcomes across CD programs or any attempts to relate such differences to systematic variations among clients or in the therapeutic approach.

Benefits and Costs of Chemical Dependency Treatment

There are no studies available on the costs and benefits or cost-effectiveness of this modality. There is some discussion of cost data, however, in Chapters 6 and 8.

DETOXIFICATION

Detoxification, unlike the previous modalities, is not a treatment for drug-seeking behavior. Rather, it is a family of procedures for alleviating the short-term symptoms of withdrawal from drug dependence (NIDA, 1981, 1983b; Kleber, 1987).[20] The major procedure is observation (because withdrawal is self-limiting and ordinarily not life-threatening, although it can be uncomfortable). There are some standard clinical indications for administering pharmacological agents during detoxification: to ameliorate severe withdrawal symptoms, to induce relaxation, to prevent seizures in the case of sedative-hypnotic drugs,[21] or to counteract severe depression.

Detoxification of different drugs involves different durations and medications. Various pharmacological agents are used for withdrawal from opiate addiction, which has been extensively studied and reported for more than 60 years. The most common detox drug is methadone, but benzodiazepines, clonidine, and some other agents also are frequently used to control withdrawal symptoms. Opiate detoxification has often been done rather slowly—over several weeks or even several months—particularly in cases in which there is a long, continuous history of dependence. Today, however, new, more rapid forms of detoxification using combinations of drugs such as clonidine and buprenormine are being tested and used in residential and outpatient settings.

---

[20] Diagnoses of abuse ordinarily do not call for detoxification procedures, although in occasional cases of abuse there is reason for 2 to 24 hours of medical observation to monitor clearing of severe intoxication or acute overdose (possibly needing emergency intervention if vital signs are poor). These treatments of single episodes of excessive dosing may be thought of as logical counterparts to detoxification from dependence, but they are not detoxification.

[21] Detoxification of barbiturates is particularly liable to involve seizures and is more likely than other drug withdrawal to need management in a supervised environment—a hospital or other residential facility with appropriate medical staff and equipment.

Detoxification of cocaine, particularly crack-cocaine dependence, has been especially difficult, but some promising approaches are now emerging. Cocaine dependence typically involves a series of binges that last from 12 to 36 hours each. These binges are usually followed by several days without cocaine use but with gradually mounting withdrawal symptoms that include mood alterations, diminished capacities for experiencing pleasure (anhedonia), and craving for cocaine. These symptoms may not abate for four to eight weeks, thus yielding another binge cycle in very short order. The critical task in detoxification is to disrupt the imminent return of the cocaine cycle.

There has been some success in the management of cocaine withdrawal symptoms and craving in ambulatory clinical trials using desipramine hydrochloride (Gawin et al., 1989a), amantadine (Tennant and Sagherian, 1987), bromocriptine (Dackis et al., 1987), flupenthixol decanoate (Gawin et al., 1989b), and buprenorphine (Mello et al., 1989), among other drugs, in conjunction with once-a-week outpatient counseling. These treatments reduced short-term rates of relapse two- to threefold for a majority of those treated. Unfortunately, most of these agents do not begin to have their major clinical effect for one to two weeks, during which outpatient dropout often occurs (in the programs in which trials have been conducted, dropout rates range from 30 to 70 percent).

Comfort, the avoidance of seizures (the most common cause of fatalities), screening and treatment of infections and other medical problems, and the achievement of a condition in which withdrawal distress is not evident are and should be the primary goals of detoxification. In these terms, current detoxification procedures for most drugs are virtually always effective if they are completed, permitting a transition to abstinence with only attenuated symptoms of withdrawal. The key to completing detoxification successfully is compliance with the detox protocol: taking medication in prescribed amounts and schedules and avoiding intervening use of the drug on which the client is dependent and any other nonprescribed drugs.

Inpatient or residential detoxification appears logically to offer better opportunities for clinicians to ensure compliance with detoxification prescriptions. There is little evidence, however, by which to judge whether this supposition is, indeed, true. Inpatient, residential, and outpatient drug detoxification have not been adequately compared to permit confident conclusions on which has the best compliance record or who belongs in which setting. On technical grounds, detoxification of most illicit drugs in most cases can occur as safely and effectively on an ambulatory basis as in a bedded setting. Hospital treatment in particular calls for justification on relevant medical grounds, such as history of seizures, concurrent conditions needing hospital care, or special cases of risk such as neonates of dependent mothers. On the basis of cost, an ambulatory detox is therefore preferable for most individuals when the medical criteria dictating inpatient detoxification are not present. These issues will be discussed further in Chapters 7 and 8.

It is crucial to underscore the fact that the goals of detoxification are quite limited. This restricted scope is mainly a product of extensive experience with the lack of longer term effects of detoxification, especially of heroin dependence. Consistently, *without subsequent treatment*, researchers have found no effects from detoxification that are discernibly superior to those achieved by untreated withdrawal in terms of reducing subsequent drug-taking behavior and especially relapse to dependence. No appreciable success in increasing rates of recovery from heroin dependence after detoxification alone has been demonstrated for different pharmacological agents or for various detoxification protocols (e.g., rapid versus slow tapering of dose). Review articles reaching this decisive conclusion include those by Resnick (1983), Newman (1983), Cole and colleagues (1981), Moffet and coworkers (1973), and Sheffet and colleagues (1976). There is much less of a literature on cocaine detoxification, but clinicians who are experienced in treating opiate dependence do not believe that short-term detoxification alone will prove any more effective with cocaine.

On the other hand, a detoxification episode offers clinicians a major opportunity to recruit clients into treatment, as the Bale team's study (1980) demonstrated (see also NIDA, 1981; Kleber, 1987). Success at recruitment may well be a more critical outcome for detoxification programs than the conventional primary goals of comfort and suppressing withdrawal symptoms. There appear to be significant variations across U.S. cities in successfully enlisting detoxification patients into treatment. Discharge data from the 1980 CODAP report indicated that only 14 percent of opiate detoxification clients were transferred or referred to further treatment, although there was substantial variation around this average: out of 62 reporting areas, 12 had transfer/referral rates lower than 5 percent, and 14 had rates greater than 25 percent. There are no studies to indicate whether such variations relate to systematic differences in clients, the treatment process, or staff performance, or to chance.

CORRECTIONAL TREATMENT PROGRAMS

The overall record of research on prison-based drug treatment programs is moderate in scope, and the findings mostly correspond to the largely negative results observed in the treatment of criminals during incarceration in hopes of reducing their recidivism (Vaillant, 1988; Besteman, 1990; Chaiken, 1989). Yet Falkin and colleagues (1990) sound a more optimistic note:

Given the current array of treatment programs (many offering only occasional counseling, drug education or other limited services), the finding of evaluation research that many programs are ineffective is not surprising. To adjudge that drug treatment is unable to control recidivism because many programs do not is to miss the crucial point that some programs have been quite successful. With the proper program elements in place, treatment programs could achieve a significantly greater reduction in recidivism than by continuing a policy of imprisonment without adequate treatment.

Their list of the elements necessary for a successful prison drug treatment program[22] is succinct:

- a competent and committed staff;
- adequate administrative and material support by correctional authorities;
- separation from the general prison population;
- incorporation of self-help principles and ex-offender aid;
- comprehensive, intensive therapy aimed at the entire lifestyle of a client and not just the substance abuse aspects; and
- an absolute essential—continuity of care into the parole period.

Three controlled evaluations of prison-based programs that incorporate these criteria are available and are discussed in the sections below. The first used three control groups: a group of program applicants (this was a voluntary program) who did not receive treatment for lack of timely openings—essentially a random selection process—and participants in two other kinds of treatment in the same prison system. The second study (also a voluntary program) used as controls an early-dropout group and an untreated group from the same prison system. The third study, sampling a very large prison/parole program with more than 1,000 admissions per year (partially voluntary), used a sophisticated case-control matching procedure involving the early dropouts from the program. All three studies collected data on the entire group entering treatment for periods of 2 to 11 years after release from confinement. Overall, the results indicate that sizable positive effects can be obtained from treatment, although the results are not unequivocal.

Stay'n Out and Cornerstone

The most recent and currently most influential study (see the discussion of Project REFORM in Falkin et al., 1990; also Frohling, 1989) is of Stay'n Out, a New York program that operates a four-unit, 146-bed prison program for male inmates and a separate 40-bed program for female inmates. The program is based on the social organization of a major therapeutic community, Phoenix House, and adapted to the prison setting; it works

---

[22] These elements could also apply to community programs, which is not surprising because many of the same clients are seen in both program settings.

closely with community-based TCs to extend treatment contact after release. Stay'n Out clients from 1977–1984 ($N = 682$) were compared with similar groups of drug-abusing and dependent prisoners. The comparison groups received either regular drug abuse counseling ($N = 576$) or milieu therapy, which is a staff-intensive congregate-residential counseling approach or quasi-TC ($N = 364$); there was also an untreated control group who applied and were waiting for Stay'n Out admission but who were not treated because there were not enough openings during their window of eligibility, the 6 to 12 months before their first parole hearing ($N = 197$). The groups were followed through 1986 (i.e., from 2 to 9 years after release from prison).

As indicated in Table 5-4, the TC group was arrested significantly less often than the other groups, with differences of 8 to 14 percentage points (which represent 22 to 35 percent reductions in rearrest rates) for men and 6 to 12 percentage points (25 to 40 percent reductions) for women. Because for every arrest, such criminally inclined individuals have generally committed hundreds of crimes (Ball et al., 1981; Johnson et al., 1985; Speckart and Anglin, 1986), these differences in rearrest rates are a valuable result. The authors indicate, however, that intergroup differences at follow-up in rates of reincarceration, rapidity of rearrest, and parole revocation were statistically or substantively negligible, except that significantly more Stay'n Out-treated women than untreated women successfully completed their parole term.

A similar controlled observational study of the Cornerstone program has been reported by Field (1984, 1989; see Table 5-5). Cornerstone is a modified TC program (a mixture of milieu therapy and TC principles) located in Oregon State Hospital in Salem. It is designed for state prisoners in the last year prior to eligibility for parole; after release, the parolees move to a halfway house that includes some therapeutic contacts. Study results indicate that prisoners in the program were convicted significantly less often than comparable parolees in the three years following release.[23]

Graduates of Cornerstone did much better at follow-up than early dropouts from the program. In the Stay'n Out study, and in several other

---

[23]The net figure in Table 5-5 for the whole Cornerstone group—that is, the 54 percent who were convicted of new crimes after release—is the yield within the combined group of dropouts (less than one month in the program) and graduates. In private communications with the Cornerstone staff, the committee was told that most dropouts from the program leave within the first few weeks; therefore, ignoring the small numbers who dropped out between the first month and graduation, for whom follow-up data have not been published, would not appreciably modify the above result. Those in the parolee comparison group, according to Field (1984:54), "do not have the chronic substance abuse histories nor the chronic criminal histories of Cornerstone graduates [and therefore] would be expected to do better at avoiding criminal recidivism than Cornerstone graduates—except, of course, for the treatment results."

TABLE 5-4 Results of Evaluation of Stay'n Out Prison Treatment Program (New York) Compared to Groups Receiving Other Treatment Modalities or No Treatment

Group (Number of Males/Females)	Percentage Re-arrested		Average Months Before Re-arrest		Percentage Reincarcerated		Percentage Not Completing Parole	
	Males[a]	Females	Males	Females	Males	Females	Males	Females
Stay'n Out (therapeutic community) (435/247)	27	18	13	12	44	c	42	23
Milieu (576/0)[b]	35	—	11	—	45	—	47	—
Counseling (261/113)	40	30	12	15	41	c	47	32
No treatment (159/38)	41	24	15	9	c	c	39	47

[a]The differences in results in this column only are statistically significant beyond the .05 level ($\chi^2 = 172$, $p < .001$).
[b]Milieu therapy was not available to female prisoners.
[c]Reincarceration data were not collected for these groups.

Source: Falkin and colleagues (1990).

TABLE 5-5   Results of a Three-Year Follow-up of the
Cornerstone Treatment Program (Oregon) Comparing
Program Graduates, Program Dropouts, and Untreated
Parolees

Group	N	Percentage Newly Convicted	Percentage Reincarcerated
Graduates of the Cornerstone treatment program	144	46	29
Cornerstone dropouts (less than one month in program)	27	85	74
Combined Cornerstone groups	171	54	36
Untreated Oregon parolees with substance abuse histories	179	74	37

Source: Field (1984).

well-regarded, well-studied voluntary correctional programs (see Falkin et al., 1990), length of stay in treatment correlated strongly with positive follow-up measures, the same result seen in community-based programs. The fact that early dropouts from prison programs are even more likely to recidivate, by every measure, than are untreated controls suggests that prison-based TCs may be more efficient than community-based programs at sorting out and excluding (or encouraging self-exclusion of) the poorest responders.

The California Civil Addict Program

A different type of correctional treatment program combines treatment in a penal institution with specialized parole supervision, including access to a variety of community-based treatment opportunities. The most comprehensive and well-studied example of this kind of program was CAP, the California Civil Addict Program, which began in 1961 (McGlothlin et al., 1977; Anglin and McGlothlin, 1984; Anglin, 1988). Two similar civil commitment programs, one federal and one operated by the state of New York, fell far short of their design goals, ended fairly quickly, and were roundly regarded as failures (Besteman, 1978, 1990; Inciardi, 1988). Even the CAP effort operated as designed only until 1969, after which much of its original character was lost, principally because the strict therapeutic rationale was overturned by the general fiscal leanness and operational leniency that overtook the California penal system during then-Governor Ronald Reagan's second term. In addition, community-based treatment programs funded largely by the federal government became available after 1970, creating attractive treatment alternatives for criminal justice agencies and clients. As discussed earlier, this expansion of treatment coincidentally presented a research opportunity to compare the results of the correctional treatment program and methadone maintenance.

CAP permitted adjudication of heroin-dependent individuals through a civil commitment procedure rather than regular criminal sentencing.[24] The first (repeatable) stop for CAP clients, once they had been committed, was a term in the California Rehabilitation Center at Corona, a medium-security prison with a large staff of psychotherapists. This period began a seven-year term of supervision, three-fourths of which, on average, was spent on parole in the community rather than in the center. (The seven-year commitment term could be terminated after three consecutive drug-free years in the community.) The community supervision component involved specially trained parole officers, smaller caseloads of only 30 parolees, and weekly drug testing (Anglin, 1988).

The conditions conducive to a case-control study were inadvertently created during the initial years of the program. The original commitment law was complex enough that legal-procedural errors were made in committing at least half of the early CAP clients. Sooner or later, most of these 1961–1963 commitments were challenged by writs of habeas corpus, and the individuals were released by court order from CAP incarceration and supervision and returned to the regular track of criminal adjudication, with credit for the time served during CAP. The overall writ-released group differed from those who continued in CAP in that many writ-releasees had less serious offenses for which the CAP commitment of seven years was a longer term than the sentence (including parole or probation) they would probably otherwise have served. On the other hand, virtually all of the continuing CAP group would probably have had longer sentences without the CAP diversion. The researchers therefore used matching procedures to select from within the writ-released group a comparison sample that was as similar as possible to the continuing group on 15 criteria, including criminal and drug histories and demographic characteristics.

During their years under CAP, individuals retrospectively reported that they reduced their heroin use (Figure 5-6) as well as total criminality while unincarcerated to levels that were half or less than half the amount reported

---

[24]As at Lexington, voluntary as well as criminal commitments to the facility were permitted. Most CAP clients, however—about 70 percent before 1970 and 93 percent afterward—had been convicted of felonies, largely for nondrug offenses such as burglary and robbery. In addition, before 1970, about 15 percent had been referred by police officers on the noncriminal basis of "believed addicted."

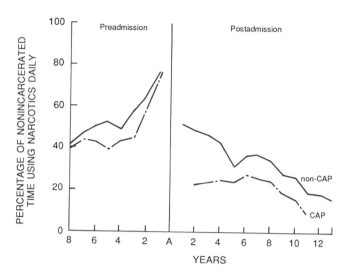

FIGURE 5-6   Effects of the California Civil Addict Program on daily narcotics use. The percentage of nonincarcerated time during which subjects reported using narcotics daily is shown for 8 pre- and 13 postadmission years. The vertical line at A denotes admission to the California Civil Addict Program (CAP). The CAP group ($N = 289$) was committed to the program for 7 years; the non-CAP group ($N = 292$) was discharged from the program by writ shortly after admission owing to procedural errors. Data for CAP year 1 are missing because this group was incarcerated nearly the whole year in the CAP facility. Source: McGlothlin et al. (1977).

by the comparison group. These reductions became apparent immediately after their release into the community, and they were sustained. The difference between CAP parolees and the comparison group on these dimensions narrowed over the next several years as more members of the writ-released group (some of them recommitted to CAP for new offenses) reduced their heroin use and other criminal behavior. By the time the continuing CAP group's parole ended, the control group was at a more nearly similar level, especially considering pretreatment (baseline) differences. The subsequent recovery paths of the two groups remained parallel.

In summary, the residential and community supervision components of CAP were evidently effective in accelerating the recovery of a significant fraction—at least half—of the treated group.

A different result of the CAP study was to examine the effects of methadone maintenance treatment during CAP supervision (Anglin et al., 1984). In 1971, as discussed earlier in the chapter, methadone programs were opened in a number of California's cities, and some members of both the CAP and the writ-released comparison group who had continued active heroin use elected to enter methadone programs. (Parole officers neither

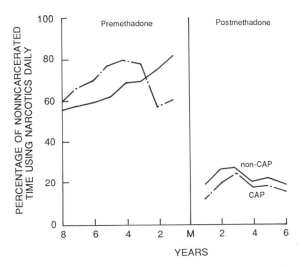

FIGURE 5-7 The effect of methadone maintenance on daily narcotics use in the California Civil Addict Program and control groups. The percentage of nonincarcerated time during which subjects reported using narcotics daily is shown for 8 pre- and 6 postadmission years. The vertical line at M denotes admission to methadone maintenance treatment. The CAP group (N = 136) entered treatment for the first time while on parole status under the California Civil Addict Program; the non-CAP or control group (N = 136) were first-treatment admissions who were not in the Civil Addict Program. Source: Anglin et al. (1981).

insisted on this option nor opposed it.) In both samples, entry to methadone had powerful effects on individuals who, by and large, had not otherwise begun recovery—effects as great or greater than those of CAP parole itself (Figure 5-7). There were no significant differences between the CAP and the comparison group in how methadone affected their heroin-seeking or other criminal behavior.

Boot Camps

A final type of prison-based treatment that has received much attention recently is the "boot camp" or "shock incarceration" (SI) concept for young offenders. This treatment constitutes a three- to six-month sentence for young offenders who are remanded to a facility employing rigorous physical exercise and a small-group organizational structure similar to Outward Bound or military training camps. A number of states, beginning with Georgia in 1983, have opened such facilities, largely as a way to reduce prison costs and improve resource management. Shock incarceration segregates young offenders, who would otherwise be mixed with the general penitentiary population (in this case, SI reduces penitentiary overcrowding) or with the general probation population (in this case, using the SI option increases the need for correctional facilities).

There are several studies under way to improve understanding of how these programs work. Boot camps vary in nature. Some are entirely militaristic environments with few if any therapeutic staff or procedures; others incorporate many drug treatment elements that the more successful prison treatment efforts display but lack still other requirements—particularly continuity of care when the individual returns to the community. Parent (1989:4,5), in a report to the National Institute of Justice, summarizes current knowledge:

Preliminary case tracking data raises questions about SI's capacity to reduce recidivism. The Oklahoma Department of Corrections used survival analysis to compare return rates of SI graduates with similar non-violent offenders sentenced to the DOC. After 29 months almost half the SI graduates, but only 28 percent of the other group, had returned to prison.

In a three year follow-up, the Georgia DOC found that 38.5 percent of their SI graduates returned to prison. For Georgia SI graduates who were in their teens when admitted to SI, 46.8 percent returned to prison within three years of release. In an earlier study, Georgia researchers found little difference in one-year return to prison rates for SI graduates, and similar offenders sentenced to prison and to a youthful offender institution. It should be emphasized that neither of these studies involved carefully constructed comparison groups.

Until evaluation results become available, policy makers should view claims of incredible success with skepticism, and should be cautious about proceeding with SI development on the basis of high hopes, preliminary data, or press clippings.

Conclusions about Prison Treatment

Prisoners with drug problems are "hard cases," but in terms of avoidable social damage, success in accelerating the recovery of even a modest proportion of them yields substantial social benefits. The limited research information on correctional treatment indicates that some programs have delivered this benefit, but many have not. The research does not clearly demonstrate why only a few prison programs have curbed recidivism, but clinical judgments about the key differences between effective and noneffective programs are consistent with the available evidence and bear repeating here.

First, clients need not be dragooned into treatment in order to enlist substantial participation in correctional programs. In the three programs reviewed here in detail, and in most well-regarded programs, entry has largely been a matter of negotiation or multilateral consent, requiring the fulfillment of certain obligations by the prospective client, program staff, and custodial authorities. The principal requirement for effective correctional treatment programs is responsiveness: the program must respond to individual client behaviors as surely as the individual must respond to clinical protocols and queries. The treatment programs have had authority to exclude clients. Mutual consent and performance are a recurrent theme, evident in the formulation of entry contracts and treatment plans, the incorporation of self-help principles and systems of earned program privileges, and roles for program graduates.

Successful correctional treatment requires clinically skillful staff who are strongly committed to their work. To maintain staff skills and commitment in the face of difficult cases is impossible without adequate material and administrative support from correctional and other authorities. Another vital element is follow-up research to let staff know what effects their efforts are having.

Treatment is not an alternative to penalties for committing violent and acquisitive crimes such as robbery, burglary, and larceny, for which offenders with drug problems are so frequently apprehended. Treatment decisions (including admission and termination) need to be made on therapeutic grounds in terms of program goals and rules; decisions in the interest of justice and custodial security must also be made by the appropriate authorities on their own merits. But decisions in either sphere must be consistent with explicit rules, and agencies must be prepared to follow through on them. Contingencies such as revocation and return to custody in the event of noncompliance with release conditions must be believable and consistently enforced.

SUMMARY AND CONCLUSIONS ABOUT TREATMENT EFFECTIVENESS

The committee is both satisfied and disappointed with the conclusions that can be drawn about the effectiveness of the major drug treatment modalities. It is satisfied that some modalities have been studied with sufficient skill and methodological integrity that conclusions can, indeed, be drawn (even though there is still much to be desired in the way of useful knowledge). It is disappointed that the same cannot be said of other modalities and that the overall state of knowledge about treatment effectiveness has not grown more rapidly in the past 5 to 10 years. Most of what is known is based on data collected between 1969 and 1981.

Table 5-6 is a succinct statement of this disappointment. Of the four major modalities, methadone maintenance has received the most extensive study, using all of the main types of treatment evaluation research techniques. Therapeutic communities have received the next most extensive assessment; outpatient nonmethadone treatments have been evaluated at a

TABLE 5-6   Comparison of Types and Strength of Evidence on Effectiveness, Numbers of Admissions, and Revenues for the Major Drug Treatment Modalities

Element	Treatment Modalities			
	Methadone Maintenance	Therapeutic Communities	Outpatient Methadone	Chemical Dependency
Evidence of effectiveness[a]				
Randomized clinical trials	**	—	—	—
Quasi-experiments[b]	**	*	—	—
Controlled observations[c]	***	***	**	—
Simple observations[d]	***	***	***	**
Annual number of admissions (in thousands)[e]	130	110	430	140
Annual revenues (in millions of dollars)[e]	200	200	300	500

[a] * = A single study of this type; ** = a few such studies; *** = studies of numerous programs with varied study designs; — = no such studies conducted.

[b] For example, the introduction of a new treatment modality, a program closing, or an incompletely randomized trial that used multivariate analysis.

[c] Studies of treatment cohorts, usually including treatment refusals and using multivariate analysis.

[d] Studies of single treatment cohorts without nontreatment comparisons and using only univariate or bivariate analyses.

[e] The source of these modality statistics is the Institute of Medicine analysis of the 1987 National Drug and Alcoholism Treatment Utilization Survey (see Chapter 6 for discussion of these admission and revenue estimates).

somewhat lower level. Chemical dependency treatment has the least extensive useful body of knowledge concerning its effectiveness.[25] Yet according to the committee's analysis of a 1987 national survey of drug treatment providers (detailed in Chapter 6), the order of expenditures for these modalities is exactly the reverse of the order of knowledge about their effectiveness.

In the final section of this chapter, the committee offers its ideas on how to go about repairing the sources of its disappointment. These ideas are presented as a series of specific research recommendations. First, however, the committee summarizes below its findings about the respective modalities.

---

[25] Correctional treatment has not been included on this chart because it is not a distinct modality. Knowledge about prison-based programs is approximately at the same level as that for community-based TCs. Detoxification also is not included because it is not considered a treatment for drug-seeking behavior in the same way as are the major modalities.

Methadone Maintenance

Methadone maintenance is a treatment for extended opiate dependence (which is usually heroin). A sufficient daily oral dose of methadone hydrochloride, which is a relatively long-acting narcotic analgesic, yields a stable metabolic level of the drug. Consumption once daily of a stable, clinically adjusted dose is not behaviorally or subjectively intoxicating and does not impair functioning or generate appreciable morbid side effects. Once a newly admitted client reaches a stable, noneuphoric "blockade" state, free of the psychophysiological cues that precipitate opiate craving, he or she is amenable to counseling, environmental changes, and other social services that can help shift his or her orientation and lifestyle away from drug seeking and related crime toward more socially acceptable behaviors.

Methadone maintenance has been the most rigorously studied modality and has yielded the most incontrovertibly positive results. However, it is also the most controversial treatment, largely on the grounds that methadone clients have "merely" switched their dependence to a legal narcotic and that some clients (the proportion varies from program to program) continue to take heroin and other drugs intermittently and to commit crimes, including the sale of take-home methadone. In the committee's judgment, these controversies and reservations are neither trivial nor compelling. The great majority of methadone clients had been consuming high levels of illicit drugs and committing other crimes (including drug selling) on a daily basis prior to admission. The issues are to what extent undesirable behaviors are reduced and positive behaviors increased as a result of methadone maintenance (in comparison to no treatment or to alternative measures), and whether enough is known about such treatment to improve poorly performing programs.

Research on methadone has demonstrated the following:

• There is strong evidence from clinical trials and similar study designs that, on average, heroin-dependent (or other opiate-dependent) individuals have much better outcomes in terms of illicit drug consumption and other criminal behavior when they are maintained on methadone than when they are not treated at all, when they are simply detoxified and released, or when methadone is tapered down and terminated arbitrarily.

• Methadone clinics have significantly higher retention rates among opiate-dependent populations than do other treatment modalities for similar clients.[26]

---

[26] It should be noted that higher retention can "load the dice" when making outcome comparisons during treatment among different modalities. Because dropouts generally show worse behavior and have somewhat poorer prognoses to begin with, a program that retains more of its initial clients, even if equal in its effect on each client, will have a lower average effectiveness on

- When assessed following discharge from methadone treatment, clients who stayed in treatment longer have better outcomes than clients who left earlier.

- Methadone dosages need to be clinically monitored and individually optimized. Clients do much better, however, when they are stabilized on higher rather than lower doses within the typical ranges that are currently prescribed (30–100 mg/day). Program characteristics such as inadequate methadone dosage levels and differences between counselors (which are not yet fully defined) are significantly related to differences in client performance while in treatment.

- Methadone treatment, when implemented at the resource levels observed in the late 1970s, provides individual and social benefits over a term of at least several years that are substantially higher than the cost of delivering this treatment, which is now $3,000 per year and which should be at least $4,000 per year to be comparable to earlier programs. The daily benefits equal the daily costs in virtually every case, even among those who continue drug taking at a lower level.

Therapeutic Communities

Therapeutic communities are residential programs with expected stays of generally 9 to 15 months, phasing into independent residence with continuing contact for a variable period. TC programs are highly structured blends of resocialization, milieu therapy, behavioral modification practices, progression through a hierarchy of occupational training and responsibility within the TC, community reentry, and a variety of social services.

Therapeutic community clients are more diverse in their drug use patterns than methadone clients because the modality is not specific to any particular class of drugs. From the 1960s to the early 1980s, a majority of TC clients were primarily dependent on heroin. In the late 1980s, cocaine dependence began to predominate in many programs. Therapeutic communities are designed for individuals with major impairments and social deficits, including histories of serious criminal behavior. The results of research on the effects of TC treatment are as follows:

- TC clients end virtually all illicit drug taking and other criminal behavior while in residence and perform better (in terms of reduced drug taking and other criminal activity and increased social productivity) after discharge than before admission. They also have better outcomes at follow-up than individuals who simply underwent detoxification or who contacted but did not enter a TC program. The length of stay is the strongest predictor

---

clients remaining in treatment. The bias fades if all admissions, not only the ones remaining in treatment, are compared across modalities.

of outcomes at follow-up, with graduates having the best outcomes at that point.

• Attrition from TCs is typically high—above the rates for methadone maintenance but below the rates for outpatient nonmethadone treatment. Typically, about 15 percent of admissions will graduate after a continuous stay; the figure is higher (20 to 25 percent) once later readmissions are considered.

• The minimum retention necessary to yield improvement in long-term outcomes seems to be several months, which covers one-third to one-half of a typical program's admissions. Improvements continue to be manifested for full-time treatment of up to one year in length.

• The benefits of TC treatment are substantial and they virtually repay the costs on a day-by-day basis, although the per diem costs are higher than for methadone maintenance: generally, about $13,000 per year—probably $20,000 for a model program—yielding somewhat lower benefit/cost ratios than for methadone but ones that still favor the use of this treatment.

Outpatient Nonmethadone Programs

Outpatient nonmethadone programs display a great deal of hetero-geneity in their treatment processes, philosophies, and staffing. Their clients generally are not opiate dependent but otherwise vary across all types of drugs. Usually, OPNM clients have much less serious criminal histories than methadone or TC clients and include more nondependent individuals. Outpatient nonmethadone programs generally provide one or two visits per week for individual or group psychotherapy/counseling, with an expected course averaging about six months.

Despite the heterogeneity of programs and their clients, the limited number of outcome evaluations of OPNM programs have generated conclusions qualitatively similar to those from studies of TCs:

• Outpatient nonmethadone clients during and following treatment exhibit better behavior than before treatment. Those clients who are actually admitted to programs have better outcomes than clients who contact but do not enter programs (and clients who only undergo detoxification). Outcome at follow-up is positively related to length of stay in treatment, and completers have better outcomes than dropouts.

• Retention in outpatient nonmethadone programs is poorer than for methadone maintenance and therapeutic communities.

• The benefits of OPNM treatment are fewer than for methadone or TCs, but the cost of the treatment, at about $1,350 for six months (about $1,800 for a model program), is low. As a result, the yields are favorable for those who stay longer than three months, and the aggregate program ratios are mildly favorable.

Chemical Dependency Programs

Chemical dependency programs generally are residential or inpatient, with a three- to six-week duration, followed by up to two years of attendance at self-help groups or a weekly outpatient therapy group. CD programs are based on an Alcoholics Anonymous (12-step) model of personal change, a belief that dependence is a permanent but controllable disability, and goals of total abstinence and lifestyle alteration. The proportion of the CD population who are drug involved is similar to the outpatient nonmethadone population in that the primary drugs are cocaine and marijuana. The modal CD client, however, is an older, socially well-supported, alcohol-dependent individual.

CD programs are often located in hospitals, but the core therapeutic elements of this modality do not require the presence of acute care hospital services. There is little evidence on whether hospital-based CD programs are more or less effective for drug problems than CD programs that are not sited in hospitals, or whether they are more or less effective than no treatment at all. Chemical dependency programs treat mainly primary alcoholism and have not been adequately evaluated for treatment of drug problems. A few follow-up studies of individuals who have completed CD treatment indicate that primary drug clients have poorer outcomes than primary alcohol clients. There are no cost/benefit analyses for chemical dependency treatment.

Detoxification

Detoxification is therapeutically supervised withdrawal to abstinence over a short term—that is, up to several months but usually five to seven days, often employing pharmacological agents to reduce client discomfort or the likelihood of complications. Detoxification is seldom effective in itself as a modality for bringing about recovery from dependence, although it can be used as a gateway to other treatment modalities.

Clinicians generally advocate that detoxification not be considered a modality of treatment in the same sense as methadone, TCs, outpatient counseling, and CD units because of its narrow, short-term focus and poor outcomes in terms of relapse to drug dependence.

Detoxification episodes are often hospital based and may begin with emergency treatment of an overdose. Much drug detoxification (an estimated 100,000 admissions annually) is now taking place in hospital beds. It is doubtful whether hospitalization (especially beyond the first day or two) is necessary in most cases, except for the special problems of addicted neonates, severe sedative-hypnotic dependence, or concurrent medical or severe psychiatric problems. For clients with a documented history of complications or flight from detoxification, residential detoxification may be indicated. Detoxification may, in the committee's judgment, be undertaken successfully in most cases on a nonhospital residential, partial day care, or ambulatory basis.

Correctional Treatment

Treatment of drug-involved prisoners is fairly common, but at least two-thirds of prison treatment programs are equivalent to outpatient non-methadone treatment—that is, periodic individual or group therapy sessions. This level of intervention is probably not intensive enough to do much for this group. The other prison treatment programs are similar to stays in a therapeutic community, including separation from the general prison population for the expected 6- to 12-month duration of the program.

Most of the prison drug treatment programs that have been studied, including specialized "boot camp" or "shock incarceration" facilities, have not been shown to reduce the typically very high postrelease rates of recidivism to drug seeking and other criminal behavior that occur among untreated prisoners. Nevertheless, a small number of well-designed controlled studies, involving prison TCs and residential programs that have strong linkages to community-based supervision and/or treatment programs, indicate that prison-initiated treatment can reduce the treated group's rate of *rearrest* by one-fourth to one-half; clear correlations are observed between positive outcome rates and length of time in treatment, just as in studies of entirely community-based modalities. The results have some anomalies and there have been difficulties in sustaining the integrity of prison-based treatment programs, but the results argue that these programs should be carefully encouraged.

* * * * *

If a single phrase could succeed in capturing most of the findings in this chapter, it would be an expression that—much like the current treatment modalities—dates from the 1960s: different strokes for different folks. No single treatment "works" for a majority of the people who seek treatment. Each of the treatment modalities for which there is a baseline of adequate studies can fairly be said to work for many of the people who seek that treatment; and enough of them do find the right treatment, and stay with it long enough, to make the current aggregate of treatment programs worthwhile.

Selection of the most appropriate treatment modality by clients or others (e.g., judges, probation officers, employee assistance counselors, family members) is constrained by poor information about programs, location/transportation issues, waiting lists at some portals and aggressive recruitment at others, and cost questions. In most locations, there is no comprehensive intake (assessment and referral) unit or agency to advise or assign applicants. (This triage feature, which was relatively common in the multimodality programs and municipal treatment agencies of the 1960s or 1970s, was often abandoned in the cost-cutting of the early 1980s.) Most of all, the search for the right program is bedeviled by variations in program quality. The signs of poor program performance (particularly of poor response to the prospective client's specific set of problems) are not readily apparent, and the general lack of reliable information about program outcomes does not offer incentives for programs to change for the better.

There is a great deal of room for improvement, and there are indications in the research literature on how to bring that about. Much of Chapters 7 and 8 is informed by the committee's reading of those indications. Before moving to the final third of the report, however, the committee considers it vital to lay out a plan for restocking and expanding the limited store of knowledge it has had to draw on so that if another group is charged with studying the treatment system 5 or 10 years from now, they will not have to be as disappointed as this body was about the knowledge gains in the intervening years. The last section of this chapter therefore presents a brief but systematic template of recommendations for a national program of treatment research.

RECOMMENDATIONS FOR RESEARCH ON TREATMENT SERVICES AND METHODS

Rebuilding the Research Base

Federal support for drug research, including research on treatment methods and services (alternatively, clinical and services research), surged during the early 1970s, declined steadily in real terms for the next decade, and began to surge again as a result of the Anti-Drug Abuse Acts of 1986 and 1988 and recent initiatives for AIDS-related research (Figure 5-8). Unfortunately, but quite predictably, the base of capable researchers declined during the decade-long period of stagnation, as scientists moved on to other fields and very few new ones entered the drug research area. The number of centers of excellence in treatment-oriented research— active programs generating sound new results on current data—declined substantially; where there were formerly close to two dozen, located in all parts of the country, there are now just a handful in a few major metropolitan centers.

The national research infrastructure must be rebuilt and the number of local centers of excellence in research on treatment methods and services increased to reverse the shortage of experienced investigators. Current funding increases are sufficient to rebuild the needed base of treatment research excellence but only if the current level is sustained for at least four or five years and expenditures are patterned during that time to ensure attention to the perennial questions that face clinicians and policymakers responsible for the system. It is critical that this base be maintained through a program of steady incremental funding changes and not be dismantled once again, a course that would leave the nation unprepared to respond quickly to whatever new epidemic of drug use might arise in the future—and the lesson of history is that some new wave *will* arise.

To evaluate and improve the adequacy and effectiveness of treatment plans and expenditures, the national services research program in particular needs rebuilding. The prospects for maintaining and improving treatment quality as well as continuing to develop more effective treatment methods depend to a great extent on treatment services research. The National Institute on Drug Abuse (NIDA), the agency most responsible for maintaining

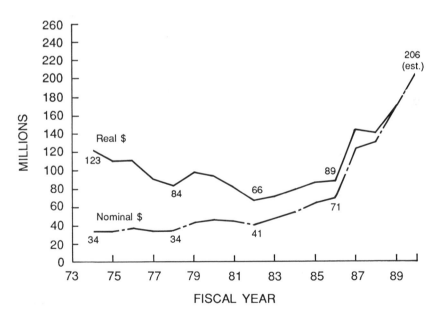

FIGURE 5-8 Annual research obligations of the National Institute on Drug Abuse (in both nominal [current] and real [1989-equivalent] dollars) for fiscal years 1974–1990. Source: National Institute on Drug Abuse, unpublished data, 1989.

treatment research, is, of course, not autonomous. Its budget and priorities are proposed by the President and disposed by Congress. Moreover, providers of drug treatment services are very much at fault for permitting and in some cases tacitly encouraging the paucity of treatment research over the past decade. Programs have been characterized too much by a fear of failure and too little by the courage of their convictions. The results of earlier treatment enterprises tell an enlightening and reasonably heartening tale, and there is little possibility of improving current therapeutic practices further without careful study of outcomes, not only in research units, with their limited patient protocols and cadre of university-based researchers, but also in all other treatment programs.

Most importantly, the advances in knowledge that came out of clinical and services research in the 1970s have not been followed up, and as a result analysts today are not better prepared to answer questions about the effectiveness, costs, and benefits of current treatment than they were a decade ago. Data systems and analytic capabilities that were designed to answer policy questions have not been well maintained. It would be a travesty of prudent governance if once again the federal government and the states were to proceed to build, or rebuild, a major instrument of national drug control policy without assuring themselves and the taxpayers that there would be timely, necessary research and evaluation to understand that instrument's performance and facilitate its improvement.

One more note needs sounding in this context. A critical longer term role is played by basic epidemiological, behavioral, biological, and neurochemical research to address such issues as the role of genetic predispositions in addiction, the factors that contribute to the plasticity of addictive behavior, the effects of social factors, and methods for reducing drug craving. The goal of such work should be to integrate the biological and behavioral sides of the drug problem. This integration will remain difficult so long as a continuing imbalance persists between substantial investments in high-quality biomedical research and meager ones in high-quality biobehavioral and psychosocial research.

Major Research Questions

The core questions that need to be addressed for the various modalities of public treatment are the following: What client and program factors influence treatment-seeking behavior, treatment retention and efficacy, and relapse after treatment? How can these factors be better managed? Treatment-seeking factors include community outreach, health promotion and disease prevention efforts such as experimental needle-exchange programs, family and employer interventions, and program intake and triage procedures. Retention and efficacy factors include optimal treatment durations and schedules, pretreatment motivations, counselor or therapist behavior, incentives and conditions of employment, clinic procedures, criminal justice contingencies, and ancillary services. Posttreatment factors include relapse prevention interventions, abstinence monitoring, and environmental reinforcement.

The questions need to be attacked in a variety of ways. Despite the difficulties of maintaining the integrity of controlled experiments in treatment programs, these studies provide the most incontrovertible evidence about comparative treatment effects, and efforts to conduct them should be strongly encouraged. A more detailed understanding of treatment processes through ethnographic and case study methods is also badly needed. This work is the basis for the design and interpretation of survey instruments. **Studies should be initiated within as well as across each major treatment modality to answer the following question: What are the relations of treatment performance (that is, differential outcomes, taking initial client characteristics into account), the content and organization of treatment (specific site arrangements, service offerings, therapeutic approaches, staffing practices), and the costs of treatment?**

Services Research

Health services research is a critical element in building treatment systems. An important foundation for services research as well as program accountability is the development, maintenance, and analysis of a system of data acquisition on treatment programs, client performance, and costs. Results from studies that use these kinds of data will permit better and more cost-effective decisions about facility characteristics, staff salary and training levels, services coordination methods, intensity of services, reasonable charges, and other components. Systems of this sort were established in the 1970s but were effectively disassembled as a matter of federal policy in the 1980s. **Treatment data acquisition systems must be rebuilt and effectively managed and utilized if the improvement of treatment knowledge and practice is to be evaluated and facilitated in the 1990s. Data on treatment effectiveness and costs should become the cornerstone of decisions about treatment coverage by public and private programs.**

NIDA, in conjunction with its sister agency, the Office of Treatment Improvement, needs to give more adequate, focused attention to the drug treatment delivery system as a whole. Stronger services research programs at NIDA are a critical complement to the research and service responsibilities of the Alcohol, Drug Abuse, and Mental Health Administration (ADAMHA). Fulfilling this responsibility requires close linkages to practice and thus some responsibility to and for service delivery. Existing legislative authority directing these linkages should be implemented fully.

The responsibilities for research coordination, however, do not stop at the boundaries of ADAMHA. Collaborative and coordinative arrangements with the National Institute of Justice, the Bureau of Justice Statistics, the National Institute of Corrections, and other relevant agencies in the Department of Justice and other federal departments should be extended beyond current levels. More extensive relationships would encourage critical technical improvements, such as the inclusion in epidemiological and treatment surveys of "linkage" items to facilitate syntheses with data from criminal justice populations. For example, treatment applicants should be asked how many emergency room admissions and arrests they have undergone during the year prior to treatment, which would not only serve to build baseline data for outcomes research but also provide calibrations with respect to the Drug Abuse Warning Network and Drug Use Forecasting data systems.

Some of the most compelling results of treatment research have come from large longitudinal studies involving thousands of clients: the DARP (Drug Abuse Reporting Program) study of a 1969–1971 national admission cohort, which included a 12-year follow-up, and TOPS (the Treatment Outcome Prospective Study), which involved a 10,000-person national sample of 1979–1981 admissions to 41 drug treatment programs in 10 cities. There is reason to believe that some findings about the treatment modalities—such as the importance of time in treatment—will prove robust in the face of changing drug markets, but others may not.

Another such national treatment sample study (DATOS, or the Drug Abuse Treatment Outcome Study) is beginning in 1990, and some smaller scale studies, such as the Drug Services Research Survey, are in process. Intervals of 10 years between entry cohorts to major studies as important as these are far too long. New study panels composed of 3-year entry cohorts (an efficient period of admission to a multiwave design) should begin at no greater than 5-year intervals.

The responsibility to study treatment services in the field generally is not met by demonstration grant programs. Demonstrations have historically functioned as a stop-gap measure to provide a new kind of service for which there seemed to be a need but no certain knowledge about how to fill it—knowledge lacking at least in part because adequate research systems were not already in place to generate it. Demonstrations are not a reasonable substitute for a strong program of treatment services research. Demonstration grants should be made only when objectives are carefully specified and independently designed and performed collaborative evaluations are funded. Collaborative clinical trials are the basis for developing standardized protocols in other forms of treatment and should be implemented as models for demonstration programs. Such a plan would allow effective programs or program components to be adequately described, replicated, and, if found useful, incorporated into certification standards.

A services research issue worth noting here is the difficulties that drug treatment programs experience in securing zoning approval for clinical facilities, a problem usually summarized as "not in my back yard" (NIMBY). This problem, of course, is not confined to siting community drug treatment programs but confronts public utilities and services of many kinds. There is currently a NIDA-sponsored market research project (Technical Assistance & Training Corp., 1989) to create technical assistance materials to overcome this "barrier" to treatment. Research support for more definitive studies of program site effects—for example, on local real estate values and criminal victimization rates—would provide a better foundation for this work.

Chemical Dependency

Chemical dependency programs are the least well studied of the drug treatment modalities. The aggressive marketing deployed by many such programs has created suspicions about them in many quarters that cannot be allayed without investments in objective treatment research and evaluation. The optimal site of delivery and length of programming, including the duration of intensive treatment and aftercare periods, and the specific therapeutic elements necessary for an effective program should be investigated more closely.

Only a few chemical dependency treatment providers have played positive roles in providing data and research opportunities for effectiveness studies. Many more need to do so to answer these questions: What is the effectiveness of chemical dependency treatment for drug-impaired clients of varying characteristics? Are there variations in program effectiveness— and if so, why? What are the actual costs and benefits of the most effective components of chemical dependency treatment?

Cocaine Treatment

The major efforts to date to investigate cocaine treatment efficacy occurred prior to the epidemiological reemergence of cocaine in the 1980s. There is reason to believe that some findings about treatment modalities— such as the importance of time in treatment—will prove robust in the face of changing drug markets, but others may not. **The infrastructure of treatment research centers decayed during the stagnation of drug research funding, and as this capability is rebuilt, it should specifically address the following questions about cocaine treatment: What are the most effective treatment elements for cocaine dependence and abuse? To what degree can** current modalities be effective for crack-cocaine? What new or existing pharmacological and nonpharmacological treatment elements can improve the clinical picture?

Women, Children, and Adolescents

The majority of individuals in treatment are adult males who are 20 to 40 years old, and their responses dominate treatment research statistics. The major findings of research to date on the effectiveness of different modalities and elements of treatment seem to apply roughly as well to adolescents and women with young children as they do to the more prevalent demographic groups (Hubbard et al., 1989). Yet the potential significance of child-bearing and child-rearing women and adolescent clients in terms of the future benefits of present treatment (or the future costs of present nontreatment) is great. Research plans in all areas need to devote special attention to differentiated knowledge about the two populations of adolescents and women with young children (including pregnant women).

It seems clear from earlier studies that women in treatment who are pregnant or have young children are especially likely to bring particular needs to the treatment system (Beschner et al., 1981; Reed et al., 1982). For example, drug-abusing or dependent women on average have poorer self-esteem than men and suffer from greater anxiety, depression, and detachment; as a result, therapists who rely too heavily on confrontative techniques may worsen such problems rather than help reduce them. Because of their child care responsibilities, long-term residential treatment in TCs may be ruled out for many women unless there are special provisions for child care. In many states, long-term TC treatment becomes doubly problematic because extended residential treatment may jeopardize family eligibility for Aid to Families with Dependent Children (welfare) or threaten the mother's custody of the children.

The federal block grant for alcohol, drug abuse, and mental health services mandates that 10 percent of the grant be set aside to provide special services for women. According to the Institute of Medicine analysis of the 1987 National Drug and Alcoholism Treatment Utilization Survey, about one-third of the more than 80,000 women in drug treatment were in programs that had at least some special services for women, although there is no further specification of the nature or extent of these services. Both clinical and services research are needed to gain an understanding of the nature and efficacy of current practices and the potential of innovations.

The state of knowledge about adolescent treatment is, if anything, even less satisfactory. The number of useful studies of adolescents is small, and most work in this area is based too heavily on studies of treatment in much earlier periods (e.g., Friedman and colleagues [1986] analyze data on adolescents in the Drug Abuse Reporting Program of the early 1970s). There are major obstacles to research on adolescents, including conceptual issues, such as discordant terminology for adolescent treatment service components, and logistical constraints, such as unmanageable requirements for obtaining parental consent.

The committee recommends that a special study initiative be undertaken by the National Institute on Drug Abuse, in conjunction with other relevant agencies of the Public Health Service, on the treatment of drug abuse and dependence among adolescents and women who are pregnant or rearing young children. The initiative should review and summarize all available sources of evidence and insight from research and clinical experience, provide as much guidance as possible for current treatment efforts, and develop a comprehensive research agenda. The agenda in turn should be pursued by research agencies of the federal government and other sources of research support and carried forward by the community of clinicians and scientists.

6
Two Tiers:
Public and Private Supply

To a person with a serious drug problem, or a referring clinician, or a parent looking for the best possible help for a troubled son or daughter, the paramount issues in drug treatment are simple and direct: what kind of treatment works best for this problem, and how easy is it to get access to the needed treatment in terms of quality, location, price, and openings? These individual concerns, repeated across hundreds of thousands of cases a year, cast a large question mark over the size, distribution, structure, and efficiency of the treatment supply system.

For analysts, these questions are articulated somewhat differently. How well does the treatment supply system now meet the need for drug treatment? What general changes in scale or structure, if any, are necessary to improve the match between the supply of treatment and the need for it? What are the most important constraints or rigidities that condition the possibility of appropriate reforms? More concisely: *Does the supply system match treatments to needs? If not, then why not, and how can it be fixed?*

In this chapter and the two chapters that follow, the committee attempts to resolve these issues. This chapter describes in qualitative and quantitative terms how the supply system is now constituted. This task was easier 10 to 15 years ago, for the system then was more uniform in its content, clients, and purposes and there was a national data collection system. Notwithstanding today's impoverished data, after thorough analysis the evidence clearly depicts the structure of the treatment system: *there are two highly contrasting tiers of drug treatment—one for the poor under public sponsorship and one for those who can pay with private insurance or out-of-pocket funds.*

The existence of two tiers of providers is not unique in social and health services. Within the general medical delivery system there are public hospitals and clinics that primarily serve the poor and underinsured and private medical centers that primarily serve the affluent and well-insured. But the drug treatment system breaks that general mold in several critical respects. The two tiers of drug treatment differ from each other not only in their sources of financing but also in their recency and origins, provider and facility characteristics, modalities and services offered, clientele served, and capacity utilized (for example, the size of "waiting lists"). Moreover, the public tier interacts extensively with the criminal justice system.

These contrasts are sharper and deeper than any of the differences that separate the two tracks of general medical care. Based on these differences and its previous analysis of treatment needs, the committee in this chapter reaches several general conclusions about the national supply system, including the relation of the public and private tiers, the nature of their major respective problems, and the general direction of needed reforms. Chapters 7 and 8 continue the discussion begun in this chapter but in greater depth.

THE TWO TIERS: AN OVERVIEW

It is useful to conceive of the treatment system as being made up of two tiers of providers. The public-tier providers are publicly owned programs or private, not-for-profit programs whose revenues are largely from government agencies. This tier includes large, multisite residential and methadone programs, but mostly it comprises small, not-for-profit outpatient clinics in about 2,000 communities across the nation. These programs primarily serve clients who are indigent or underinsured. This system of care had its origins in the wars on crime and poverty of the late 1960s and early 1970s, and it was (and is) in many ways an adjunct to the criminal justice system.

The private tier is made up of privately owned providers (both for-profit and not-for-profit programs) that serve clients who have private health insurance or sufficient financial resources to pay for drug treatment. The private tier has developed mainly from hospital units that originally focused almost entirely on medically directed inpatient treatment of alcoholism. Yet the characteristics of these programs are changing as outpatient care and aftercare become more important. This tier is growing rapidly, and the total revenues received by its providers are beginning to approach the total revenues of providers in the public tier. Within the private tier, the ranks of for-profit providers are growing more rapidly than the number of not-for-profit providers.

There is very little overlap in providers and limited overlap of clientele between the two tiers. On the one hand, people with private health insurance rarely choose to be treated initially by programs that serve the indigent population. On the other hand, public subsidies often are not large enough to cover the charges of private-tier providers. There are a few programs—especially residential not-for-profit facilities—that straddle the two tiers, but they are dwarfed in number by those clearly belonging to one tier or the other.

Financing Differences

No data sources currently available permit a comprehensive description of the two tiers. Nevertheless, the tiers are sharply distinguishable in data collected in the 1987 National Drug and Alcoholism Treatment Utilization Survey, or NDATUS.[1] The axis that most clearly divides the two tiers of treatment is source of revenue. Closely correlated with these tiers are radically higher levels of reimbursements for private clients, modest differences in the nature and richness of delivered care, and disparities in accessibility of services, with a much greater chance that applicants to the private tier can gain immediate admission to treatment.

Figure 6-1 shows private revenues as a percentage of total revenues by type of treatment facility and ownership. The figure clearly shows that all types of for-profit providers serve primarily clients who are covered by private health insurance or who pay their own fees; these providers gain about 80 percent of their revenues from these two courses. Government-owned providers clearly serve clients who are covered by government programs.

---

[1] The most recent editions of the survey, in 1982 (NIDA, 1983a) and 1987, each came shortly after dramatic changes in the public financing system. First came the switch in FY 1982 to federal block grants, the major effect of which was to reduce federal treatment funding virtually overnight by 25 percent. The second major change was the 1986 Anti-Drug Abuse Act, which reversed the earlier trend and increased federal dollars for drug treatment by 20 percent.

Several cautions are in order regarding the 1987 estimates. First, there is evidence from state reports (Butynski and Canova, 1988) that the response rate to the 1987 NDATUS may have been as low as 70 percent of all programs. Prior NDATUS efforts were reported to have had response rates of better than 95 percent. Second, financial data were omitted by almost 15 percent of responding programs. Thus, the estimates of treatment delivery and funding are conservative. (How conservative cannot be known unless nonresponse analysis is performed by the original survey contractor.) Moreover, this survey focused only on provider units specializing in drug and alcohol treatment. Probably not included in the NDATUS were such providers as community hospitals that deliver symptomatic treatment (detoxification) in scattered units and private practitioners—psychiatrists, psychologists, and social workers—who do not work in formally identified specialty service units. The 1987 data reported here are based on original analyses of the 1987 NDATUS data tape supplied to the committee by NIDA.

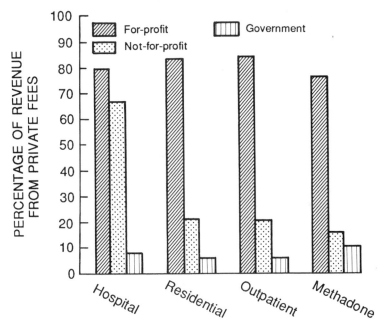

FIGURE 6-1 Defining the two tiers: private fees as a percentage of total revenues, by ownership and facility type. Source: Institute of Medicine analysis of the 1987 National Drug and Alcoholism Treatment Utilization Survey.

Not-for-profit organizations are in the middle but are clearly differentiated by type of facility. More than 66 percent of the revenues of programs that are based in not-for-profit hospitals come from private sources. About 20 percent of the revenues of all other types of not-for-profit providers come from private sources; the remaining 80 percent of their revenues come from public contracts, grants, and reimbursements.

Table 6-1 presents information, divided into the two tiers, on clients, facilities, and service intensity among the providers responding to the NDATUS in 1987. The private tier comprises all for-profit providers plus private not-for-profit hospitals; the public tier comprises all other not-for-profit facilities plus government-owned programs. Private-tier providers received 41 percent of the reported drug treatment expenditures while treating 22 percent of the clients; public-tier providers received 59 percent of total revenues and treated 78 percent of the clients. The average revenue per client admitted to a private-tier program was $2,450, compared with $1,240 per public-tier admission. The primary factor in this difference in revenues is the locus of services offered in the two sectors. About 83 percent of the revenues received by the private tier were generated by hospital-based programs, in contrast to 9 percent in the public tier. Moreover, inpatient and residential revenues per client in private-tier facilities were three to four times greater in private- than in public-tier facilities, although average outpatient revenues per client were nearly identical (Figure 6-2).

The programs of private-tier providers were more service intensive than those of public-tier providers. In the private residential and inpatient setting, there were 7.2 clients per counselor, compared with 9.7 clients per counselor in the public setting. Although the number of clients per counselor in the outpatient setting was more nearly similar for both tiers, private-tier clients were seen more often. However, without adjusting for group versus individual therapy and for the size of the groups, data not available from the NDATUS, these findings concerning personnel ratios must be viewed cautiously. Finally, although much more expensive, the duration of treatment tends to be somewhat shorter in private- than in public-tier facilities. The net impact of these differences vis-à-vis quality of care is difficult to assess because the two systems serve quite different types of clients, and those differences probably extend to client therapeutic needs.

TABLE 6-1   Comparison of Selected Characteristics of the Public and Private Tiers of Drug Treatment

Characteristic	Total	Private	Public
Annual admissions (in thousands)	848	212.4	636.0
Current census (in thousands)	263	47.5	215.9
Capacity (in thousands)	329	72.2	256.5
Capacity utilization	80%	66%	84%
Additional capacity	25%	52%	19%
Revenues (millions of dollars)	1,312	521	791
Revenue per admission	1,550	2,450	1,240
Facilities	5,121	1,275	3,846
Hospitals	960	801	159
Residential	990	76	914
Outpatient	2,765	331	2,434
Methadone	334	67	267
Corrections	72	0	72
Clients per counselor			
Inpatient	9.1	7.2	9.7
Outpatient	38.5	37.3	38.8
Outpatient appointments/week	1.7	1.9	1.65

Source: Institute of Medicine analysis of the 1987 National Drug and Alcoholism Treatment Utilization Survey. Data were provided by the National Institute on Drug Abuse.

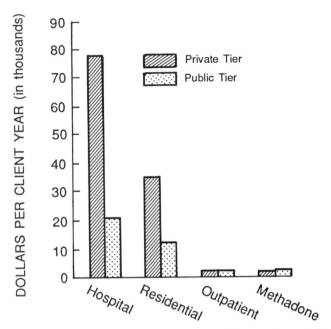

FIGURE 6-2 Two tiers of cost: estimated revenues per client year in each tier, by facility and tier. Source: Institute of Medicine analysis of the 1987 National Drug and Alcoholism Treatment Utilization Survey.

Client Differences

Compared with private-tier clients, public clients have longer histories of drug taking, are more likely to have taken more types of drugs, are less likely to be employed or engaged in other socially conventional activities, are more likely to have major social deficits (e.g., education), and are more likely to have records of criminal activity and involvement with the criminal justice system. These differences are evident in all of the major studies of public-tier clients, including the Drug Abuse Reporting Program, or DARP (Sells, 1974a,b); CODAP, the Client-Oriented Data Acquisition Process; and TOPS, the Treatment Outcome Prospective Study (Hubbard et al., 1989), when contrasted with multiprogram studies of private-tier clients (e.g., the Chemical Abuse/Addiction Treatment Outcome Registry, or CATOR, as reported in Hoffmann and Harrison [1988] and Comprehensive Care Corporation [1988]).

Most of the clients served in the public tier have many deficits such as diminished general health, poor education, and family breakdown. These deficits may be due to their drug problems, or they may predate such problems and exacerbate them. Public-tier providers thus need to have a variety of services at hand to accomplish their therapeutic goals. As a consequence, their staff requirements may well be higher than those of private-tier providers, and the staff patterns shown in Table 6-1 probably mask deep-seated differences in the program resources available to achieve their therapeutic objectives.

Capacity Differences

In 1987 there was considerable excess capacity in the nation's drug treatment system. (The extent of capacity utilization in the two tiers is shown in Table 6-1 and Figure 6-3.) Capacity utilization varies by type of program and by tier. In general, there is considerable excess capacity throughout the private tier and much less in the public tier. There is excess capacity in hospital-based programs but little excess capacity in methadone programs. Nationwide, public methadone programs reported about 5 percent excess capacity—quite a narrow margin as these programs often have unexpected dropouts and chronic staff shortages. The excess capacity is not evenly distributed across the country. Programs in cities and states are virtually full, with long waiting lists. Moreover, excess capacity, particularly in the private tier, does not necessarily mean that there is currently idle or underused staff and space. Rather, it indicates providers' willingness to expand and accept additional clients and to increase staffing and other program inputs appropriately.

THE GROWTH OF THE NATIONAL TREATMENT SYSTEM

Trends in Client Numbers and Provider Characteristics

The characteristics of the national treatment system have changed over time. Most of the data come from the NDATUS series, which has been conducted by the National Institue on Drug Abuse (NIDA) since 1976. The basic trends are shown in Figure 6-4.

In 1976 there were approximately 229,000 individuals in treatment on a daily basis. The majority were in outpatient nonmethadone programs. The next largest group was in methadone maintenance, followed respectively by residential and hospital programs. Enrollment in the residential and outpatient nonmethadone modalities declined steadily from 1976 through 1982, although in some areas of the country, residential treatment enrollment was stable even in the face of dwindling funds. In the subsequent five years, however, residential and outpatient nonmethadone enrollment rebounded dramatically; in contrast, methadone maintenance enrollment remained fairly stable. The methadone census peaked at 80,000 in 1977,

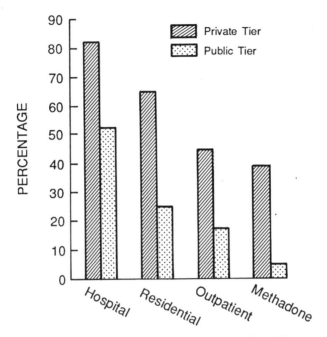

FIGURE 6-3 Additional available treatment capacity in the national drug treatment system by facility type, as a percentage above current client census. Source: Institute of Medicine analysis of the 1987 National Drug and Alcoholism Treatment Utilization Survey.

declined to 68,000 in 1980, and increased to 72,000 in 1982 and to 82,000 in 1987.

In light of the great national concern about drugs and crime, it is surprising to observe that formal drug treatment in correctional settings canvassed by the NDATUS fell steadily from 9,100 clients in 1977 to 6,200 in 1982. This figure was nearly unchanged in 1987, even though the number of inmates had more than doubled during the five-year period. A Bureau of Justice Statistics survey (Innes, 1988) estimated that more than 30,000 state prison inmates were receiving drug treatment in 1986, many of them evidently in programs not recognized and included in the 1987 NDATUS. It is likely that these additional inmates were reporting on drug-specific problems discussed during the course of general prison counseling, education, or medical services.

The most radical changes were in the hospital census, which declined from 5,500 in 1976 to below 3,000 during 1978–1982 and then rebounded to 10,600 in 1987. When the drug treatment system was built up in the early and mid-1970s, hospital-based care was judged to be no more effective in most cases than residential care (or, for many clients, than outpatient

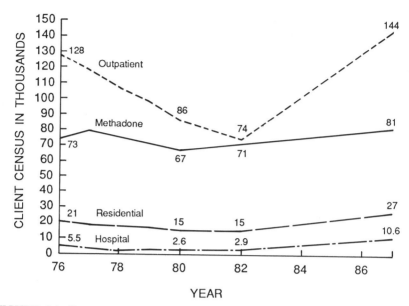

FIGURE 6-4 Drug treatment client census by treatment modality, 1976–1987. Sources: National Institute on Drug Abuse (1976–1980, 1983a) and Institute of Medicine analysis of the 1987 National Drug and Alcoholism Treatment Utilization Survey.

care) in protecting health or promoting recovery, but hospitals were clearly much more expensive (Strategy Council on Drug Abuse, 1975; Besteman, 1990). Therefore, the use of federal drug treatment funds was restricted to medically complicated detoxification; they could not be used for any hospital-based rehabilitation treatment. By October 1987, however, total enrollment in hospital-based detoxification still was only 3,369 clients, but hospital-based inpatient rehabilitation treatment had grown exponentially and was being delivered every day to 7,279 patients.

The parallel trend is in the number of hospitals newly reporting specialty treatment units for drug problems. This type of facility increased from 350 in 1982 to 960 in 1987 and reported a total of 180,000 admissions of individuals for drug problems (21 percent of total 1987 admissions). Five out of six of these hospitals were in the private tier.

Another recent trend is away from programs that mainly treat drug problems and toward units that treat both alcohol and drug problems. Prior to 1982 the majority of drug treatment programs treated drug clients only. This situation has now changed dramatically. The vast majority of programs (80 percent) now treat both drug and alcohol problems. Since the first survey to make the distinction, the 1979 NDATUS, specialty units treating only drug problems have decreased in number from 2,000 to 1,000.

A last major change is in the balance of ownership of programs. The number of government-owned programs has changed little, going from 950 in 1982 to 1,020 in 1987. But private for-profit programs multiplied from 159 units with 9,800 clients (daily count) to 730 units with 29,000 clients. Private not-for-profit units grew from 1,900 to 3,400 programs, with an almost proportionate increase in clientele. Thus, drug treatment facility growth has been largely in the private tier, especially among hospital-based combined drug and alcohol (chemical dependency) units.

In 1987 most of the programs (2,750) in the drug treatment system offered outpatient nonmethadone treatment as their primary modality. Nearly 1,000 hospitals, another 1,000 residential (nonhospital) programs, 330 methadone maintenance outpatient programs, and 72 correctional facilities with specialty drug treatment programs completed the drug abuse treatment system. The total enrollment of 263,000 persons in 1987 was 50 percent greater than in 1982, although only 20 percent larger than in 1976, the first year of the NDATUS. About 848,000 persons were admitted to drug abuse treatment in NDATUS programs during the 12 months preceding the census date, October 31, 1987. A total of 263,000 persons were currently enrolled in drug treatment as of October of that year. Treatment was provided by 5,100 different specialty facilities at an annual cost of $1.3 billion. Additional health care was undoubtedly provided by general health care providers (hospitals with no specialty units, physicians in their offices), but this care was presumably symptomatic in nature (treatment of emergency overdoses, accidents, or infections) and did not constitute efforts to rehabilitate drug abuse or dependence as such.

The vast majority (225,000, or 86 percent) of clients in drug treatment during October 1987 were being treated on an ambulatory basis—either methadone maintenance or outpatient nonmethadone treatment—although previously they may have received inpatient or residential services. The backbone of the public drug treatment system was 3,100 primary ambulatory programs that admitted 506,000 clients in 1987 and had 194,000 clients as their static population number (including a small number temporarily in hospital and residential beds). The 1,950 hospital and residentially based programs in the system admitted 303,000 clients during 1987 and had a static enrollment of 62,000 clients; however, 50 percent of these clients were enrolled in their outpatient (including aftercare) services. Nonhospital residential facilities served 27,000 persons, and hospital inpatient wards, 10,600 persons. Hospital and residential revenues, however, were substantially greater than ambulatory and outpatient receipts.

There were more clients in drug treatment in October 1987 than at any previously recorded date. The 5,100 programs reporting to the NDATUS for 1987 were the largest number ever recorded, up from only 3,000 in 1982.

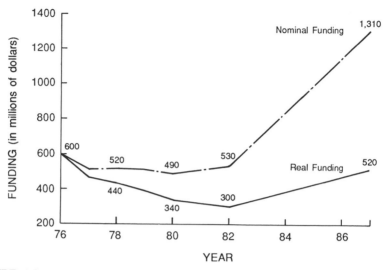

FIGURE 6-5 Drug treatment system funding for 1976–1987 in nominal and real 1976 dollars. Sources: National Institute on Drug Abuse (1976–1980, 1983a); Institute of Medicine analysis of the 1987 National Drug and Alcoholism Treatment Utilization Survey.

Trends in the Funding Base

The specialty drug treatment sector had revenues of $1.3 billion in 1987 (based on the NDATUS), which is sharply above the total system funding of $530 million in 1982 and $500 million to $600 million per year in the 1976–1980 period (Figure 6-5). Yet in terms of real dollars or purchasing power, funding of the national treatment system has seriously deteriorated since the first NDATUS. Adjusting for inflation by using the medical price index, total 1976 funding was worth 15 percent more than total 1987 funding (Figure 6-5). On a per-client basis the real value of funding decreased about 21 percent from 1976 to 1987.[2]

The erosion in funding is further indicated in data on funding per client in single-modality treatment programs from 1976 through 1987 (Figure 6-6). Although the nominal dollar values indicate growing revenue per

---

[2] Inflation adjustment might be performed with the consumer price index (CPI) rather than the medical price index (MPI), but the latter is more realistic because treatment system personnel are hired in the medical labor market. In 1982 the NDATUS (NIDA, 1983a) found that drug program staffs were composed of physicians (3 percent), clinical psychologists (5 percent), social workers (7 percent), nurses (9 percent), counselors (35 percent), other medical and direct care personnel (17 percent), and medical administrators and support staff (24 percent). When the CPI is used for inflation adjustment, real system revenues are 9 percent higher in 1987 than in 1976, and funds per client year are nearly identical.

client over the period, in real terms there was a decrease. The outpatient nonmethadone and the methadone maintenance revenues per client declined by about one-third. The decrease in real expenditures, however, does not necessarily extend to the private tier. In the one meaningful series in which a comparison of modalities in each tier across time is possible, residential treatment per client in the public tier was funded in 1987 at 15 percent below the 1976 level after adjusting for inflation, whereas the private-tier equivalent was about 150 percent higher.

Sources of Treatment Dollars

Underlying the shifts in clients and providers were substantial changes in who paid for treatment (Table 6-2). In 1976 the federal government paid for at least 43 percent of drug treatment (NIDA, 1978), and state and local governments paid for 48 percent. The rest of the funds came from private fees and donations. Since that time, private payments for drug treatment services have increased dramatically and represent the most fundamental financial change in the system, largely corresponding to the increasing treatment of drug problems in private hospital facilities. Even within governmental funding, there has been a distinct trend away from grant funding and toward more use of fee-for-service reimbursements.

In 1987, contracts and vendor reimbursements from states and local governments ($483 million) were the most important sources of revenue

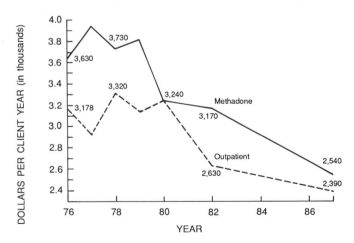

FIGURE 6-6 Annual funding per client year in methadone and outpatient nonmethadone programs during 1976–1987 (in 1987 dollars). Sources: National Institute on Drug Abuse (1976–1980, 1983a); Institute of Medicine analysis of the 1987 National Drug and Alcoholism Treatment Utilization Survey.

TABLE 6-2   Funding of the National Treatment System, 1976–1987, by Year and Final Source of Funding (in millions of dollars)

Source	1976	1977	1978	1979	1980	1982	1987
NIDA/ADAMHA[a]	160.8	119.3	131.6	143.7	127.6	79.4	11.2
Other federal agencies	88.3	50.0	47.4	48.5	44.8	46.1	36.3
State[b]	206.0	177.3	164.5	147.7	133.8	165.4	355.3
Local	77.5	51.2	58.1	43.5	39.9	41.4	64.1
State/local fee-for-service reimbursements	0.0[c]	0.0	0.0	3.2	10.7	16.6	74.3
Welfare/social services	0.0	0.0	25.9	21.6	20.2	22.4	55.8
Public third party	0.0	0.0	0.0	49.5	44.5	62.2	139.5
Private third party	0.0	0.0	0.0	11.2	20.0	43.5	348.1
Client fees	0.0	0.0	17.6	17.2	21.3	35.6	157.3
Other	70.8	112.9	73.0	24.6	23.8	21.1	69.8
Total	603.4	510.7	518.1	510.7	486.6	533.7	1,311.7
Total in 1987 $	1,519.1	1,173.3	1,098.1	990.7	851.0	755.0	1,311.7
Revenue per client in treatment	2,500	2,200	2,400	2,500	2,700	3,100	5,000
Revenue (in 1987 $) per client in treatment	6,300	5,000	5,100	4,900	4,700	4,400	5,000

[a]National Institute on Drug Abuse/Alcohol, Drug Abuse, and Mental Health Administration.

[b]Incorporating federal disbursements (e.g., block grant funds) administered by state authorities.

[c]From 1976–1978, cells reported as "0.0" were included in the "Other" category.

Source: For 1976–1980, data were taken from the National Institute on Drug Abuse reports of data from the National Drug and Alcoholism Treatment Utilization Survey (National Institute on Drug Abuse, 1976–1980). For 1982 data, see National Institute on Drug Abuse (1983a). The figures for 1987 were derived from the Institute of Medicine analysis of the 1987 National Drug and Alcoholism Treatment Utilization Survey.

for drug treatment providers. These monies, however, incorporated federal block grant funds administered by the states. Block grant outlays in FY 1987 are estimated to have been about $110 million, or half of the $220 million available for alcohol and drug treatment (Butynski and Canova, 1988) after the 20 percent set-aside for prevention. State and local governments thus spent about $373 million of their own appropriations for drug treatment, compared with $110 million in federal block grant monies. Programs reported the receipt of another $47 million in federal categorical contracts, $139 million from Medicaid, Medicare, or other public insurance, and $56 million for welfare and social service payments (e.g., housing and food allowances for clients in residential environments). The exact federal share of these later payments is uncertain, but it is assumed to be about 50 percent because the federal contribution to Medicaid is a minimum of 50 percent. Medicare (which is all federal dollars) has historically experienced a small number of claims for drug treatment.

In sum, state and local government expenditures on drug treatment from all sources were approximately $470 million, or 37 percent of total NDATUS expenditures, and the federal contribution was about $250 million, or 19.5 percent of the total (Figures 6-7a and 6-7b). About 36 percent of government treatment expenditures in 1987 (up from 16 percent in 1979) came from public insurance payments (primarily Medicaid), welfare/social

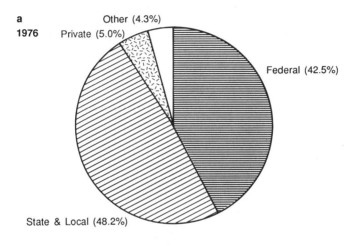

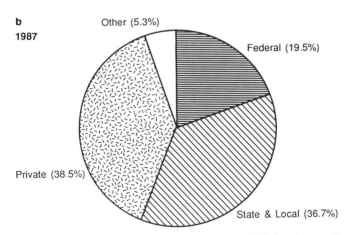

FIGURE 6-7 (a) Funding sources for drug treatment in 1976 (total expenditures: $603 million). Source: National Institute on Drug Abuse (1976–1980). (b) Funding sources for drug treatment in 1987 (total expenditures: $1.311 billion). Source: Institute of Medicine analysis of the 1987 National Drug and Alcoholism Treatment Utilization Survey.

services payments, and local/state government fee-for-service reimbursements. Nongovernmental revenue constituted a large share of total system funding in 1987. With $348 million from private insurance and $157 million from client out-of-pocket payments, private reimbursements totaled $505 million, or 38.5 percent of all revenues.

Trends in Federal Funding

Federal funding has played a major role in shaping the drug treatment system. Nominal federal funding grew from $40 million in FY 1969 to a peak of $300 million in FY 1974; it stabilized at $250 million to $290 million between 1975 and 1980, then rapidly declined to $160 million in 1982 before again growing to $190 million in 1986 and to $370 million in 1987 and 1988 (Figure 6-8). Final figures for 1989 and tentative figures for 1990 are not yet certain, but they are likely to be comparable to those of the late 1970s. These shifts up and down are even more dramatic after adjusting for inflation.

Federal treatment monies directed toward community-based treatment come primarily from Alcohol, Drug Abuse, and Mental Health Administration (ADAMHA) categorical and block grant funds (Table 6-3). These figures also demonstrate the magnitude of fluctuations in federal funding for publicly provided treatment between 1980 and 1990.

It is important to consider the role of treatment in the federal anti-drug abuse strategy. From 1969 to 1975, the federal government put more

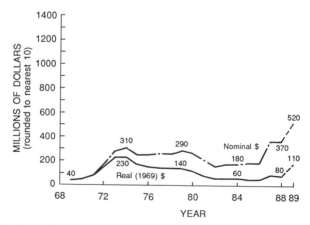

FIGURE 6-8   Federal drug treatment expenditures during FY 1969–1989 (in nominal and real 1969 dollars). Source: Nominal drug expenditure data from the Strategy Council on Drug Abuse (1975 and later years), White House Office of Public Affairs (1988), and Office of National Drug Control Policy (1989). Price deflators were provided by the Bureau of Labor Statistics.

of its anti-drug abuse resources into treatment than into criminal justice or prevention activities. That pattern has now changed. In 1989 criminal justice efforts received an estimated $2.7 billion, compared with $680 million for prevention and $520 million for treatment (Figure 6-9 and Table 6-4).

In summary, the nation's drug treatment system began to erode after 1976. Although the private tier grew steadily all through the 1980s and the public tier has been increasing since the middle of that decade, the drug treatment system is still notably weaker and smaller than it was in 1976 in aggregate funds and in resources per client served. Sources of overall

TABLE 6-3   Federal Appropriations (in millions of dollars) for Drug, Alcohol, and Mental Health Treatment Provided Through Alcohol, Drug Abuse, and Mental Health Administration (ADAMHA)-Administered Categorical and Block Grants, 1980–1989

Year	ADMS[a] Block Grant	ADTR Supplement[b]	Estimated Portion for Drug Treatment[c]
1980	625[d]	—	256
1981	543	—	136
1982	428	—	107
1983	468	—	117
1984	462	—	92
1985	490	—	98
1986	468	—	93
1987	508	163	167
1988	487	156	160
1989 (est.)	765[e]	—	260
1990 (tent.)	1,133[f]	—	448

[a] Alcohol, drug, and mental health services (ADMS).

[b] Alcohol and drug treatment (ADTR) supplemental 1987–1988 appropriations.

[c] Approximately half of the ADMS block grant was for drug and alcohol treatment. All of the ADTR monies were for drug and alcohol treatment. Congress instituted a 20 percent set-aside of the block grant funds for prevention services in 1984. Approximately half of the block grant substance abuse treatment funds have been spent on drug treatment. Statutorily, *not less than* 35 percent of the substance abuse monies could be spent on either drug or alcohol treatment.

[d] In 1980 this figure was an aggregate of categorical grant programs for alcohol, drug, and mental health services. In later years these funds were collapsed into the ADMS block grant.

[e] The 1989 appropriation of $805.6 million was effectively reduced to $765 million by a 10 percent set-aside for data collection, technical assistance, and services research.

[f] Adding the 1990 tentative set-aside of 5 percent yields the actual block grant total ($1.192 billion).

Source: Unpublished data from the ADAMHA Office for Treatment Improvement.

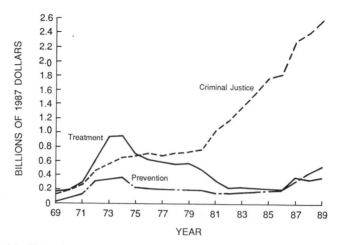

FIGURE 6-9   Federal anti-drug abuse funding for FY 1969–1989 (in 1987 dollars). Source: Nominal drug expenditure data from the Strategy Council on Drug Abuse (1975 and later years), White House Office of Public Affairs (1988), and Office of National Drug Control Policy (1989). Price deflators were provided by the Bureau of Labor Statistics.

support for the treatment system have changed materially. The governmental share—particularly that of the federal government—has declined, whereas private reimbursements have been growing. Even with the recent large increases in funding through the Anti-Drug Abuse Acts of 1986 and 1988 and the emergency ADAMHA appropriation for FY 1990, federal support for treatment in inflation-adjusted dollars is still well below the level achieved in 1973–1974.

CONCLUSION

The most important feature of the nation's drug treatment supply system is its very clear division between two tiers of providers that differ in financing, origins, clientele, capacity utilization, and modalities. There is a public tier of mostly outpatient and residential programs for indigent clients, many with serious criminal records and other social deficits, that is about 20 years old; and there is a smaller private tier of mostly hospital-based programs for middle- and upper-class clients, which is effectively about 10 years old.

The 1987 NDATUS, although a limited and imperfect instrument of observation, gives the clearest available picture of the two tiers. Its data show a private tier composed of 1,275 treatment providers, all of whom were receiving at least half (on average, more than three-quarters) of their revenues from client fees or private third-party reimbursements. More than

800, or 63 percent, of these private-tier providers were in-hospital programs (both for profit and not for profit); about 25 percent (334) were outpatient programs; and the remaining 11 percent were about evenly divided between residential and methadone programs.

The public tier revealed by the 1987 NDATUS comprised 3,846 providers receiving on average just below one-fifth of their revenues from client fees or private reimbursements. More than 2,400 (63 percent) of these programs were outpatient facilities (largely private, not-for-profit contractors); 24 percent (914) were residential facilities; and the remaining 13 percent were divided among methadone programs (267), government hospitals (159), and correctional programs (72).

The private tier treated 22 percent of all reported admissions and received 41 percent of system revenues; it averaged $2,450 per treated client, double the $1,240 average in the public tier. This cost difference was largely attributable to two factors. Most private-tier (but relatively little

TABLE 6-4 Federal Anti-Drug Abuse Expenditures (in millions of dollars) for Treatment, Prevention, and Criminal Justice: Obligations for Fiscal Years 1969–1989 Provided in Nominal and Inflation-adjusted Figures

Year	Nominal Dollars[a]		Criminal Justice	Real 1987 Dollars[b]		Criminal Justice
	Treatment	Prevention		Treatment	Prevention	
1969	40	10	40	160	20	120
1970	50	20	60	190	70	180
1971	80	50	90	290	130	260
1972	170	110	170	600	310	460
1973	280	140	210	950	350	540
1974	310	160	280	960	360	640
1975	250	110	320	700	230	660
1976	250	110	360	620	210	700
1977	260	110	370	590	200	670
1978	260	110	420	560	190	720
1979	290	120	470	560	190	730
1980	270	140	550	480	190	770
1981	210	120	810	330	150	1,030
1982	160	120	980	230	150	1,180
1983	180	140	1,190	240	160	1,370
1984	180	150	1,420	230	170	1,560
1985	190	180	1,670	220	190	1,780
1986	190	190	1,760	200	190	1,830
1987	370	320	2,290	370	320	2,290
1988	370	450	2,490	340	440	2,400
1989	520	680	2,660	450	630	2,460

[a]Nominal drug expenditure data are taken from Strategy Council on Drug Abuse (1975 and later years), White House Office of Public Affairs (1988), and Office of National Drug Control Policy (1989).

[b]Price deflators were provided by the Bureau of Labor Statistics.

public-tier) treatment takes place in hospitals, which are more expensive than other settings; moreover, the average per diem charge in private-tier hospital programs is about four times as high as the average charge in public-tier hospital programs. There is also a threefold average differential between the costs of private and public nonhospital residential programs. Only the outpatient (methadone and nonmethadone) programs were similar in cost in the two tiers.

The level of per diem support per client in the public tier fell substantially from the mid-1970s to the mid-1980s, although there has been a notable recovery in the past three years. The actual cost of delivering treatment has not declined; rather, the intensity and breadth of program services and the experience levels of public-tier staff have been reduced. The public tier was originally built, staffed, and trained in the early 1970s largely with federal dollars, under an explicit plan to steadily reduce the federal contribution and increase state and local dollars in proportion. Something like this has occurred, but the federal decline has been much more pronounced than the state and local increases. This pattern is attributable to a general shrinkage in public services and a more specific shift back toward the criminal approach to drug problems, rather than to patterns or trends in the severity of the drug problem—the epidemiological trends in dependence during the early part of this period were stable and in the latter part have been rising.

Private drug treatment was a small, nearly invisible presence throughout the 1970s but then began exponential growth after 1980. This growth largely involved increasing delivery of drug treatment in preexisting or newly opening alcoholism treatment units, which began to see increasing numbers of alcohol/drug and drug-only (mostly marijuana and cocaine) clients among their insured clientele; some programs also began aggressive efforts to reach more such patients as the incidence of alcoholism stopped growing during the 1980s. The extension of alcoholism treatment capacity to drug treatment occurred in the public tier as well and is manifest in the sizable increase in the self-designation of NDATUS treatment units as combined alcohol/drug providers. There was also a large expansion of private methadone programs as political opposition to methadone maintenance combined with budgetary pressures to close down existing public methadone clinics.

How well does the treatment system match current demand and the estimated need for services? In the 1987 NDATUS, reports of additional treatment capacity (which the committee has interpreted to mean idle capital assets, adequate licensing and use permits, and access to additional personnel comparable in training to those already employed) was highest (more than 50 percent above the current census) in private and public hospitals and in private-tier residential facilities; it was lowest in public-tier methadone and outpatient facilities. There were substantial regional differences in public-tier capacity; consequently, some areas of the country are sorely pressed for public-tier residential treatment as well.

The two tiers are so differently configured that it is not sensible, in the committee's judgment, to try to engage more private-tier capacity on a large scale for public use. There is a need for expansion of the public tier—but with an important reservation. The current resource intensity of many public-tier programs is marginal at best. Expansion will reduce and dilute this intensity unless careful countermeasures are taken. The need for more resource-intensive treatment appears at least equal in importance to increases in capacity. Rigorous data on the clinical effectiveness of more intensive resources per patient are too sparse to permit certainty or precision on this point, but the most sensible course, in the committee's judgment, is to divide increased public resources between improving the quality of services, facilities, and staff skills and increasing the capacity for new admissions. A high priority should also be assigned to creating data resources and analyses that will permit a close look at the relation of service intensity, quality, and treatment outcomes.

Although the rise in severe cocaine problems has meant reductions in opiate drug use in some areas, overall this trend has added to rather than undercut other drug problems such as heroin dependence. Because methadone maintenance—provided at adequate levels and with supporting services—is the most rigorously validated treatment for heroin dependence, there is good reason to put additional resources into this modality in areas of the country where need and demand for it are strongest, keeping in mind the general principle of improving treatment resource intensity in parallel with capacity. The private tier may be capable of offering methadone treatment as efficiently as the public tier, although the scarcity of evaluation research on private-tier methadone treatment warrants serious caution.

7

Public Coverage

The question of whether there should be a large-scale system of publicly supported drug treatment was answered affirmatively in the 1970s. That answer has been reaffirmed in the past few years, and the committee's analysis to this point has not raised any fundamental new doubts. With the existence and legitimacy of the public tier no longer at issue, the questions for public coverage are instead ones of management objectives and techniques. The task of this chapter is to consider the present system of public coverage in light of the needs, wants, and demands placed on it and to make appropriate recommendations for improvement.

First, it is necessary to frame the fundamental policy questions that those responsible for public coverage of drug treatment should address—a critically important endeavor. Even when some of the answers can only be provisional, approximate, or resolvable by public debate and political negotiation, asking the right questions is essential in order to assemble relevant evidence and give rational shape to the decision-making process.

Policy has to do with ends and means. The committee sees three questions under each of these categories. In deciding on the ends of treatment policy, the questions are as follows:

- What are the fundamental principles that justify public coverage of drug treatment? Or, whose treatment should public funds cover, and why?
- What priorities should guide the current expansion of public coverage?

● What is the optimal level of public spending to implement these priorities?

The committee identifies as principles that public coverage should seek to remedy treatment constraints that arise from inadequate income and to reduce external social costs, particularly those relating to crime and family role dysfunctions. Such efforts often require actively inducing people to seek treatment through a variety of methods, as well as seeking mechanisms to increase retention (e.g., legal coercion, outreach efforts, enhanced social services). Four specific priorities flow from these principles and conform to the committee's empirical analysis: reduce admission delays, improve program quality and performance, reach out to young mothers, and treat more criminal justice clients. This chapter outlines three progressive strategy options for public decision makers to consider: a core spending strategy, an intermediate plan, and a comprehensive option.

The priorities and expenditure patterns recommended in this chapter should not be implemented without reconsidering the adequacy of present means for managing the public tier. These considerations divide into three instrumental questions:

● What should be the respective state and federal roles in public coverage of drug treatment?
● What are the most appropriate financial mechanisms for providing public support—essentially, to what degree should the emphasis be on direct service programs versus public insurance?
● What disciplines or controls should be in place to ensure that public expenditures for drug treatment are appropriate and effective?

State governments have played the major role in financial administration and quality control of drug treatment in recent years. Now, however, the federal government, in pumping major new funds into treatment, is reasserting its earlier leading role. It should take this opportunity to rebuild important directional and accountability mechanisms and to prepare the ground for later introduction of a larger share of public insurance financing. (However, public insurance financing will never obviate the need for direct service support of critical program elements such as outreach and integration with nonhealth services.) Routine outcome measurement, training and technical assistance, gatekeeping functions, and performance contracting will be the keys to upgrading drug treatment and introducing it permanently into the mainstreams of health and human services.

THE PRINCIPLES OF PUBLIC INTERVENTION

Twenty-five years ago, publicly supported drug treatment in the United States was confined to the provision of certain therapeutic amenities at four correctional facilities. Each site admitted hundreds of drug-abusing and dependent individuals in a given year; most of them were convicted of narcotics violations, but some of them were volunteers requesting treatment. Two of the facilities were large federal prison-hospitals, at Lexington, Kentucky, for the eastern United States and at Fort Worth, Texas, for the West; the others were specialized rehabilitation prisons operated by the two most populous states at Rikers Island, New York, and Corona, California.

The challenges of financing and managing public-sector treatment have changed markedly since that time. Instead of four prison treatment sites, there are several thousand public-tier programs in communities and institutions in every state, treating well over 600,000 annual admissions and interacting with federal institutes, state offices, county agencies, elected officials, local bureaucracies of criminal justice, education, welfare, and health care organizations, and occasionally even private insurers. The issue certainly is not whether there will be large-scale public support for treatment but how much, what kinds, and for whom.

The reasons why society has become interested in treating illicit drug abuse are neither strictly hard-headed nor purely idealistic but rather a combination of the two. These reasons have moved the public not only to permit treatment of illicit drug abuse and dependence in community settings but also to enhance the amount of treatment taking place by substantially reducing the price that the majority of individuals pay for treatment to well below the cost of providing it—often, in fact, to nothing.

To better understand the logic by which the government arrives at the "right" level of support, it is necessary to grasp firmly the specific rationale for these public subsidies. The reasons for supporting public treatment fit comfortably within the realm of conventional justifications for other public health measures, but that is a very broad realm, indeed (Institute of Medicine, 1988a). In the case of public drug treatment, there are important specific emphases that ought to be made explicit.

External Costs

Individuals who can be clinically identified as meeting the criteria for drug treatment (whether or not they are interested in treatment to help extinguish their drug-seeking behavior) generally impose serious burdens on other members of society. The harm to victims of violent crime, the damages to the well-being and future prospects of the individual's family, the risk of transmitting hepatitis or HIV infection, and other such burdens are called externalities, or external costs. The problem with external costs is that, unlike the self-imposed consequences of actions, they do not automatically discipline or instruct the individual, which is usually the way harmful behavior is corrected.

Solutions to external cost problems ordinarily take one of two forms. One form is to reassign these costs to the individuals who produce them through selective taxes or confiscations, civil liability, or the imposition of criminal sanctions such as fines or incarceration. Taxing and confiscating the proceeds of illicit drug-related behavior have proved to be difficult and frequently haphazard endeavors; moreover, the individuals who originally impose the external costs are often too poor to pay commensurate civil or criminal fines. Determining an appropriate fine for transmitting serious and even deadly diseases is beyond nearly anyone's capacity. With legislatively mandated sentencing, the consequent sanction for such individuals has increasingly become jail or prison—the individual is made to pay a liberty price as a "just desert." What this measure emphasizes is less the burden of harm to individual others and more the moral weight of the drug offense; and it is a moral calculus that assigns the exaction due—the criminal's "debt to society."

Nevertheless, this price may be considered unsatisfactory in at least two ways. In the first instance, the penal strategy generally does not fully reassign the social costs because society has to pay a substantial price to impose deprivations of liberty on unwilling individuals. Second, to date, imprisonment has not had enough of the desired effect: individuals who have paid the price of incarceration have all too frequently (at the rate of about three felons out of four) come out of prison and reimposed the same criminal burdens on society.

There is also a third dissatisfaction. Society is uneasy about the strictly criminal approach to drug consumption. However broad the consensus on maintaining criminal penalties, particularly for trafficking offenses, the historical streams of libertarian and medical ideas continue to affect the nation's collective thinking. Although clearly in the minority, there are respectable voices questioning the entire wisdom of drug laws, even from within the bastions of the criminal justice system. In contrast, no such voices rise in dissent regarding laws that proscribe homicide, sexual assault, robbery, or grand theft (auto).

These shortcomings of the criminal approach, in particular, the first two, led originally to the development of the public tier of treatment. As a result of studies in public-tier programs, which are reviewed in Chapter 5, there are now reasonable grounds to believe that at least some modalities of treatment do in fact reduce the external costs of drug abuse and dependence in greater measure than the cost of the treatment itself. Moreover, in doing so, treatment provides some benefits that drug-abusing and drug-dependent individuals themselves seek (although it often takes a substantial amount of exterior pressure or interior misery—or both—to bring them to that point).

This last statement brings up the second mode of dealing with externalities (the first being to reassign the external costs): design positive incentives to induce the persons who are producing external costs to stop. Incentives are a carrot that often accompanies the stick of penalties. The committee's review in Chapter 4 indicates that the treatment motivations of drug-abusing and drug-dependent individuals are usually ambivalent, with some degree of desire for recovery, some degree of pressure to avoid drugs, and some degree of desire and compulsion to continue seeking drugs; in other words, applicants show an interest in the benefits of treatment mixed with hostility toward its constraints. Under these circumstances, the money price of treatment may for some fraction of individuals play a pivotal role in determining whether treatment is sought or how much treatment is utilized. For relatively inexpensive treatment such as outpatient care, a partial subsidy may make a difference; for relatively expensive residential or inpatient treatment, the cost is high enough that a subsidy may be critical to whether an individual actually receives treatment.

A complication enters here, namely, the relationship between public and private benefit. If both the individual and society would benefit from the individual's positive response to treatment, then who should pay for it? One approach is to say that the answer should depend on the proportions of public and private benefit; a second is to express a strong preference for maximizing private payments (for example, through sliding-scale fees); a third strategy is to put the fullest onus on public payment. To be completely efficient in the use of public funding, one would want to lower prices *discriminately*. No one who is prepared to purchase treatment on his or her own at its market price (the cost of production plus markups, reserves, or profit margins, adjusted to competition) should be subsidized. Subsidies should go only to those who would purchase treatment at some below-market price, and the amount should be only what is necessary in each case to assure the purchase.

If the external costs of untreated drug consumption (which, on average, treatment can be expected to reduce significantly) exceed the costs of treatment by a large amount and there are individuals who need treatment but do not want it even at zero cost, then the public might even find it optimal to create a "negative price." A negative price is an inducement to enter and stay in treatment that exceeds the minimum cost of helping clients to extinguish drug seeking. The extreme case of a negative price is cash inducement: paying people to enter treatment. A more palatable alternative is incentives in kind, such as amenities that are not strictly needed for treatment (even though some may in fact prove to make treatment more effective)—for example, attractive facilities, free coffee, or assistance in dealing with a variety of other social, medical, or psychological problems.

Intrinsic medication effects may fulfill this incentive function. For example, clinically optimal levels of either methadone or naltrexone "block" the euphoric effects of any other opiates. But the very mild analgesic properties of stabilized methadone doses, in contrast to the virtually complete lack of perceptible effects of naltrexone maintenance, constitute a positive inducement, which may help to explain why methadone maintenance typically retains a substantial percentage of clients whereas naltrexone retains very few.

In summary, the combination of high external costs and a reluctant clientele may lead society to want not only to provide treatment for illicit drug abuse and dependence at a reduced cost but even to provide some selected inducements, at least to some potential clients, that go beyond the cost of bare-bones treatment. (A more technical analysis of the issue of treatment demand and pricing is sketched in Figure 7-1.)

Income Constraints

Whether or not the external social costs equal or exceed—and hence begin to efficiently justify—treatment expenditures, there is a second major reason for public support of treatment: the problem of income constraints, or the fact that some people are simply too poor to afford the cost of treatment even if they are very interested in obtaining it. In some respects, society has taken a broad ethical position on income constraints, namely, that there are certain goods and services that should never be denied to anyone on the grounds of inadequate income. Generally, these goods and services fall into one of two categories: items that everyone needs at some minimum level but that most people can afford (e.g., food and shelter) and items that only a few people (relatively speaking) might need very badly at any one time but that most cannot afford at all or without undergoing some severe degree of hardship—for example, major medical care.

Drug treatment appears to belong in the second category. In these kinds of cases, the government has both encouraged the formation of private compacts (using tax incentives and regulatory guarantees) to help the individual in need—employer-sponsored health insurance is the prime example—and has entered directly into the sponsorship of such arrangements, most prominently in the Medicare program. But private insurance and Medicare share the characteristic that eligibility for these forms of coverage depends on making (or having made) ongoing contributions to an insurance pool through regular premiums that are matched by an employer and/or deducted from a steadily incoming paycheck.

This form of coverage is inapplicable to individuals who do not belong to a private group health insurance plan and are too young (or otherwise lack qualifications) for Medicare eligibility. At a minimum, this group includes an estimated 31 million individuals who are without any health insurance (Moyer, 1989; cf. Chollet, 1988). It may also include an additional

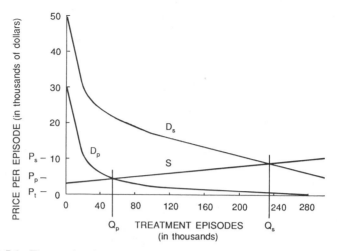

FIGURE 7-1 The market for drug treatment showing private and public demand. The great force of external cost considerations affects the whole market for treatment. If treatment episodes are expected to provide benefits to the public beyond those to the recipient by reducing the external costs of untreated drug problems, then that expectation should be reflected in the market by raising the demand schedule for treatment. In other words, at any given price, the amount of treatment demanded should be greater than just that sought by individual clients. This increase in the demand for treatment, which results from including the benefits to the general public, implies that the socially optimal amount of treatment is greater than the amount that would be provided in a completely private treatment market.

This principle is illustrated in conventional economic terms in the figure, which is hypothetical but modeled on realistic assumptions. The purely private market for treatment is represented by the downward-sloping demand curve D_p and the supply curve S. Their intersection shows the average price, P_p, and total quantity, Q_p, of drug treatment episodes that would be delivered in the private marketplace if the government did not intervene. The public benefit from treatment dictates that the social demand for treatment, curve D_s, is higher than the purely private demand for treatment, curve D_p, and the quantity of treatment desired at any price is accordingly greater. When the social value of treatment is recognized in the demand schedule D_s, the socially optimal amount of treatment is indicated by the intersection of the new demand curve and the supply curve. The socially optimal quantity of treatment Q_s is greater than the quantity delivered in the private market Q_p. To achieve utilization of treatment at the socially optimal level Q_s, subsidization of treatment must be undertaken (by means of governmental or philanthropic subsidies) to make up the difference between P_s, the price of inducing the socially optimal level of treatment, and P_t, the average price that many potential clients would actually be prepared to pay for that many episodes of treatment.

13 million people covered by Medicaid plans and 48 million with private health plans that lack specified coverage for drug treatment services. These 61 million people are covered for emergency services (e.g., drug overdoses) and treatment of physical sequelae of drugs; many would probably be covered for some types of treatment of drug problems under general plan

provisions; and some could afford to pay drug treatment costs out of pocket. In the committee's judgment, however, a large proportion of the 61 million individuals in this country without specified coverage for drug treatment are not covered by their health insurance for appropriate drug treatment in the event they were to need it.

There are, in other words, at least 31 million and possibly 92 million individuals for whom insurance coverage of drug treatment may be unavailable when it is needed; absent stronger data, the approximate midpoint of this range, 60 million, is a reasonable figure to use. For many of these individuals, the out-of-pocket costs of treatment are formidable, particularly for residential or hospital treatment. The committee hazards the further estimate that one-third of the 31 million individuals who are uninsured and one-half of the 30 million who are insufficiently covered might be able to afford outpatient treatment out of pocket. This still leaves roughly 35 million individuals who could not do so and who would qualify as indigent with regard to buying any form of drug treatment. For residential treatment, the committee's estimate of the number who would be considered indigent rises to 60 million.

If society does not want to see drug treatment denied to persons in this group as a result of income constraints, the standard solution is to develop a scheme of differential pricing, which enables the relatively indigent person to pay a below-market price for treatment through a government subsidy or service program, contingent on an accurate determination of his or her level of income or wealth. The income criterion could be graduated according to circumstances; the guiding principle is that the price of treatment should be brought below whatever threshold rules out the individual being able to purchase the needed treatment or at which paying for treatment would create undue hardship. In many cases, using this guideline means the price must be effectively zero.

Positive Response to Treatment

There is a third principle besides external costs and income constraints that is worth mentioning: the treatment should do good; that is, the client should respond well. Of course, some do not. There are public clients who never achieve significant reductions in their drug-seeking and other criminal behavior (when the latter is present to begin with) during treatment. When those who are not responding well leave treatment, their departure cannot be called an effective result. Yet it does achieve the virtue of efficiency, in that no further money is wasted. When the public (or any other third party) is paying the bill for treatment, the most troubling problem is individuals who neither modify their behavior positively *nor* leave treatment.

There are not many such people, particularly in the more intensive and demanding programs and modalities. For the most part, people who stay in treatment do well as long as they are in it, and they either drop out or are discharged when their behavior deteriorates and therapeutic corrections (if the program makes them) are unsuccessful. This is not to say that most people in treatment are absolutely crime and drug free but that unmistakable improvement over pretreatment conditions is very much the day-to-day norm.

In principle, there should be no coverage of individuals who are not expected to respond positively to treatment. But prognostic precision is simply not acute enough to draw bright exclusionary lines. Even previous treatment failure is no sure guide because the route to recovery often leads through several such misfires.[1] In drug treatment, *as in virtually all medical care for severe, chronic conditions*, the limited capacity to accurately predict individual responses dictates that this principle be applied sparingly, usually on a retrospective rather than prospective basis, therefore erring on the side of treating too many rather than too few. In practice, denial on the grounds of expected nonresponse is exercised very little at the point of admission; instead, it is a judgment made by clients (through voluntary attrition), by clinicians (through discharge decisions), or by third parties such as police officers (by arresting violators of the law).

Balancing Treatment Needs and Cost Concerns

With declining budgets the norm from the mid-1970s until fairly recently, one must assume that there will be continuing budget constraints on drug treatment dollars. It is difficult to believe, despite notable recent budget increases by the federal government and a few states, that the day may come when public treatment funds overshoot the need for treatment. Ideally, to make the best decisions with limited budget dollars, one should look at every individual for whom a legitimate argument for public support could be made, evaluate the strength of the argument in each instance in terms of relative costs and benefits, and apply a triage or optimizing procedure to achieve the most efficient distribution of limited funds—that is, to get the greatest return on the investment of each treatment dollar. This triage would apply not only to whether an individual needed treatment but also to how intensive (and expensive) a treatment is needed for optimal results.

However, to calculate precisely for each drug-abusing and dependent

---

[1] Treatment programs do in fact exclude some people whose personal history is unpromising. However, these negative prognostic signs are attended to mostly out of a desire to minimize the risks that nonresponding behavior will disrupt other clients or endanger the clinical setting—for example, programs are leery of admitting individuals who are chronically assaultive or known as large-volume drug traffickers.

individual the extent of attributable external costs, the ability to pay, the relative strengths of the desire for and hostility toward treatment (including the potency of exterior and interior pressures), and the probabilities of response to the various treatment options is a complex and demanding assignment. The specific information needed about individual and program performance, the cost to collect and evaluate it, and the sheer conceptual challenge are all extensive, and there would be unavoidable residual uncertainties about the results, in light of the current and foreseeable state of the prognostic arts.

Instead of trying to exact the last ounce of efficiency by fine-tuning the structure of price subsidies, some simpler rules of thumb may be (and generally are) employed. For example, ability to pay is usually determined by a preset income maximum that for convenience may be equivalent to local standards for welfare (and Medicaid) eligibility; copayments, if required, are graduated according to very broad income levels, and external cost and motivational issues are seldom explicitly considered in determining direct charges to patients (although they may be very important in admission and treatment planning decisions). Income is obliquely taken as an index of external costs in that low-income drug-abusing and dependent individuals are considered very likely to resort to criminal activities to pay for their drugs.

The committee believes it is clear that external cost and income considerations are already firmly incorporated into public decisions about the coverage of drug treatment. The external costs, particularly in terms of violent crime and increasingly in terms of harm to young children's lives, have been uppermost in importance. These considerations have been reinforced by the second type of concern—that treatment should not be appreciably less available to the poor than to the well-off and well-insured because it is mostly poor individuals who commit violent crimes and whose children are least protected from neglect or abandonment. There is a further overtone of concern (an echo of the 1960s War on Poverty) that general conditions of racial and income inequality might help cause and perpetuate drug problems and retard recovery, further reinforcing the urgency of public intervention.

The principal decision criterion in public coverage is and should be to make publicly subsidized treatment available to those who are doubly needy—those who most need treatment according to clinical criteria and who most need financial help to afford it.[2] Generally, having a serious

---

[2] Exact titration of the inability to pay, so as to marginally reduce public payments to those who are partially able financially, may be expensive and may reduce the desirable incentives that help draw reluctant individuals into treatment; in other words, the resulting revenue gains from copayment requirements may not be worth it. However, the introduction of means-based copayment requirements for long-term outpatient treatment, such as methadone maintenance, would make sense once stabilization of behavior had occurred. Similarly, a payback principle in kind or in

need for treatment stands as a guarantee or, at least, makes it quite probable that external costs are present; moreover, the less the individual's legitimate financial capacity, the greater these external costs are likely to be. In general, the principle of covering the needy should be applied not only to all those who readily seek treatment but also to all others who can by legitimate means be induced to seek it. Considerations of external costs further argue that there is reason to create incentives beyond minimal coverage of bare-bones programs. Just as the external costs of crime justify negative incentives—coercion by the criminal justice system, which may be helpful in steering individuals toward treatment—these costs justify positive incentives to some degree, provided they can induce greater motivation and better retention in treatment. The external costs of poor job performance and parental deficiencies may justify positive incentives as well, given that criminal justice coercion of drug-abusing and dependent individuals who are steadily employed or taking care of children, or both, may be impractical or unlikely.

In summary, the committee recommends that the principle of public coverage be to provide adequate support for appropriate and timely admission, completion, or maintenance of good-quality treatment for individuals who cannot pay for it, either fully or partly. Public coverage should be invoked whenever such individuals *need* treatment, according to the best professional judgment, and *seek* treatment, or can be *induced* through acceptable means to pursue it, assuming there is some probability of positive response.

FROM PRINCIPLES TO PRIORITIES

Chapter 3 concluded that the aggregate need for treatment in the United States at any one time in 1988 involved about 2.5 million drug-dependent individuals and 3 million more individuals who were at least abusing drugs. Chapter 6 indicated that the 1987 survey of treatment providers found about 260,000 clients in treatment at that time, with total annual admissions numbering 850,000. Even allowing for an incomplete count of providers, it is clear that the need for drug treatment according to relevant diagnostic criteria exceeds the number of annual admissions by a substantial amount.[3]

---

dollars for successful graduates of therapeutic communities or other programs may also make sense; the prevalence of supportive "alumni groups" and "thirteenth-steppers" reflects this idea.

[3] Of course, there are also dynamic considerations: 4 million young people newly enter the prime onset period each year, and an unknown number leave the drug scene. Appendix 7B contains some additional comments on the need for dynamic analysis.

Given the preponderant number of treatment applicants who already seek help from the public tier, their generally low income, the prevalence of criminal histories among individuals needing treatment, and the substantial excess of supply over demand in the private tier (even allowing that this last situation has something to do with cost-containment pressures), the committee estimates that between 60 and 80 percent of those needing treatment for illicit drug abuse and dependence belong in the public tier. The apparent excess of current need for treatment over annual admissions is on the order of 2 million to 3 million individuals.

This disproportion between the need for treatment and the number of people receiving treatment seems inconsistent with indications that more potentially usable treatment resources are on hand in some states (and in some programs in other states) than are being utilized. Much of the disproportion is attributable to the circumstance that needing treatment is not the same as wanting it or being able to pay for it, either individually or with assistance. But bringing these elements into better balance is not a simple task. For one thing, despite the recent large increases in federal appropriations for treatment, there is clearly not enough money actually available as yet in the field to implement the principles summarized above. And even if the budgetary commitment to that end were firm, creating actual effective treatment capacity will take time, trial and error, and hard work. Priorities must be established. Where should new monies and energies go first?

This choice is clearly a matter of informed judgment. In light of the principles articulated above and the current status of the public treatment system, **the committee's recommendation is that priority be given to the following:**

- **closing the most obvious regional gaps in coverage—that is, reducing delays in admission as evidenced by waiting lists for treatment;**
- **improving the average quality, performance, and retention rates of existing modalities by raising the level of service intensity, personnel quality, and experience; by having programs assume more integrative roles with respect to related services; and by instituting systematic performance monitoring and follow-up;**
- **expanding treatment through more aggressive outreach to pregnant women and young mothers, those for whom it promises the greatest potential reduction in external social costs; and**
- **further expanding community and institutionally based treatment services to provide treatment to drug-abusing and dependent individuals under criminal justice supervision.**

Eliminate Waiting Lists

There are individuals who want treatment now as it is currently offered but who are stymied by the constraints on its availability. The best estimate of the number of such individuals comes from a survey of 43 states conducted by the National Association of State Alcohol and Drug Abuse Directors (NASADAD) in September 1989, which indicated that 66,000 individuals were awaiting treatment admission. This figure is equivalent to more than a quarter of the total daily enrollment in public-tier programs.

The 1988 Anti-Drug Abuse Act included a one-time grant program providing $100 million for the reduction of waiting lists. Because this is a one-time allocation, many programs have been leery of applying for the funding: the implication of expanding admissions is to commit to additional space and staffing, and such a commitment would fly in the face of the nonrenewability of these funds. Programs that have waiting lists have found that when they are able to accelerate admissions as a result of expanded capacity, they attract even more applications. The committee believes it is more realistic to consider current waiting lists a minimum estimate of the sustained size of additional interest in treatment and therefore to anticipate a continued increase in service requirements that is at least equal to current waiting lists.

Improve Treatment

The upgrading of program performance and quality levels is intrinsic to the other priorities and would be needed even if expanded treatment admissions were not an objective. The recent diminution of treatment program resources from the middle 1970s to the late 1980s hobbled many programs' capacity to provide treatment as effectively as the state of the art permitted. Research findings about large variations in program performance and the consistent importance of retention in predicting outcome all support the need to upgrade per capita funding, quality, and retention levels in treatment.

The evidence on the specific components of drug treatment effectiveness and attractiveness is beguiling but slender. One must depend to a large extent on a few careful studies done in methadone programs, on the judgment of experienced clinicians, and on organizational common sense. Some of the personal characteristics, skills, or procedures followed by individual drug counselors make a measurable difference in their clients' performance. Other professionals can usually detect or recognize these qualities (although in the absence of definitive studies, they differ in how to describe them), and there is a market for good therapists whose talents have been honed on difficult cases, such as drug-dependent criminals. Traditionally, clinical staff in public programs are attractive recruits for private practices or agencies that offer higher pay and a less demanding clientele.

Moreover, staff who are overloaded with cases and working in organizations that are underendowed with positive incentives sometimes "burn out": they may simply lose their enthusiasm and effectiveness or actually leave the program. Incentives and tools for upgrading clinical practices, which were a critical part of the agenda of public-tier programs in the early 1970s, have been casualties of retrenchment; in particular, periodic retraining and technical assistance and well-designed systems of performance monitoring diminished and nearly disappeared in the 1980s.

The chronic inability of public programs in recent years to keep caseloads within reason and to attract or retain the best counselors is a fundamental problem that more per capita funding can help solve. The same solution applies to reversing the erosion of clinical tools and service intensity. A prominent program need is to be able to afford more frequent and more accurate random drug tests whose results are available quickly. Of at least comparable importance is the systematic multidimensional assessment of client needs and the provision, where indicated, of vocational, educational, and specialized psychiatric and medical services; these services may be provided either by incorporation of such capacities into the program or by referral (particularly, funded referral) to other service agencies *and systematic follow-up with them*. For example, treating cocaine requires increased use of physicians, nurses, and pharmacists to monitor the early stages of treatment because emerging therapies for cocaine dependence often incorporate transitional medications that, until much greater experience has accumulated, will continue to need individualized prescribing.

The upgrading of staff abilities and morale and the modest but critically needed renovation of decrepit facilities and furnishings have multiple significance. Good morale and decent facilities increase the attractiveness of treatment programs and thus their ability to recruit and retain effective staff and effectively motivated clients. Most critically, the competence, quality, and continuity of care givers may well be a critical element in explaining the differential effectiveness of treatment programs.

Reach More Young Mothers

The committee attaches high priority to treating expectant mothers and single women with young children. The external costs of drug abuse and dependence among this group are especially worrisome because these children's present and future welfare depends so heavily on their mothers' welfare. High risks of drug problems and other severe dysfunctions inhere in children of parents who are abusing or dependent on illicit drugs.

Consequently, the committee values children's welfare on both an equity basis—they obviously have very limited ability to help themselves because of their physical immaturity, lack of personal income, and inexperience—and in terms of the future social costs that it is strongly suspected these children will bear.

Site visits by the committee demonstrated that it is especially hard for expectant women or single mothers of young children (and often, women are both) to receive intensive residential treatment, and sometimes even to maintain regular outpatient schedules, because of child care needs and other medical and social problems. The committee believes that any initiative to bring more of these women into treatment must also emphasize services that will help them find safe, decent dwellings in which to live and productive activities for themselves and their children.

The problem of pregnant women who take illicit drugs has received a great deal of attention recently. Although no study has specifically examined the number of expectant mothers in drug treatment, applying the roughly 10 percent annual fertility rate for women demographically similar to those currently in treatment indicates that about 30,000 expectant women receive some drug treatment each year—very few of them in programs with a primary focus on and special services for pregnant women. The committee estimates that 105,000 pregnant women a year need treatment. There is no basis to believe that treatment of these women would be appreciably more or less effective than for other adult clients. But even if the distribution of results is the same as for others in terms of extinguishing drug-seeking behavior, that outcome would be worth pursuing more intently because of the external costs to the children.

Reaching more pregnant women will require active and expensive outreach. One demonstration outreach project in Harlem, New York (Brown, 1988), cost $850 per expectant mother enrolled in prenatal care, an expenditure completely apart from the cost of drug treatment and prenatal care services as such. Pregnant women are likely to require relatively more intensive residential treatment than most clients owing to the special risks they pose to their babies and their aversion to treatment. For pregnant women with older children and other single women in treatment, onsite care for dependent children is a critical treatment-related need. It is often a major obstacle to enrolling and staying in intensive residential or day treatment because very few programs at present have onsite child care. Despite the stories of abandonment and grave concerns voiced (most often by male professionals) about the "destruction of the maternal instinct" by cocaine dependence, most mothers will not stay in treatment for long if it means separation from their children.

Induce More Criminal Justice Clients to Accept Treatment

In 1985 about 25 percent of public-tier clients in 14 states were under probation or parole supervision; extrapolated to the national level, this percentage translates into a census of 55,000 or about 160,000 annual admissions of community-based criminal justice clients. In addition, 30,000 to 50,000 prison inmates were in treatment—although these estimates include less specialized counseling, education, and mutual self-help group meetings. These figures indicate a 10 to 20 percent rate of treatment among criminal justice clients who need treatment.

These individuals constitute the group whose imposition of high external costs represents the primordial raison d'être of the public tier. Because of the flooding of criminal justice channels during the past decade and a half, the induction into drug treatment of suitable, younger criminal justice clients has lagged behind the rates achieved in the 1970s. Yet a central lesson of Chapters 3, 4, and 5 is that treatment, far from being antithetical to the criminal justice system, is complementary to it, sharing its principal goals and offering a resource that may permit more efficient use of enforcement, correctional, and judicial facilities and resources. Although there is no way to substantiate this impression, the committee deems it plausible that the erosion of resource intensity and surveillance capacity within treatment programs during the period of retrenchment in the 1980s contributed to the increasing pressure on the criminal justice system, particularly from probation and parole violators.

THREE STRATEGY OPTIONS

The public tier is now on a rapid expansion course, largely as a result of decisions at the federal level. This expansion began in a moderate way with the 1986 Anti-Drug Abuse Act, gained momentum with the 1988 Anti-Drug Abuse Act, and accelerated even more dramatically with the emergency supplemental appropriation to the alcohol, drug abuse, and mental health services (ADMS) block grant and related demonstration authorities late in 1989 (see Table 6-3). The Office of National Drug Control Policy, which was legislatively authorized and established in March 1989, has been assigned a leading role in national strategic planning for drug treatment (as well as enforcement, interdiction, and prevention), whereas the Alcohol, Drug Abuse, and Mental Health Administration (ADAMHA) in September 1989 consolidated the block grant and many of the treatment demonstration authorities in the Office of Treatment Improvement, which has not yet received congressional ratification.

To date, however, there is no settled, detailed plan for this expansion course, although the January 1990 National Drug Control Strategy does identify eight national drug treatment funding priorities[4] and budget figures for fiscal years 1991–1993. Congress has shaped the block grant and demonstration appropriations through 1986 and 1988 amendments to the ADAMHA authorization codes, but that process is incomplete; a set of 1990 amendments that are currently under committee consideration may entail more sweeping changes in the structure of the federal money streams and targets.

To inform and provide a common reference point for these policy formulation processes, the committee has developed three detailed strategy options based on the priorities it recommends for adoption:

• **A core strategy, to deal with existing waiting lists, remedy deficiencies in program quality and management, and implement modest program initiatives for young women with children. The core strategy would exceed 1989 levels of public-tier operating support by about $1 billion, plus $0.5 billion as an additional one-time investment for staff training and facilities construction and renovation.**

• **A comprehensive strategy, adding to the core plan a substantially greater induction of criminal justice clients and a more ambitious plan for treating drug-abusing and drug-dependent mothers; this comprehensive plan would, in the committee's judgment, provide the optimal level of public treatment resources. The comprehensive plan would entail an annual operating increase over 1989 levels of about $2.2 billion, plus a $1 billion one-time investment.**

• **An intermediate strategy following between the core and comprehensive approaches. The intermediate proposal would cost about $1.6 billion, plus a $0.8 billion one-time charge.**

To estimate the amount of new public financing needed to carry out each of these strategic options, the committee made some key assumptions about such parameters as capital costs, training expenses, the number of individuals who could be induced into treatment at various levels of effort, and the costs of improving treatment performance. The costs and expected numbers of clients to be served are summarized in Table 7-1.

---

[4] The eight priorities are as follows: increased availability and quality in drug treatment; additional vocational counseling, training services, and aftercare for recovering addicts; improved and expanded outreach and treatment services for pregnant women and drug-affected infants; expanded availability of treatment services within correctional institutions; development of innovative approaches to drug treatment, including drug treatment campuses and special programs targeted toward adolescents and pregnant women; expanded fellowship and grant programs for drug treatment professionals and staff; establishment of the Office of Treatment Improvement within the Department of Health and Human Services to focus on drug treatment quality and effectiveness; and enhanced treatment research, including expanded data collection, medications development, and evaluation of current treatment methods (Office of National Drug Control Policy, 1990:28).

TABLE 7-1   Three Strategy Options for the Public Tier of Drug Treatment: Estimated Incremental Costs and Client Projections Relative to 1989

Cost Element	Strategy Type		
	Core	Comprehensive	Intermediate
Annual Costs[a]			
Reduce waiting list	330.0	330.0	330.0
Restore funding	412.5	412.5	412.5
Counselor training	19.6	30.1	24.9
Performance data	75.9	112.8	94.4
Expectant mothers			
Outreach	18.8	112.5	56.3
Treatment	87.9	263.7	175.8
Child care	45.9	77.5	61.7
Probation/parole	0.0	660.0	330.0
Prison	0.0	156.3	78.1
Total	990.6	2,155.4	1.564.5
One-Time Investments[a]			
Expand residential facilities	278.8	746.2	512.5
Renovate residential facilities	90.0	90.0	90.0
Renovate outpatient facilities	118.1	118.1	118.1
Train new staff	33.2	116.8	75.0
Total	520.1	1,071.1	795.6
Number of clients served[b]			
Average daily census[c]	387	607	497
Total annual admissions[d]	1,012	1,505	1,258

[a]In millions of 1989 dollars.

[b]In thousands.

[c]The average daily client census in 1987 was 212,000; it was estimated at 275,000 in 1989.

[d]Total annual admissions to public-tier treatment in 1987 were 636,000; total admissions for 1989 were estimated at 815,000.

Source: See Appendix 7B for calculations.

The dollar amounts are defined in terms of increases over estimated 1989 public outlays by state, federal, and local agencies; the detailed calculations required to arrive at these figures are provided in Appendix 7A. It should be noted that the data supporting the costs and results of proceeding along any of the recommended option lines have many uncertainties. As relevant data collection processes are improved and analytical research performed, the models underlying these cost estimates will, over time, be capable of adjustment.

The Core Strategy Option

The core option focuses on three of the four priorities noted earlier: reduction of waiting lists, improvement of treatment quality, and dedicated efforts to treat expectant mothers and provide onsite child care for other parents of young children.

The $330 million estimated cost of the waiting list reduction is based on increasing the daily treatment enrollment by 66,000, which corresponds to the estimate of the NASADAD survey of 43 states in September 1989. The committee calculated the cost of these additional treatment spaces assuming that per capita funding would be restored to 1977–1979 levels and that this restoration would increase retention rates by about 10 percent. There is also funding allotted for one week of specialized annual training or equivalent staff development programming for every clinician and budgeting to implement a comprehensive treatment performance monitoring system that includes intake, discharge, and postdischarge/follow-up data collection and analysis on a sample basis.

Also included in the core strategy option is the cost of outreach directed toward pregnant women who need treatment and targeted increases in treatment capacity appropriate for this group, with an aim to reaching 25 percent of the committee's annual untreated prevalence estimate, which is 75,000 women. Finally, the plan includes an allocation for child care for women in public residential programs, including pregnant women with older children.

The estimated $1 billion incremental operating cost of the core option nearly doubles estimated 1989 public outlays for treatment; in addition, there is a need for one-time investments in new facility acquisition and construction, long overdue renovation of older clinical sites, and initial training for new staff. The committee considers these supports to be critically important in avoiding dilution of the effectiveness of other efforts to upgrade treatment quality. This one-time set of expenditures need not be made in a single year; however, it cannot be stretched over more than three years without creating a bottleneck in terms of effective treatment capacity.

Comprehensive and Intermediate Strategy Options

The comprehensive option requires approximately double the operating increment and one-time outlay of the core plan. Virtually all of this difference is accounted for by two particular initiatives and their implications for staffing, facilities, and related services. One of these initiatives is a large-scale push to induct into treatment many more individuals who are under criminal justice supervision. Although many waiting list clients and some of the pregnant women to be added to treatment censuses under the core plan are under criminal justice supervision, there would not be enough of them under the core expansion to make an appreciable difference in the operations of the criminal justice system—that is, to build up the complementarity that the courts and correctional agencies need to improve the management of their own responsibilities. The committee projects an increase in daily treatment enrollment of 132,000 parolees and probationers, which would bring annual admissions to a figure that exceeds half of all those estimated to need treatment. In the committee's view this increase probably pushes to the outside limit the number of criminal justice clients who can be induced or pressured into entering treatment under existing coercive structures.

The committee also projects enrolling 50,000 prisoners in new comprehensive yet drug-specific programs. Although this figure is double the highest current estimate of prisoners in treatment, it may well be that the actual number of people in recognizable drug treatment modalities is much smaller, making this in fact a very large increment—again pushing the outside limit of what is possible. Although prisoners might seem an easy lot simply to order into treatment—a truly captive audience—it is evident that there are many older prisoners who have tried treatment more than once before and do not like it. It is constitutionally dubious and hazardous to correctional safety to try to increase greatly the amount of coercion used on people who are already in prison. The most fundamental disciplinary sanction in prison is length of time left to serve, but under mandatory release legislation, court orders to limit overcrowding, and the multiple tensions that stain the social order of these "total institutions," manipulation of this sanction to serve any imposed purpose must follow a cautious path.

The committee has set the number of expectant mothers to be reached and treated in a comprehensive strategy at 57,250, or three-quarters of the number estimated nationally to need treatment but who are not now receiving it. This figure also seems to be an outer possible limit, a view conditioned by the formidable difficulties that prenatal outreach programs have experienced in trying to induce less severely impaired and dysfunctional populations to enter prenatal care programs, which make far fewer demands on time, concentration, motivation, or level of organization than drug treatment would.

The intermediate option needs little additional comment. It basically splits the difference between the core and comprehensive strategies, adopting a more conservative level of effort than the comprehensive strategy to induce the criminal and maternal populations to enter treatment.

PUBLIC INTERVENTION IN THE 1990s

Whatever strategy options or levels of expenditure emerge in the next few years, three basic issues will need to be faced by those responsible for organizing and managing the publicly funded treatment system.

- The first issue is how responsibilities should be allocated among the different levels of government and especially between the two levels that have taken the major responsibilities for financing public treatment: the federal government and the states.
- The second issue is which financial mechanisms should be used. The fundamental choice lies between two models that have dominated public support of health care services and certain other welfare services: the public health insurance approach and the direct service approach. Public insurance is a commitment to the individual from the government to reimburse certain kinds of treatment costs wherever the individual incurs them (within certain limits). In direct service the government arranges to support particular providers directly, who are then open to serve any individuals meeting stipulated criteria for the receipt of subsidized care.
- The third issue is what kinds of controls, disciplines, and incentives should be used to ensure that specific expenditure decisions will be appropriate and effective. The concerns here are fiscal prudence, cost containment, and quality assurance and control.

The committee believes that the most informed judgment on how to resolve these issues effectively must begin with a careful consideration of the lessons of the recent past, namely, how these types of questions were handled in the period of the last "war on drugs" and its aftermath in the 1970s and during the block grant period of the 1980s.

Federal and State Roles in the 1970s

The high point of centralized federal command of the drug treatment system was the early 1970s, the period of SAODAP—the Special Action Office for Drug Abuse Prevention (Table 7-2; also see Chapters 2 and 6 and Besteman, 1990). SAODAP negotiated directly with local treatment providers to set them up to provide treatment or to "buy" their waiting lists through increased funding. It specified the nature of the treatments to be delivered, set reimbursement rates based on those specifications, provided technical assistance to program managers, and organized and delivered clinical and management training to treatment staff. It also created a nationally standardized Client-Oriented Data Acquisition Process (CODAP) that was capable of monitoring the performance of treatment programs in terms of admission characteristics, retention, and patient status at discharge.

Nevertheless, it was clear to the federal managers that close supervision of a national system that was rapidly growing and had already passed 100,000 daily clients (treatment slots) was really beyond the scope of a small, albeit powerfully positioned federal agency. As rapid growth outstripped SAODAP's capacity to maintain oversight, the strategy was to "seed and cede"; that is, build community programs to what seemed an appropriate size and then turn over their further supervision and the responsibility for financial support largely to other authorities, predominantly at the state level.

The devolution of the national treatment system to 52 state-level systems (the 50 states plus Washington, D.C., and Puerto Rico) advanced sharply in 1975, when virtually all of the treatment and prevention authority of SAODAP (which was then being disestablished) was fully transferred to the National Institute on Drug Abuse in the Department of Health, Education, and Welfare. NIDA converted all direct contracts with treatment providers into grants, which implied less federal direction and greater autonomy for the treatment programs. At the same time, additional resources and authorities were directed to "single state agencies" designated to take over most of the management responsibilities for administering federal funding for treatment; by 1981 nearly 90 percent of federal support to community-based treatment was routed through the state agencies, mainly in the form of statewide formula grants.

Between 1975 and 1981, federal support for drug treatment services flagged, initially under pressure of the 1974–1975 recession and climbing federal deficits. Nominal federal treatment dollars remained relatively stable from 1976 through 1980, which, in the face of unprecedented inflation, meant that federal support for the system was steadily decreasing. Federal funds were generally available to the state agencies on the basis that states had to at least maintain their own current levels of appropriation for treatment, although no specific matching-type provisions were involved once the conversion from program-level support to using the state agencies as intermediaries had taken place.

The 1980s: Block Grants

The 1981 Omnibus Budget Reconciliation Act (OBRA) accelerated state control of the national treatment system and completed the transition of NIDA's mission to one of purely research and educational functions. All community-based categorical funding was consolidated within a block grant that covered alcohol, drug, and mental health services—the ADMS block grant, which was administered by NIDA's parent bureau, ADAMHA. The total ADMS funding for each state was reduced by 25 percent from the previous year's equivalent funding (the official rationale for this reduction being that the system would be that much cheaper to manage after consolidation; state officials, among others, considered this rationale not even remotely plausible), and the division of funds among the states was frozen at the previous year's proportions of the equivalent funding. The block grant did not require any particular state contribution, but it continued to

TABLE 7-2 Chronology of Major Policies Toward Drug Treatment

Year	Event/Policy
1930s	Federal prison hospitals are opened at Lexington and Fort Worth.
1962	California and New York addiction initiatives—These measures authorized pretrial civil commitment to treatment; an integral component was intensive, long-term, community-based supervision.
1966	Narcotic Addict Rehabilitation Act—This legislation authorized federal pretrial civil commitment, voluntary self-commitment, and federal support of community-based supervision/treatment through a grant-in-aid program; it constituted the foundation for the future federally funded grant-in-aid program.
1967	The City of New York proposes expanding a small network of methadone clinics to 25,000 slots.
1969	An investigative new drug (IND) application is made for methadone by the National Institute of Mental Health. This allowed methadone programs to be established under the umbrella of mental health centers as part of the process leading to full Food and Drug Administration (FDA) approval of methadone maintenance in 1972.
1971	Executive Order 11599 establishes the Special Action Office for Drug Abuse Prevention (SAODAP) designed to organize, direct, and evaluate the federal drug treatment effort.
1972	The Drug Abuse Office and Treatment Act (P.L. 92-255)—Congressional authorization is given for SAODAP; the act also provides a major increase in support for community-based treatment, authorizes formula grants for directing funds to states, and requires the designation of a responsible state agency for submission of a state drug abuse treatment plan.

1972	The federal government "buys up" waiting lists of local treatment agencies to expand the treatment system.
1973	The National Institute on Drug Abuse (NIDA) is established to collect under one roof all of the disparate treatment and prevention services (funding, technical assistance, system monitoring, training, etc.) and research functions.
1975	NIDA converts the statewide services contracts to grants, which provides the states with important resources and authority in managing local treatment contracts. SAODAP is terminated.
1981	Omnibus Budget Reconciliation Act—This legislation ends categorical grants, converting them to block grants and reducing federal effort by 25%. All federal support for community-based treatment is now funneled through block grants; states assume all responsibility for managing the treatment system, including technical assistance, quality assurance, and training. NIDA staffing level greatly reduced. Federal support declines over the next several years, from about 40% to about 20% of total treatment funding.
1986	Alcohol and Drug Abuse Amendments of 1986 (Title IV of the Anti-Drug Abuse Act of 1986)—This legislation renews the federal commitment to treatment, approximately doubling federal funds through supplemental block grant appropriations and new demonstration authorities.
1988	Comprehensive Alcohol Abuse, Drug Abuse, and Mental Health Amendments Act (Title II of the Anti-Drug Abuse Act of 1988)—This act continues the federal commitment to treatment and provides for increased federal involvement in monitoring of the system, as well as one-time grants for waiting list reduction.
1989	An emergency appropriation is attached to the Transportation Bill; it supplements the block grant, adding half as much again to the annual substance abuse treatment and prevention allocation.

require that states not use the new no-strings federal funding to supplant state support for the same functions—basically putting a floor under state support for total ADMS functions.

As the federal role in treatment, outside of basic and clinical research, was reduced to certifying 52 Treasury vouchers, the states acquired virtually sovereign responsibility for the shape and vitality of the public tier. This responsibility included deciding how much drug treatment would be provided out of the combination of ADMS funds and state appropriations, allocating monies among programs and localities, maintaining or revising treatment protocols and staffing and other requirements, monitoring program performance, delivering technical assistance and training services, and setting reimbursement rates. Many states, however, redirected money for these purposes, as well as authority and responsibility, to their constituent counties.

Federally managed data systems that had monitored treatment were discontinued, leaving only a semblance of national information about how treatment dollars were being spent and to what effect. There was, for example, a 5-year interregnum in the survey of treatment providers (NDATUS), an end to the national client research sample (TOPS), and closing down of the client data requirements (CODAP), although some states elected to retain elements of the CODAP system and provide data summaries to NIDA.

Federal appropriations to the block grant fund changed modestly between 1982 and 1986, and federal inflation-adjusted support declined further. State appropriations generally increased, however, depending on local economic conditions and the severity of the state's drug problem. In aggregate, state and local funds by 1987 were about double the federal contribution (see Figure 6-7b). During this period Congress instituted several categorical set-asides and minimum proportions for types of services within the block grant—for example, a 35 percent minimum expenditure each for drug and alcohol treatment—which marginally narrowed state autonomy in spending block grant funds.

With the Anti-Drug Abuse Act of 1986 came a significant boost in federal support for treatment, nearly doubling the federal funding nominally allocated to drug treatment, adding an alcohol and drug abuse treatment and rehabilitation (ADTR) block grant on top of the ADMS grant, and implementing other increases as well. The act specified that a combination of the size of the population and documented estimation of the need for treatment would be used to determine the allocation per state. The legislation indicated Congress's concern over the lack of data on the national treatment system by setting aside 1 percent of block grant funds for collecting evaluation data and requiring states to develop and submit plans for their anticipated use of block grant funds and evaluation of the impact of the additional treatment funds provided through the ADTR. Yet there was no federal response contingent on such plans or evaluations. The federal office could not really question or disapprove state plans, and there was no mechanism of accountability, that is, no way to determine whether the plan was followed or what the results were. There was no fundamental change in the organization or management of the system.

The Anti-Drug Abuse Act of 1988 further increased federal appropriations and began to rebuild some national analytical capacities and flexibilities. It added more categorical set-asides mandating how the money could be spent, again cutting into state autonomy. These set-asides included a requirement that 20 percent of the substance abuse part of the grant be allocated to prevention activities, 20 percent of the total be spent on women, and at least 10 percent of the drug portion be spent on treating problems involving intravenous drugs. With this act came a congressional mandate for the Department of Health and Human Services to set aside 5 to 15 percent of the grant to collect data about the operation of the national treatment system and give ADAMHA authority to resume making unmediated demonstration and service grants to local programs and governments, without regard to the block formulas for state-by-state division of funds. There was a one-year appropriation for the purpose of grants to reduce waiting lists. The 1988 act also created the new Office of National Drug Control Policy, with broad coordinative authority over federal budgets and activities.

At the end of 1989 an additional appropriation, attached to a major transportation bill, increased the alcohol and drug block grant appropriations by nearly 50 percent over the 1988 levels. However, a series of proposed accompanying changes in specific authorization levels were not passed. Despite the concern of Congress evidenced in the 1986 and 1988 acts over the state of the treatment system, and despite various perceived efforts to improve information and tighten federal control, the balance of responsibility between state agencies and the federal government has not materially changed from the roles each assumed in 1981.

The 1990s: Appropriate Shifts in Federal and State Roles

The committee has recommended—on the grounds of reducing external costs and helping the poor—that drug treatment be made universally accessible and even attractive when it is clinically appropriate. To achieve this objective, it seems necessary now, as it was in the early 1970s, for the federal government to undertake a major near-term expansion of its financial commitment to drug treatment. This expansion is clearly a responsibility that Congress and the Bush administration have agreed is appropriate, although there are differences with regard to what this commitment should be in dollar terms and some uncertainty about how best to organize the effort. With the new increases in federal funding, it is appropriate that there be a realignment of the federal role. But unlike the situation during the SAODAP era, there is now in place a series of well-developed state administrative capabilities and a large base of public treatment on which to build. Further building will require that federal executive authority be deployed again but with a much more complicated agenda than in the earlier period.

In carrying out this expansion, the committee believes that two major considerations—management tasks for the federal government—pertain:

• federal drug treatment funds must be spent efficiently and coordinated effectively with other elements in the "war on drugs," including related social, health, rehabilitative, and correctional services; and

• the drug treatment system must be clearly linked with other forms of state and federal cooperation to assure the integration of drug treatment with other health and welfare services.

The first management task applies in the short term—the next three to five years. The committee has serious doubts that the block grant system and its current spending formulas are the best way to use federal authority under the current circumstances. It seems unwise to simply pump major funding increases through the current mechanisms without revising the distribution of authority so that greater responsibility and accountability requirements can flow along with greater sums of money. This task can be fulfilled best, in the committee's judgment, by a strong federal program of categorical spending—the direction in which the block grants are already moving as categorical spending floors, set-asides, and data requirements are attached to them. The federal program, however, needs to have as much flexibility on the management level as possible to permit the responsible federal offices to adapt rapidly to the varying needs and administrative environments of states and their localities. Without that flexibility, it is difficult to see how the federal offices can be responsive and be able to facilitate the states' responses to such priorities as treating more women and criminal justice populations and creating performance improvement factors and measurement systems.

The financing mechanism that appears most appropriate for achieving these managerial tasks in the near term is neither block grants hedged in with formulas nor federal demonstration grants to providers but rather categorical support of treatment programs administered through state agencies by a mechanism like the former statewide services grants or contracts used in the 1970s. The state agencies in turn should develop cooperative agreement-type mechanisms to ensure the involvement of and coordination with appropriate units of state and local government and community-based programs. The importance of state agency coordination and accountability was recognized by ADAMHA in allocating a substantial evaluation factor (20 points out of 100) to "umbrella grant" proposals for the waiting list funds authorized in the 1988 Anti-Drug Abuse Act.

Cooperative agreements can be multilateral, involving multiple levels of government. When the SAODAP expansions of federal funding occurred and money began going directly to providers, the federal office found that it could not expect to expand its staff enough to monitor these programs successfully but had to seek intermediaries—the state agencies—for this task. Because the states were already directly involved in managing the system, they compensated for some of the decline in federal support that occurred in the early 1980s and in fact became a substantially larger source of funds than the federal government.

In lieu of fixed formulas for the allocation of funds received by the states (which, as most recently revised, are based on population weighted somewhat by degree of urbanization), **the committee recommends that state agencies be required to submit plans that analyze the conjunctions and mismatches among the most current epidemiological information and known treatment capabilities; it further recommends that the states propose annual spending patterns that reflect this information.** Formally defined and state-certified addiction treatment programs, and not individual practitioners, should continue to be the recipients of public grants and contracts for addiction treatment. In addition, a portion of the federal dollars must go into technical assistance and data system building to ensure at the state, local, and program levels that this planning effort will have a factual basis.

As performance data systems come on line, data should be reported in the following period to indicate whether actual spending details depart from the plan, and why, with analysis, explanation, and adjustment in the subsequent plan. The focus initially needs to be on improvement and response rather than punishment (such as shifting federal funds to mechanisms that bypass state or local intermediaries), but the objective of coming into line with performance standards should apply without much delay. An independent analysis of each state's performance with respect to its planning goals and control of resources should be developed and submitted in a report to Congress on an annual or biannual basis.

Taking a longer term view, the general pattern of federal initiatives has been to pour money into categorical programs, then consolidate those programs to reduce the natural accretion of paperwork requirements on recipients and to cap or reduce federal expenditures. Direct categorical funding is the best way to build service capacity rapidly, but historical experience shows that only by making a transition from narrower categorical programs to broader spectrum funding can quality programs be maintained at suitable service levels. The risk in direct categorical support is that recipients and intermediaries will not move toward a self-sustaining, self-adjusting system. When the federal government reduces its funding and direct management involvement, as it inevitably will, the tasks of coordination, accountability, and adjustment may suffer, to the detriment of beneficiaries and the public interest.

Therefore, a longer term goal (the next 5 to 10 years) must be kept in view from this point forward in building up the treatment system: namely, to move the mechanisms for funding drug treatment away from central reliance on direct service support and toward consolidation with the mainstream of health care financing for low-income populations, which is the Medicaid system. During the 1980s the growth of private health insurance coverage for drug treatment brought the private tier and its insured clients into the mainstream of health dollars, and although this movement has not been complete, fully efficient, or without troubles in various respects (as discussed in Chapter 8), it has unquestionably improved accessibility to treatment for those covered by private insurance. It is time to stimulate a similar process across the board with Medicaid.

In Appendix 7C, the committee provides a more detailed discussion of the current Medicaid system—in particular, its eligibility and coverage policies. Currently, however, there is ongoing discussion and reconsideration of Medicaid, as there is of the overall character of health care financing, and it would not be sensible therefore to prescribe too finely for a system that is meant to emerge 5 to 10 years from now. Yet these discussions should take careful note of the conclusion of the appendix discussion: **in the committee's judgment, if Medicaid is to assume a consistent role across the board in financing the public tier of drug treatment, federal legislation governing Medicaid must be materially altered so as to address drug treatment needs. Such legislation should delineate new eligibility criteria, the kinds of services and providers eligible for reimbursement, and minimum reimbursement levels.**

It is clear that adequate drug treatment benefits under Medicaid would diminish the need for direct service support of drug treatment programs, particularly if broader eligibility for Medicaid were to emerge for presently ineligible indigent populations. Nevertheless, even if completely universal insurance coverage were achieved, there would still be a need for direct support of public-tier programs to offer outreach and other important adjunctive services to the many individuals for whom low income is not the only barrier to seeking and responding well to treatment.

Transitional Steps Toward the Year 2000

There are five steps that would be particularly useful as incentives toward this transition and that would not compromise the efficiency of the direct service support mechanism. The first is to require all parties to cooperative agreements, grants, or contracts involving federal funds to develop and display evidence of progress toward the long-term goal of increasing the receipt of funds from the Medicaid system—for example, by facilitating the registration of clients eligible for Medicaid benefits and by meeting relevant accreditation standards familiar to Medicaid, such as those of the Joint Commission on Accreditation of Healthcare Organizations or the Commission on Accreditation of Rehabilitation Facilities. Those respective accreditation organizations, by the same token, need to be pressed when developing standards to explicitly recognize and incorporate knowledge of the public tier of drug treatment providers and their procedures.

The second useful step is to begin stipulating matching requirements rather than maintenance-of-effort requirements for increases in grant support to the states. By determining the matching ratio with the same formula used to determine Medicaid matching, the incentive to states to use Medicaid structures will be increased, and the disincentive—having to match every new Medicaid dollar but being able to get more block grant dollars without increasing state appropriations—will be removed.

The third step is for the federal government to require state Medicaid programs to include drug treatment as part of the standard package of benefits offered to all current (and any newly added) Medicaid-eligible persons. The drug benefit package should cover methadone treatment, outpatient nonmethadone treatment, and residential treatment in state-accredited freestanding (nonhospital) as well as hospital-affiliated residential facilities and outpatient programs. No special copayments or limitations—that is, no copayments or limits not generally applicable to medical/surgical benefits—should be applied to drug treatment.

It is appropriate, however, to impose referral and utilization controls to ensure that unrestricted self-referral does not lead to the abuse of services. These controls, and particularly limitations on inpatient services, should conform to those described below. For those states with private insurance mandates for drug treatment insurance coverage, the Medicaid drug treatment benefit should be at least as comprehensive as (which does not mean identical with) the mandated private insurance benefit.

The fourth step, which applies not only to Medicaid but also to the entire range of health and human services programs, is to reduce gross inconsistencies in the way drug problems are handled in eligibility determinations for Medicaid, Aid to Families with Dependent Children, Medicare,

Supplemental Security Income, and other income maintenance, education, and housing assistance entitlement programs. These inconsistencies create a bureaucratic nightmare for the drug treatment programs and state agencies that draw on more than one such source of funds—which most of them try to do. The responsible federal agency should analyze definitional inconsistencies among federal programs and lay out a plan to minimize resulting problems.

The fifth step is to develop a thoroughgoing system of public utilization management. Many of the components of such a system were developed in the SAODAP period but were subsequently disestablished. Moreover, a substantial portion of the utilization management efforts now under way to control costs in the alcohol/drug/psychiatric and the general medical/surgical benefit areas of Medicare and private health insurance are quite similar to the controls instituted by SAODAP.

Utilization Management

Utilization management describes arrangements to define access to effective treatment while keeping costs at efficient levels (Gray and Field, 1989). Good utilization management works to ensure that a fully appropriate and needed range of services is used and that different service components are coordinated. The most fundamental principles of such management are that access to and utilization of care should be controlled and managed on a case basis by "neutral gatekeepers" or central intake personnel (although the central intake function may need to be dispersed geographically). These personnel should be regulated by certification standards and undergirded by time-limited, performance-accounted licenses and contracts.

Client assessment, referral, and monitoring of progress in treatment should be reviewed (or performed) independently of the treatment provider. These personnel should have appropriate clinical credentials that include the understanding that longer residential and outpatient durations are strongly correlated with beneficial results among public clients. **Effective utilization management should recognize that drug abuse and dependence are chronic, relapsing disorders and that for any one client, more than one treatment episode may be needed and different types of treatment may need to be tried. The gatekeepers should have access to ongoing performance evaluation results and responsibility for implementing specific cost-control objectives.** As with the implementation of planning and performance accounting on a large scale, the central intake function should focus initially on improvement and response and not punishment. Yet here, too, the principle of coming into line with performance standards must apply without much delay.

There should be rigorous preadmission and concurrent review of all residential drug treatment admissions, and especially of hospital admissions, and concurrent review of outpatient treatment. Unlike the objective in utilization management of acute hospital care for most medical conditions, which is basically to hold inpatient lengths of stay to a minimum, the objective for drug treatment services should be to increase client retention in appropriate, cost-efficient treatment settings.

The major cost-control concern in this area is the use of high-cost treatment when lower cost alternatives could be as effective. This hazard attaches principally to acute care hospital inpatient services for detoxification or rehabilitation treatment. Utilization management is a highly appropriate way to check this hazard because no modality of drug rehabilitation treatment as such requires continuous, onsite access to acute care hospital services. However, if other criteria (as specified below) dictate hospitalization, drug treatment may begin in an acute care setting and continue elsewhere or shift to more appropriate cost rates when acute care requirements end.

The scientific basis of utilization management of drug treatment is at present rudimentary, but intake specialists should at least be required to demonstrate an understanding of diagnostic criteria and effectiveness findings for drug treatment programs. A rigid limit on the number or duration of treatment episodes permitted to individuals is inadvisable; a better method is to employ clinical judgment about the client's probability of responding positively to treatment.

The public tier has generally not been heavily invested in hospital-based drug treatment, and this should continue to be the case—but not as a matter of rigid exclusion. **The committee recommends that hospital-based drug services be reimbursed at the same level as nonhospital residential treatment rates, unless there is evidence that a client specifically requires continuing acute care hospital services. Hospital-based drug detoxification should only be covered in the event of medical complications such as those noted below or the lack of appropriate residential or outpatient facilities nearby. Indications for hospital-based inpatient drug detoxification are the following:**

- **serious concurrent medical illness such as tuberculosis, pneumonia, or acute hepatitis;**
- **history of medical complications such as seizures in previous detoxification episodes;**
- **evidence of suicidal ideation;**
- **dependence on sedative-hypnotic drugs as validated by tolerance testing (therapeutic challenge) to determine the appropriate length of stay; and**

  • history of failure to complete earlier ambulatory or residential detoxification versus completion in inpatient settings.

As perhaps the most important and immediately needed utilization management requirement, the committee recommends that all drug treatment programs receiving public support be required to participate in a client-oriented data system that reports client characteristics, retention, and progress indicators at admission, during treatment, at discharge, and (on a reasonable sampling basis) at one or more follow-up points. There should be periodic, independent investigation on a sampling basis of the quality and accuracy of the data system or systems, and the systems should be designed to dovetail with ongoing services research and data collection in other government agencies and units concerned with drug problems. (For example, there should be attention to "linkage" questions about numbers of arrests and emergency room visits for comparability with the Drug Use Forecasting [DUF] and Drug Abuse Warning Network [DAWN] systems; see the discussion of research needs in Chapter 5.) Certification for public support should be time limited and based on performance—especially client retention and improvement—rather than on process standards. Performance is to be demonstrated by outcome evaluation, and the standards of performance adequacy should be informed by past and ongoing treatment effectiveness research on retention and outcomes.

THE SPECIAL CASE OF VETERANS' COVERAGE

The Department of Veterans Affairs represents a special case of public coverage. The VA is a potential provider of health care for 26.9 million surviving veterans of military service—more than 10 percent of all U.S. citizens. However, its total outlay for medical and hospital care in 1988 was $10.3 billion, which is less than 2 percent of total health expenditures. Although all former military personnel are nominally eligible for treatment in VA health facilities, all hospital, nursing home, and outpatient care provided through the VA is now rationed on a priority basis. Of first priority are category A veterans (41 percent of the total veteran population), those with primarily service-related injuries or health problems who are receiving VA pensions or who have low incomes. Category B veterans (7 percent of veterans) have low incomes but no service-connected disabilities. Category C veterans (52 percent) have higher incomes; they are last in priority and must make copayments to receive VA care. In the first year (FY 1987) of these standards, 95 percent of admissions to VA facilities were from category A; only 2 percent each were from categories B or C. Although there are 11 million veterans eligible for VA health services, in FY 1989 only 3.3 million of them requested health services of one kind or another.

The VA operates a system of 172 general medical facilities that include 56 inpatient drug abuse programs, mostly chemical dependency modalities but some modified therapeutic communities, and 66 outpatient drug abuse programs. About one-sixth of outpatients in the VA system are on methadone maintenance. Although this system is accessible (though not always convenient) to most veterans for purposes of nonemergency inpatient treatment, it entails commutes of several hours or more for some veterans, which is not suitable for outpatient treatment. (The VA can arrange and pay for veterans to be treated in public programs under certain circumstances.)

The VA drug treatment programs delivered 560,000 inpatient days of care to 17,250 individuals and 919,000 outpatient visits to 19,800 individuals in FY 1988. In addition, 18,800 individuals with primary diagnoses of drug dependence received other kinds of inpatient treatment in general medical or psychiatric wards, and 2,050 received care in nonspecialty outpatient clinics. (There is an unknown degree of overlap among these populations in different treatment settings.) The VA system probably treats more individuals than the public tier in any state except California or New York. But is this level of service high enough? There is reason to think it is not.

Drug problems among veterans have been a significant issue for about 20 years. Approximately 8.2 million men and women served during the Vietnam combat period, of whom nearly 40 percent were actually stationed at some time in southeast Asia. A study of personnel returning from duty in Vietnam in 1973 found that 43 percent had consumed illicit drugs there. Consumption rates declined dramatically, however, upon their return home, and only 10 percent reported any use in the first six months or more after returning; 4 percent reported more-than-weekly use for a month or more (Robins et al., 1974). A more recent study found drug abuse or dependence in about 1.5 percent of veterans who served during the Vietnam War era, which would equal about 125,000 veterans of that era in need of drug treatment (Robins, 1974).

The Treatment Outcome Prospective Study (Hubbard et al., 1989) closely examined the military experience and discharge status of 11,200 clients admitted to drug treatment programs in 10 major cities during 1979–1981 and found that 14.5 percent of all admissions were veterans with honorable, general, or medical discharges (another 2.7 percent of admissions had dishonorable discharges). Very similar proportions were seen across different modalities and in different cities. Even in Philadelphia, which has a major VA methadone treatment program that was not included in the TOPS sample, eligible veterans constituted 15 percent of TOPS methadone admissions. Virtually all of these individuals had incomes low enough to make them eligible for category A or B status under the VA priority system.

Applying the 15 percent proportion to the 640,000 admissions to public-tier treatment programs in 1987 suggests that 90,000 to 100,000 admissions to these public treatment programs were veterans eligible to receive treatment from VA facilities. Even if one assumes that the proportion of veterans entering drug treatment in the late 1980s was substantially less—let us say, one-half or even two-thirds less—than the number in 1979–1981, that still totals 30,000 to 45,000 veteran admissions to the public tier. It appears very likely that a large proportion of eligible category A or B veterans were receiving drug treatment outside of the VA system, perhaps as many as were treated inside it.

No study has closely examined whether large numbers of veterans are in fact still entering public programs instead of VA programs. Neither is it clear whether these veterans had attempted unsuccessfully to gain admittance to VA treatment programs or whether veterans today are unsuccessful in gaining admittance. It is only strongly suggested by the available data that the VA may not be serving a major proportion of veterans who are eligible for and need drug treatment. In the past several years the VA has targeted drug programs for drastic budget reductions in order to meet overall fiscal limitations. At the very least, outpatient or residential drug treatment services—furnished directly by VA facilities or by contract—should be made available to meet the needs of former inpatients.

CONCLUSIONS

The committee has developed recommendations regarding the public coverage of drug treatment in light of some explicit principles that justify public coverage, and these principles in turn suggest specific priorities for the expansion of the public tier that is now under way. The committee identified as principles that public coverage should seek to reduce external social costs—in particular those relating to crime and family role dysfunctions—recognizing that this objective often requires actively inducing people to seek treatment, and that it should remedy constraints arising from inadequate income.

Public coverage should provide adequate support for appropriate and timely admission, as well as completion or maintenance, of good-quality treatment for individuals who cannot pay for it (fully or partly) whenever such individuals *need* treatment, according to the best professional judgment; whenever they *seek* treatment; or whenever they can be *induced* through acceptable means to pursue it, assuming there is some probability of positive response. The committee estimates that 35 million individuals qualify as indigent with regard to private purchase of any form of drug treatment; that is, they are neither adequately insured nor able to pay out of pocket for appropriate forms of specialized treatment if needed and thus would have to rely on public services. For residential drug treatment, the committee's estimate of those who are unable to afford it if needed rises to 60 million.

The resources needed to achieve the general goal of public coverage represent a major increase in public support for treatment, and even under the current conditions of extraordinary public concern about the drug problem and the possibility of commensurate appropriations, everything cannot be done at once. Priorities for treatment thus need to be defined. The committee's recommendations on priorities for public-tier expansion are the following:

• end delays in admission when treatment is appropriate, as evidenced by waiting lists;
• improve treatment (by raising the levels of service intensity, personnel quality and experience, and retention rates of existing modalities; by having programs assume more integrative roles with respect to related services; and by instituting systematic performance monitoring and follow-up);
• expand treatment through more aggressive outreach to pregnant women and young mothers; and
• further expand community-based and institutionally based treatment of criminal justice clients.

It is possible to estimate the amount of new public financing needed to meet these priority objectives, although to do so, key assumptions must be made about such parameters as capital costs, training expenses, and the number of individuals who could be induced to enter treatment at various levels of effort. The committee judges that the amount needed to upgrade and expand the drug treatment system, beyond current spending rates, is $2.2 billion in annual operating costs (plus $1.1 billion in one-time costs) for a comprehensive plan, $1 billion annually (plus $0.8 billion up front) for a core plan, or $1.6 billion annually (plus $0.5 billion in up-front costs) for an intermediate plan. Because the data supporting the costs of the recommended strategies are uncertain, it is essential that relevant data collection be developed very quickly and its products analyzed as soon as possible.

The committee's recommended strategies lead to a consideration of needed changes in how to manage the public tier. These issues divide into the following: the roles and interrelations of the states, the federal government, and public-tier providers; the most appropriate shorter and longer term financing mechanisms for providing public support (direct service programs versus public insurance); and the controls needed to make the most effective and efficient use of public funds.

State governments have played the major role in financial administration and quality control of drug treatment programs in recent years, but there has also been cyclical movement between state and federal leadership. The federal government originally built most of the public tier of providers and then transferred responsibility for regulating and supporting this tier largely to the states; it is now moving back into the lead role. This expansion of federal support should be accompanied by more active, centralized direction and control of treatment resources.

At present, both direct service grants or contracts and reimbursement through Medicaid (and similar programs) play some part in supporting the public tier. Direct program support is much larger and will continue to grow as the federal grant and demonstration programs expand. Emphasis on direct service is an appropriate model for directed system building, but long-term system maintenance may be better served by a proportionately greater use of public insurance financing supplemented by direct service grants to ensure critical program elements such as outreach and integration with nonhealth services. The ground should be prepared to "mainstream" drug treatment more fully, incorporating it into public health care financing for the poor, that is, Medicaid.

Under either support mechanism, the protection and stimulation of program quality, efficient operation, and appropriate utilization are crucial. Utilization criteria and regular outcome analysis should be more generally deployed in drug treatment systems. Central intake functions based on clear clinical criteria, performance measurement and contracting, and outcome analysis are critical components of a system of treatment performance disciplined by information and incentives.

In the special case of drug treatment for low-income veterans, enough evidence has accumulated to provoke concerns that the VA may not be providing an adequate range of services. There is probably a need to expand VA outpatient drug treatment programs, and the adequacy of the VA residential system needs comprehensive evaluation.

APPENDIX 7A
BASELINE AND STRATEGY OPTION CALCULATIONS

Baseline Comparison Values

All cost estimates for the committee's three strategy options are based on the most recent data available at the end of 1989 concerning the size and financing of the public treatment system. According to the National Drug and Alcoholism Treatment Utilization Survey compiled in late 1987 and early 1988 (see Chapter 6), the public tier of community-based drug treatment providers treated at least 636,000 clients during 1987, had 212,000 individuals enrolled in treatment in October 1987, and had annual revenues of $800 million. This tier includes a very small proportion (less then 10 percent) of privately reimbursed clients and revenues. (In addition, a very small number of publicly financed clients were treated by private-tier providers.)

These baseline values are biased downward somewhat because the 1987 survey was incomplete (some providers did not respond at all or responded only partially) and resources and clients increased between 1987 and 1989. In a number of the projection components of the strategy options (e.g., costs of training, renovations, expansion of treatment facilities), 1987 baseline values are used for estimation. To the extent that these values are below the actual 1989 values, the committee's projections underestimate future resource requirements.

The committee imputed a provisional set of 1989 estimates for the public tier of providers, pegging expenditures at $1.1 billion, the number of clients currently in treatment at 275,000, and the number of clients treated during the past year at 815,000. The imputation is based on partial information about increases in funding and clients served. Expenditures in public-tier treatment in 1989 were at least $1.1 billion, based on extrapolating the 17 percent annual increases in public drug plus alcohol treatment funding reported by state drug and alcohol agencies between 1985 and 1988 (Butynski and Canova, 1989, and prior years). According to the same source, the number of drug clients treated increased by about 20 percent annually; these authors, however, attribute an unknown proportion of this increase to improvements in the comprehensiveness of state data systems (for example, including clients treated in community mental health centers). The committee therefore has imputed a 13.3 percent annual client increase (two-thirds of the apparent annual change, allowing for a small inflation adjustment).

CORE STRATEGY OPTION

Annual Recurring Costs

Eliminate waiting lists

Increase daily treatment enrollment by 66,000 (survey of 43 states in September 1989 by NASADAD shows minimum need of 66,000 slots).

Fund at new rate per client in treatment—$5,000 per client in treatment, or $1,860 per client treated (based on increased resources per client and retention).

Keep current mix of residential and outpatient treatment.

66,000 × $5,000 = **$330 million**

Restore funding per client to 1976–1979 level

Increase reimbursements per client by 25%.
Expect client retention to increase by 10%; therefore, admit same number of clients per year, with current census increasing by 10%.
Keep current mix of residential and outpatient treatment.

($1.1 billion × 1.25 × 1.10) − $1.1 billion = **$412.5 million**

Staff training

Assume minimum of 26,000 staff in 1989.
Assume 39,200 total staff in future, which equals 26,000 staff in 1989 divided by 275,000 clients in 1989 times 377,900 clients in future times 1.1 for increase in staffing intensity.
Assume annual training expense of $500 per staff person (average 5 days/year at $100 per day).

26,000 × $500 = **$13 million, first year**
39,200 × $500 = **$19.6 million, subsequent years**

Program/client performance monitoring system

Assume 815,000 annual public-tier clients in 1989.
Core scenario treats 196,600 more clients annually.
Estimate $25 per client for client reporting at intake, during treatment, and at discharge.
Assume postdischarge follow-up performed on 25% of public clients.
Estimate $200 per client tracked and interviewed to perform follow-up assessment after discharge.

(815,000 + 196,600) × [$25 + (0.25 × $200)] = **$75.9 million**

Active outreach to expectant mothers

Assume active outreach to drug-using expectant mothers reaches 18,750 at a cost of $1,000 each (about the cost per expectant mother reached in a demonstration outreach in Harlem, NY, cited in Institute of Medicine report on neonatal care [Brown, 1988]).

18,750 × $1,000 = **$18.8 million**

Treat 18,750 expectant mothers

Assume half of recruited expectant mothers participate in 6 months of therapeutic community treatment ($12,500 per year plus 25% increase), and half get 6 months of outpatient treatment ($2,500 per year plus 25% increase; costs documented in Chapter 6).

[9,375 × ($12,500 × 1.25) / 2] + [9,375 × ($2,500 × 1.25) / 2] = **$87.9 million**

Children of mothers in residential programs

Assume 25% of the 28,600 public residential clients are female (Institute of Medicine analysis of 1987 NDATUS).

Assume residential treatment given to 10.6% of waiting list (same as the proportion of 1987 NDATUS public clients in residential programs) but only 25% of those entering will be female.

Of 18,750 additional expectant mothers treated per year, half get residential care of average 6 months.

Assume 22.5% of women have one or more children, and these average 2.5 children each (communication from R. L. Hubbard, special analysis of TOPS data).

Assume domiciliary child care costs of $500 per child/month, or twice the cost of inexpensive day care ($6,000/year).

[(28,600 × 1/4) + (66,000 × 0.106) × 1/4) + (18,750 × 1/2 × 1/2)] × 0.225 × 2.5 × $6,000 = **$45.9 million**

One-time Capacity Expansion/Improvements

Residential capacity expansion

Increased length of stay requires additional 2,250 beds.
Waiting list expansion requires 7,000 beds.
Expectant mothers expansion requires 4,688 beds.
Assume construction cost of $20,000 per client space (from Donald McConnell, executive director of the State of Connecticut Alcohol and Drug Commission; alternative estimate of $26,000 per client space from David Mactas, president of Marathon House in Rhode Island).

(2,250 + 7,000 + 4,690) × $20,000 = **$278.8 million**

Repair existing residential facilities

Assume cost of repairing space in use is 20% of cost of building (0.20 × $20,000 = $4,000 per bed).

Assume 22,500 public-tier residential beds in use in 1987.

22,500 × $4,000 = **$90 million**

Repair existing outpatient facilities

Assume 189,000 enrolled in public-tier programs.
Assume repair costs of 20% of upgraded annual cost, which equals $2,500
per client year times 1.25, or $3,125.

189,000 × 0.20 × $3,125 = **$118.1 million**

Train additional staff

Assume minimum of 26,000 staff in 1989.
Assume requirement for 13,300 additional staff, which equals 26,000 staff in
1989 divided by 275,000 clients in 1989 times 377,900 clients in future
times 1.1 for increase in staffing intensity.
Assume $2,000 per additional staff for first 10,000 (assumes most with some
prior experience or related training in drug problems) and $4,000 per
each additional staff (minimal or no closely related experience or
training).

10,000 × $2,000 + 3,300 × $4,000 = **$33.2 million**

COMPREHENSIVE STRATEGY OPTION

Annual Recurring Costs

Eliminate waiting list

Same as under core option. **$330 million**

Restore funding per client to 1976–1979 level

Same as under core option. **$412.5 million**

Staff training

Assume minimum of 26,000 staff in 1989.
Expect 60,200 total staff in future, which equals 26,000 staff in 1989 divided
by 275,000 clients in 1989 times 578,600 clients in future times 1.1 for
increase in staffing intensity.
Assume annual training expense of $500 per staff.

26,000 × $500 = **$13 million, first year**
60,200 × $500 = **$30.1 million, subsequent years**

Program/client performance monitoring system

Assume 815,000 annual public-tier clients in 1989.
Compromise scenario treats 689,600 more clients annually.
Estimate $25 per client for client reporting at intake, during treatment, and at discharge.
Assume postdischarge follow-up performed on 25% of public clients.
Estimate $200 per client tracked and interviewed to perform follow-up assessment after discharge.

(815,000 + 689,600) × [$25 + (0.25 × $200)] = **$112.8 million**

Aggressive outreach to expectant mothers

Assume aggressive outreach to drug-using expectant mothers reaches 15% with increasing cost per expectant mother reached (18,750 reached at $1,000 each plus 18,750 reached at $2,000 each plus 18,375 reached at $3,000).

18,750 × $1,000 + 18,750 × $2,000 + 18,750 × $3,000 = **$112.5 million**

Treat 56,250 expectant mothers

Assume half of recruited expectant mothers participate in 6 months of therapeutic community treatment (currently $12,500 per year, funding upgraded by 25%), and half get 6 months of outpatient treatment (currently $2,500 per year, funding upgraded by 25%).

(28,125 × $12,500 × 1.25 + 28,125 × $2,500 × 1.25) / 2 = **$263.7 million**

Children of mothers in residential programs

Same as under core option except 56,250 expectant mothers treated per year.

[(28,600 × 1/4) + (66,000 × 1/4 × 0.106) + (56,250 × 1/2 × 1/2)] × 0.225 × 2.5 × $6,000 = **$77.5 million**

Comprehensive probation emphasis on treatment

Increase daily treatment enrollment of probationers or parolees by 132,000 (double the waiting list number).

Fund at new rate per client in treatment—$5,000 per client in treatment, or $1,860 per client treated.
Keep current mix of residential and outpatient treatment.

$$132,000 \times \$5,000 = \textbf{\$660 million}$$

Comprehensive prison treatment

Increase daily prison treatment enrollment by 50,000, or twice the compromise goal (average treatment retention, 6 months).
Assume $3,125 per treatment year delivered in prison.

$$50,000 \times \$3,125 \,/\, 2 = \textbf{\$156.3 million}$$

One-time Capacity Expansion/Improvements

Residential capacity expansion

Increased length of stay requires additional 2,250 beds.
Waiting list expansion of 25% requires 7,000 beds.
Criminal justice system expansion also adds 50% (14,000 beds).
Expectant mothers expansion requires 14,060 beds.
Assume cost of $20,000 per additional space (discussed above).

$$(2,250 + 7,000 + 14,000 + 14,060) \times \$20,000 = \textbf{\$746.2 million}$$

Repair existing residential facilities

Same as under core option. **$90 million**

Repair existing outpatient facilities

Same as under core option. **$118.1 million**

Train additional staff

Assume minimum of 26,000 staff in 1989.
Assume requirement for 34,200 additional staff, which equals 26,000 staff in 1989 divided by 275,000 clients in 1989 times 578,600 clients in future times 1.1 for increase in staffing intensity.
Assume $2,000 per additional staff for first 10,000 (assumes most with some prior experience or related training in drug problems) and $4,000 per each additional staff (minimal or no closely related experience or training).

$$10,000 \times \$2,000 + 24,200 \times \$4,000 = \textbf{\$116.8 million}$$

INTERMEDIATE STRATEGY OPTION

Annual Recurring Costs

Eliminate waiting list

Same as under core option. **$330 million**

Restore funding per client to 1976–1979 level

Same as under core option. **$412.5 million**

Staff training

Assume minimum of 26,000 staff in 1989.
Expect 49,800 total staff in future, which equals 26,000 staff in 1989 divided by 275,000 clients in 1989 times 478,300 clients in future times 1.1 for increase in staffing intensity.
Assume annual training expense of $500 per staff.

$26,000 \times \$500 = $ **$13 million, first year**
$49,800 \times \$500 = $ **$24.9 million, subsequent years**

Program/client performance monitoring system

Assume 815,000 annual public-tier clients in 1989.
Compromise scenario treats 443,100 more clients annually.
Estimate $25 per client for client reporting at intake, during treatment, and at discharge.
Assume postdischarge follow-up performed on 25% of public clients.
Estimate $200 per client tracked and interviewed to perform follow-up assessment after discharge.

$(815,000 + 443,100) \times [\$25 + (0.25 \times \$200)] = $ **$94.4 million**

Aggressive outreach to expectant mothers

Assume aggressive outreach to drug-using expectant mothers reaches 18,750 at $1,000 each plus 18,750 additional at $2,000 each.

$18,750 \times \$1,000 + 18,750 \times \$2,000 = $ **$56.3 million**

Treat 37,500 expectant mothers

Assume half of recruited expectant mothers participate in 6 months of therapeutic community treatment (currently $12,500 per year, funding upgraded by 25%), and half get 6 months of outpatient treatment (currently $2,500 per year, funding upgraded by 25%).

(18,750 × \$12,500 × 1.25 + 18,750 × \$2,500 × 1.25) / 2 = **\$175.8 million**

Children of mothers in residential programs

Same as under core option except 37,500 expectant mothers treated per year.

[(28,600 × 1/4) + (66,000 × 1/4 × 0.106) + (37,500 × 1/2 × 1/2)] × 0.225 × 2.5 × \$6,000 = **\$61.7 million**

Modest probation/parole induction

Increase daily treatment enrollment of probationers or parolees by 66,000 (equal to prior increase to admit waiting list).
Fund at new rate per client in treatment—\$5,000 per client in treatment, or \$1,860 per client treated.
Keep current mix of residential and outpatient treatment.

66,000 × \$5,000 = **\$330 million**

Modest prison treatment

Increase daily prison treatment enrollment by 25,000.
Fund at \$3,125 per treatment year delivered in prison (assumed as equal to annual funding of outpatient because residential costs are already covered by prison).

25,000 × \$3,125 = **\$78.1 million**

One-time Capacity Expansion/Improvements

Residential capacity expansion

Increased length of stay requires additional 2,250 beds.
Waiting list expansion of 25% requires 7,000 beds.
Criminal justice system expansion also adds 25% (7,000 beds).
Expectant mothers expansion requires 9,375 beds.
Assume annual cost of \$20,000 (see core estimates).

(2,250 + 7,000 + 7,000 + 9,375) × \$20,000 = **\$512.5 million**

Repair existing residential facilities

Same as under core option. **\$90 million**

Repair existing outpatient facilities

Same as under core option. **$118.1 million**

Train additional staff

Assume minimum of 26,000 staff in 1989.

Assume requirement for 23,750 additional staff, which equals 26,000 staff in 1989 divided by 275,000 clients in 1989 times 478,300 clients in future times 1.1 for increase in staffing intensity.

Assume $2,000 per additional staff for first 10,000 (assumes most with some prior experience or related training in drug problems) and $4,000 per each additional staff (minimal or no closely related experience or training).

$$10,000 \times \$2,000 + 13,750 \times \$4,000 = \textbf{\$75 million}$$

APPENDIX 7B
MODELING FUTURE TREATMENT NEEDS AND EFFECTS

All of the strategy options presented here involve prospective resource requirements and expenditures over the next three to five years. How long such needs will last is a very important question, but unfortunately there is no solid base on which to ground the answer. The goal of early aggressive initiatives is obviously to reduce current and future problems and requirements for drug treatment and enforcement expenditures in the future.

Although there is evidence that drug treatment reduces the treated individual's likelihood of future drug use and criminal activity, this evidence must be incorporated into a systematic epidemiological model of drug consumption across the population, considering factors that affect onset, progression, duration, recovery, and relapse, as well as the respective effects of prevention, enforcement, and treatment. A dynamic model is required that predicts the potential need for treatment services over time contingent on alternative public policies. One might hypothesize that a "status quo" policy of limited availability of treatment with current prevention and enforcement policies would produce a gradually increasing need for treatment. "Legalization" of currently illicit drugs could result in dramatic increases in the clinically defined need for treatment (although legalization proponents contend this tendency to increase need would be offset in terms of economic costs and perhaps clinical criteria as well by reduced criminal activity). Intermediate anti-drug policies (treatment, prevention, and enforcement) could be expected to progressively reduce the need for treatment over time relative to the status quo of limited treatment availability. The alternative scenarios represent fears and desires regarding the effectiveness of drug policy; what is required is sophisticated analysis and modeling of the effects of different anti-drug policies on the number of drug users, their legal and criminal behaviors, and their need for treatment.

Although rudimentary dynamic models of heroin and cocaine use have been developed (Levin et al., 1975; Hunt and Chambers, 1976; Gardiner and Schreckengost, 1987; Homer et al., 1988), no one has yet produced a model that incorporates all drugs or simulates the effects of public policy variables (prevention, treatment, and enforcement). Consequently, the strategy options described earlier in this chapter must be considered short- to medium-term estimates, and judgments about more distant future requirements must be left in abeyance at present.

APPENDIX 7C
MEDICAID

Although the ADMS block grant has been the principal federal mechanism to support the public drug treatment system during the 1980s, the public health insurance plans, Medicaid and Medicare, have devoted a notable amount of resources and attention to drug treatment in recent years. Coverage by Medicaid is the major alternative to grant and contract mechanisms as the way to provide public coverage.

Medicaid is the major mechanism of public health care financing for low-income people in the United States who by and large cannot afford individual private health policies and do not hold jobs that include employer-sponsored group plan coverage—with the obvious exception of the large group of people with low incomes who receive their primary health coverage from Medicare.[5] The Medicare population of 32 million is mostly over 65 years of age and is relatively peripheral with regard to the kinds of drug problems that most engage public concern. Therefore, Medicare is not a key element in considering public-tier funding.[6]

---

[5] In addition, certain large populations depend on health programs of the Department of Veterans Affairs and the Department of Defense (DoD) for access to drug treatment. Generally, the committee has not considered populations covered by the specialized programs of DoD—military personnel and dependents—as part of this study, except insofar as VA programs were discussed earlier in this chapter.

[6] To put the point more concretely, illicit drug abuse and dependence are not major cost factors in Medicare, nor do Medicare clients figure prominently in the financing of drug treatment programs. In 1983, for example, there were 4,451 general hospital admissions of Medicare clients with a primary diagnosis of drug dependence or abuse—0.04 percent of the 10 million annual Medicare hospital admissions. (By comparison, there were 53,019 Medicare admissions with a primary diagnosis of alcoholism [Harwood et al., 1985].) In 1987, drug treatment programs of all modalities reporting to states admitted only 1,300 clients aged 65 and older (Butynski and Canova, 1988).

A few states now use Medicaid on a fairly extensive basis to support drug treatment services, and it has some role in nearly all states. Enough states increased their use of Medicaid during the 1980s that, according to the NDATUS results, from 1982 to 1987 public third-party reimbursements (which are primarily Medicaid) more than doubled. Yet despite the significant use of Medicaid in a few states, there are powerful limitations on what it now can and cannot do for the population without private insurance. To see why, it is necessary to review briefly the way Medicaid coverage policy is determined and its limitations with respect to eligibility and services.

Coverage Policy Determination Under Medicaid

Medicaid is a cooperative federal/state program regulated by federal law but administered by state officials; under it the states have a great deal of autonomy, including the simple option not to participate. The federal government pays half or more of the costs of Medicaid program claims in a state on a matching formula basis, with the match coming from state appropriations. The match varies from 1:1 to 3:1 (federal:state funds), depending on a mathematical formula that is set for each state based on its poverty and income characteristics. The federal government sets certain minimum requirements (in terms of whom a state must consider eligible and what services and procedures its program must cover) for classification as a "participating state," that is, to receive federal matching dollars.

Beyond these minima, states have substantial options to cover more people or services on their own, and the federal government will continue to match these expenditures on the same basis as the required coverage. Federal regulations permit reimbursement of most services delivered in the major drug treatment modalities, but they do not require states to cover most of them. As a result, there is no consistency across states in who gets covered for drug treatment or in what kinds of drug treatment services are reimbursed.

In 1987 the NDATUS found that third-party public payments to reporting providers were $139 million, or nearly 11 percent of total reported revenues (Table 7C-1). Third-party public reimbursements included Medicaid, Medicare, and some payments by insurance programs for military families using nonmilitary treatment services. It is probable that most of the reported revenues were Medicaid dollars, among other reasons because the majority of these reimbursements were in just three states that make significant use of Medicaid for drug treatment: New York, California, and Pennsylvania, which accounted for nearly $90 million out of the $139 million in revenues. (These states have quite different approaches, however, and the large dollar flow in California is attributable to that state's large size rather than to an unusual level of commitment to this financing mechanism.) Without more detailed information, which no one has yet assembled, it is impossible to know to what extent different factors account for the very large differences in state coverage, factors such as eligibility requirements, the nature of services covered, the reimbursement rates established by the different states, underlying needs for treatment, and adequacy of alternative financing mechanisms.

Eligibility

The Medicaid system was the primary health insurance protection during some part of 1986 for 20.6 million citizens under the age of 65 (Chollet, 1988; U.S. Department of Commerce, 1988); in comparison, 32.4 million persons in this age group were estimated to be living in poverty (U.S. Department of Commerce, 1988). The reason for this evident gap is that, although federal requirements hold that certain disadvantaged persons and family configurations are categorically qualified for Medicaid coverage, the states still have enormous discretion in setting the income-based standards for eligibility within these categories.

All state plans must cover individuals who qualify for Supplemental Security Income, which includes blind, permanently and totally disabled, and aged (over 65) individuals with low annual incomes and total assets. These standards qualified 6.3 million persons in 1986, of whom 3.1 million each were aged and disabled, for reimbursement by Medicaid of services not covered by Medicare. Probably the major significance of this population's eligibility is that Medicare will not pay for nursing home care but Medicaid will, and nursing home claims now account for more than two-thirds of all Medicaid payments, limiting the capacity of this system to deal with other kinds of health problems.

Most Medicaid beneficiaries (15.5 million) are eligible for Medicaid assistance owing to their receipt of Aid to Families with Dependent Children (AFDC), which is another federal/state cooperative program. AFDC eligibility is based on a categorical qualification plus an income standard established by the individual states. It always covers single-parent families, pregnant women, and young children in two-parent families *provided* their household of residence has an income below a financial "standard of need" that is usually configured in terms of a percentage of the federal poverty line. States may at their option cover as "medically needy" categorically eligible persons in households with incomes somewhat *above* the AFDC standard (that is, individuals who cannot receive AFDC). But most states have used their great latitude in establishing the standard of need to set the income level of AFDC eligibility, and thus Medicaid eligibility, at a percentage somewhat if not substantially (e.g., 35 percent) below the poverty line.

TABLE 7C-1 Third-Party Public Revenues by State in 1987 as a Percentage of Public State Total Revenues and of National Third-Party Public Payments

State	State Revenues		Third-Party Public Payments	
	Third-Party ($000s)	Total ($000s)	Percentage of State Total	Percentage of All National
Alabama	644	6,987	9.2	0.5
Alaska	16	3,366	0.5	0.0
Arizona	948	24,328	3.9	0.7
Arkansas	354	2,641	13.4	0.3
California	17,779	256,530	6.9	12.8
Colorado	3,753	18,458	20.3	2.7
Connecticut	1,797	20,832	8.6	1.3
Delaware	5	1,352	0.4	0.0
District of Columbia	17	7,306	0.2	0.0
Florida	2,446	61,729	4.0	1.8
Georgia	478	24,288	2.0	0.3
Hawaii	22	4,730	0.5	0.0
Idaho	5	1,429	0.3	0.0
Illinois	1,227	40,484	3.0	0.9
Indiana	1,092	17,391	6.3	0.8
Iowa	1,118	11,553	9.7	0.8
Kansas	498	6,443	7.7	0.4
Kentucky	1,161	7,745	15.0	0.8
Louisiana	1,880	13,967	13.5	1.4
Maine	245	3,459	7.1	0.2
Maryland	3,031	27,837	10.9	2.2
Massachusetts	642	20,300	3.2	0.5
Michigan	1,613	36,408	4.4	1.2
Minnesota	2,337	25,772	9.1	1.7
Mississippi	115	1,769	6.5	0.1
Missouri	500	15,103	3.3	0.4
Montana	9	1,786	0.5	0.0
Nebraska	146	4,725	3.1	0.1
Nevada	21	2,971	0.7	0.0
New Hampshire	196	5,637	3.5	0.1
New Jersey	788	32,797	2.4	0.6
New Mexico	610	6,363	9.6	0.4
New York	58,773	250,382	23.5	42.2
North Carolina	1,337	18,848	7.1	1.0
North Dakota	725	6,486	11.2	0.5
Ohio	6,209	59,123	10.5	4.5
Oklahoma	527	8,227	6.4	0.4
Oregon	223	10,918	2.0	0.2
Pennsylvania	14,190	69,845	20.3	10.2
Puerto Rico	0	10,127	0.0	0.0
Rhode Island	28	5,115	0.5	0.0
South Carolina	431	7,263	5.9	0.3
South Dakota	0	778	0.0	0.0
Tennessee	1,016	9,279	10.9	0.7
Texas	4,856	64,341	7.5	3.5

Continues on next page

TABLE 7C-1   *(Continued)*

State	State Revenues		Third-Party Public Payments	
	Third-Party ($000s)	Total ($000s)	Percentage of State Total	Percentage of All National
Utah	220	6,828	3.2	0.2
Vermont	73	917	8.0	0.1
Virginia	1,531	28,653	5.3	1.1
Washington	1,275	11,474	11.1	0.9
West Virginia	249	2,941	8.5	0.2
Wisconsin	2,023	18,200	11.1	1.5
Wyoming	48	1,762	2.7	0.0
Total United States	139,227	1,308,013	10.6[a]	100.0

[a]This figure is an average rather than a sum.

Source: Institute of Medicine analysis of the 1987 National Drug and Alcoholism Treatment Utilization Survey.

The federal statutes for Medicaid allow states the option of covering certain additional individuals who do not fit the mandatory categories: older children, two-parent intact families, single adults, and childless couples. Very few states have taken up these options, which would bring Medicaid much closer to being a form of universal coverage for low-income people. As a result, probably the largest segment of drug-abusing and dependent individuals—young, single, adult males—are categorically ineligible for Medicaid.

Aside from eligibility as such, actual registration for Medicaid can be a problem. In New York, where Medicaid standards are relatively inclusive, drug treatment programs routinely check whether new clients are certified or prima facie eligible for public assistance, which virtually ensures Medicaid eligibility. Uncertified but eligible clients may complete application forms (kept handy by admission units) at the time of initial program contact and submit them by mail. In contrast, application for Medicaid coverage in most states must be made in person at a central office.

Coverage Provisions

The federal guidelines for minimum benefits do not specifically deal with drug treatment. Federally required Medicaid services primarily include inpatient and outpatient hospital services and physician services. Although these services are sometimes necessary to treat some kinds of drug problems and to deal with such sequelae or complications as trauma, AIDS, and other infectious diseases, the primary components of drug abuse treatment are psychosocial services (counseling, social work, psychotherapy), pharmacotherapy (medications such as methadone, buprenorphine, or desipramine), and residency in a therapeutic milieu. Coverage for counseling services, prescribed medications, and residential treatment outside of hospital wards is not required but is left to the discretion of the states, along with the rates at which these elements are reimbursable.

There is no systematic study available of state Medicaid coverage for specific drug treatment services. A number of states do reimburse selected types and amounts of relevant services, most commonly (based on the committee's site visit information) physician examinations at admission (but generally at a rate equal to a conventional outpatient office visit rather than a multiphasic examination appropriate for an individual potentially severely compromised by drug abuse or dependence), methadone prescription (but generally at a rate that does not cover the cost of meeting federal regulations to run a lawful maintenance clinic), and services of psychiatrists or licensed clinical psychologists (but not other counseling professionals). Emergency hospitalization for drug overdoses is generally covered, but treatment in residential programs is rarely reimbursed.

These selective reimbursements have been sufficient to allow a few states with relatively wide eligibility and generous benefits, such as New York, Pennsylvania, and Colorado, to draw on Medicaid as the source of more than 20 percent of all provider revenues. (In New York, moreover, public assistance-eligible clients in residential programs may also receive reimbursement under the Home Relief and Food Stamps programs, which helps to defray residential program expenses.) In many other states, however, drug treatment providers receive almost no Medicaid support.

The Current and Future Status of Medicaid Coverage

In theory, the Medicaid system could cover many drug-abusing and dependent individuals because the clients served by the public tier are mostly indigent and that population is the group Medicaid was designed to serve. Yet the future role of Medicaid is undefined. In a few states, it is an important underpinning of the treatment system; in others, its effect is negligible. **In the committee's judgment, if Medicaid is to assume a consistent role across the board in financing the public tier of drug treatment, federal legislation governing Medicaid must be materially altered so as to address drug treatment needs. Such legislation should delineate eligibility criteria, the kinds of services and providers eligible for reimbursement, and minimum reimbursement levels.**

There are interesting precedents for Medicaid financing of drug treatment. The AIDS crisis is leading to new federal and state initiatives that extend Medicaid coverage to populations not previously included. In California, individuals diagnosed with AIDS or AIDS-related complex are categorically eligible for Medicaid coverage, whether or not they are eligible under other categories. If they qualify in terms of the income criterion, these individuals may receive Medicaid reimbursement for covered hospital and physician services.

In a related precedent, many states are using their Medicaid systems to disburse $30 million in federal formula grant funds for purchase of the prescribed AIDS medication AZT. These one-time emergency grants had no federal attachment to Medicaid, but many states have found it efficient and convenient to use their existing Medicaid billing, administrative, and disbursement systems to spend and document these funds, even though the medication is purchased largely by individuals who are not otherwise categorically eligible or are not recipients of Medicaid coverage. This experience demonstrates that existing Medicaid reimbursement mechanisms can be adapted to manage other reimbursements that are parallel to but not part of Medicaid under present state criteria.

Finally, and most pertinently, recent legislation (P.L. 100-360) requires states to provide Medicaid coverage to pregnant women and their infants who meet or exceed the federal poverty level by up to 35 percent. This provision is limited to health services related to pregnancy and to conditions that threaten the well-being of the infant. Maternal drug abuse certainly threatens the health of the infant, but whether this provision leads to the induction of such women into appropriate forms of care remains to be seen. The committee's recommendations regarding expanded outreach to this population could be partially—and increasingly over time—supported through Medicaid reimbursement for those eligible.

8

Private Coverage

Although the public tier admits the great majority of drug-abusing and drug-dependent individuals who receive treatment each year and their treatment is paid for mainly with public funds, there is a private tier of treatment providers as well that serves a significant proportion of the individuals seeking treatment and that uses an even larger proportion of treatment funding. Most of the support for the private tier depends on insurance reimbursements, and most private health insurance in the United States is obtained through employer-sponsored health insurance plans. Moreover, most if not all of the premium is treated as a fringe benefit rather than a part of wages or salaries. As a result, health insurance purchases are constrained in ways that purchases of other consumer goods, such as food, cars, or housing, are not.

Employers, whether private firms or public agencies, are the primary payers on behalf of their employees and immediate families. Consequently, employers have a major influence on and financial responsibility for the extent and nature of insurance coverage for drug treatment. This influence is especially felt when the benefit package is not developed by collective bargaining agreements, which give workers greater leverage over the terms of coverage. Although employer-sponsored health insurance was developed originally in bargained (that is, union-management) contracts, most employees are not represented by unions. This chapter therefore considers the provision of coverage largely from the perspective of employers vis-à-vis employees and insurers.

The chapter first discusses the logic of private coverage by health insurance and out-of-pocket payments. In Chapter 7 the committee estimated the number of individuals who would probably need to rely on the public system for coverage in the event they sought drug treatment. Here, the discussion simply reviews the principle that treatment effectiveness, cost, and the price sensitivity of potential consumers of treatment jointly contribute to determining the socially optimal level of private coverage.

The next issue is the actual extent of private coverage. There are data to respond to this question, but they are less than satisfactory. The first source of information is ostensible coverage, that is, the written details of health insurance policies or comparable health plan benefits. Surveys of coverage provisions, however, are generally limited to medium- and large-scale employers. Moreover, this information, although useful, is of uncertain application because actual coverage may vary under the same ostensible provisions. The usual survey practice is to index coverage according to whether drug treatment benefits are explicitly defined. But the written provisions may understate that coverage if the plan implicitly considers drug dependence to be just another standard medical diagnosis. In that case, without making specific reference to it, the plan would cover drug treatment to the full extent that any other health services delivered by recognized therapeutic professionals are covered. On the other hand, the plan may overstate coverage because the coverage policy does not play out in practice, owing to the denial of certification to drug treatment seekers by managed care personnel, retrospective denial of benefits by utilization review personnel, or a refusal to make referrals.

The second source of data on coverage is claims experience, from the point of view of insurers paying or of providers receiving these payments. Regarding claims payments, there are many anecdotes and short-term trend statistics for particular companies, but this information is virtually always in terms of combined alcohol/drug or alcohol/drug/mental health benefit utilization. The committee has been unable to access or assemble any systematic payer-based data on claims payments for drug treatment that are reasonably representative of national experience. From the provider end, the various National Drug and Alcoholism Treatment Utilization Survey (NDATUS) efforts are good indicators of provider insurance receipts despite some weaknesses in that data base (see Chapter 6). Unfortunately, the NDATUS has been too sparse (only two surveys since 1980) and too limited in its queries to yield a detailed picture of changing private coverage experience.

Explicit coverage certainly expanded in the 1980s, and the NDATUS indicates that insurance payments expanded as well, but there is no way to peer deeply enough into the overall process to be completely certain of the relationship. For these reasons, this chapter lays out the available information but proceeds cautiously to conclusions.

An important issue in the drug and alcohol treatment fields concerns the setting of treatment services, especially inpatient versus outpatient and hospital versus nonhospital residence. The committee could be considered to be basically agnostic regarding the specific setting of care, but it is far from indifferent to quality and cost considerations. The quality of care offered under private coverage is not easy to assess because so much of it is provided in the outpatient nonmethadone and chemical dependency modalities, about which the effectiveness data (not to be confused with effectiveness as such) are, respectively, highly variable and poor.

Managed care personnel are conversant with and justify certification and review decisions based on research reports that are virtually all alcohol specific. Although it is true that chemical dependency treatment for alcohol or drug problems is similar and that there is some suggestion that it may be less effective for drug than for alcohol problems, this information is a weak reed on which to rest clinical care decisions. One can understand the rationale of payers that, absent outcome data, general medical care providers such as hospitals at least employ a credentialing and quality management system with which payers are familiar and in which they have some confidence.

Moreover, medical necessity exists in some cases in the form of serious psychiatric disturbances or somatic illnesses, and it is best to err on the side of safety—although that margin has become much less elastic since the advent of managed care. Nevertheless, the committee believes it would be far better to insist that drug treatment providers begin to provide solid outcome data as a basis for recruitment and reimbursement. This policy is not only in the treatment buyer's interests but also in the interests of the providers—more and more sellers will find it worthwhile if not necessary to participate in evaluation research to reestablish credibility with the private coverage community.

Cost management is at the core of most health care issues today, and drug treatment is no exception. It is important to remember that cost-containment schemes have proven much more successful at curbing utilization rates for expensive services such as hospitalization than at reducing unit costs. Nevertheless, there is clearly an opportunity if not a necessity to curb the unit costs of private care for drug treatment.

The final private coverage question concerns state mandates for drug treatment. In 19 states, the law requires private insurance to include drug treatment as a covered service. These statutes are an offshoot of the movement since 1970 to mandate private insurance coverage of alcohol treatment. Considered in their own right, the committee does not find a strong case for the value of further such mandates in other states or at a national level. In part, the lack of impetus for additional required coverage can be ascribed to data that show that drug treatment coverage is now much more extensive than the mandates would suggest; in part, it is because mandates have such a narrow application. In the competitive environment of private health coverage, in which commercial indemnity insurers, third-party administrators of self-insured company plans, Blue Cross/Blue Shield carriers, and health maintenance organizations are fighting for market share, mandates that apply only to some of these segments hobble their competitive position in ways that seem inefficient and inequitable.

THE LOGIC OF PRIVATE COVERAGE

The rationale behind mandating private health insurance coverage of drug treatment parallels the argument for public coverage: even among the privately insured population, there are negative external costs to drug abuse and dependence that may be reduced by drug treatment, and access to treatment is influenced by the price of treatment. Coverage of drug treatment by private insurance can make the effective price of treatment, at the time it is needed, significantly lower (for example, 80 percent of inpatient or residential costs may be covered) than if the full costs of treatment had to be paid out of pocket. This lower price means that more insured people who need treatment will seek it.

From society's perspective, insurance should reduce the effective purchase price of treatment for individuals who need it to the point that the insured population purchases the socially optimal amount of treatment. The socially optimal amount of coverage depends on both the effectiveness of treatment in reducing external costs, its own costs, and the sensitivity of drug abusers to the price of effective treatment. The greater the social benefits from treatment, the greater should be the coverage rate (the share of costs paid by insurance). The greater the sensitivity of drug-abusing and dependent individuals (who create negative external costs) to the price of treatment, the greater should be the rate of coverage by insurance.

The sensitivity of drug abusers to the price of treatment may also depend on their income and wealth and on the relative cost of the treatment. For a wealthy family, the price of treatment may be quite secondary, whereas a lower income family may find price to be a major factor. Similarly, a cost of $1,500 for a typical treatment episode of average effectiveness may have quite different implications than a cost of $7,000. Access to expensive treatment is more likely than access to inexpensive treatment to be sensitive to insurance coverage.

There has been no systematic, empirical economic study of private demand for privately supplied, competitively priced treatment or of the responsiveness of private demand to the price of treatment. It is known that, corresponding to the increase in private insurance coverage for drug treatment (effectively reducing the cost of treatment to insured drug abusers), the private treatment sector appears to have grown dramatically. Employer-provided private insurance coverage for drug treatment was held by 43 percent of employees in medium-sized and large companies in 1983 (Morrisey and Jensen, 1988) but had increased to 74 percent in 1988 (Bureau of Labor Statistics, 1989a). During this period a number of states enacted mandates requiring private health insurance policies to cover drug treatment.

In 1982 the private, for-profit drug treatment industry included 159 programs with 9,800 clients in treatment; by 1987 it had grown to 735 programs with 30,000 drug abuse clients in treatment. Private insurance reimbursements for drug treatment (defined as such by treatment providers and thus not contingent on whether benefits were explicitly covered under a drug treatment clause) increased from $43.5 million in 1982 to $348 million in 1987. Client out-of-pocket reimbursement grew from $35.6 million in 1982 to $157 million (National Institute on Drug Abuse, 1983a; Institute of Medicine analysis of the 1987 NDATUS). It is not known, however, what proportion of the 1982 insurance reimbursements and client fee payments went to private-tier programs.

In contrast to residential and outpatient nonmethadone treatment, methadone treatment has a significant private demand that is not subsidized by private insurance reimbursements. Out of $200 million in total methadone clinic revenues, client out-of-pocket payments made up 20 percent. Within the $22 million private, for-profit methadone treatment system, $17 million, or more than 75 percent of revenues, were from client out-of-pocket payments.

The private tier predominantly treats clients who are ineligible for public coverage because of their level of income. In the absence of insurance coverage, these clients would have to pay for treatment out of pocket. Because the private treatment sector expanded so significantly in parallel with the growth of insurance coverage for drug treatment, it seems reasonable to suppose that whether potential drug treatment clients actually enter treatment is in fact quite sensitive to the price of treatment.

THE EXTENT OF PRIVATE INSURANCE COVERAGE

More than 150 million persons are covered by private health insurance coverage, the vast majority as a benefit of their employment (Chollet, 1988; Moyer, 1989). The focus of this section is the degree to which this coverage extends to drug treatment. The details of health insurance coverage have been studied periodically by the Bureau of Labor Statistics (BLS) during the 1980s, primarily through surveys of insurance provided to employees of medium-sized and large firms and state and local governments. The drug treatment coverage afforded to privately insured employees of the federal government has also been examined recently by the Office of Personnel Management. These studies constitute the source material for the following discussion. The major limitation on these detailed coverage data is that they do not include small, nongovernment employers, who employ half of the labor force.

As discussed in Chapter 7, it is possible that in some cases drug treatment is reimbursed in the absence of explicit coverage. A claim for treatment under a drug diagnosis, submitted by an appropriately licensed practitioner or accredited medical or rehabilitation facility, may simply be accepted without question; alternatively, it may be submitted under the guise of a different diagnosis that is clearly covered (e.g., a psychiatric disorder such as severe depression, alcohol dependence, or a physical abnormality). It is difficult to determine the extent to which either practice occurs, particularly the latter.

It has been said that alcoholics were treated in the past, despite the absence of explicit coverage or formal alcohol treatment programs, by simply employing different diagnoses within the general medical population. This statement cannot be disproved, but it is difficult to credit. Certainly, many alcohol-dependent individuals received medical treatment at times, but most medical practitioners had no training in alcohol treatment (versus the treatment of, for example, gut ailments resulting from excessive alcohol consumption). The initial growth spurt of chemical dependency providers occurred largely after explicit coverage emerged in a number of key states and company plans, and its arc of growth has echoed the spread of explicit coverage. Nevertheless, the bar to treatment was probably much more the lack of formal programs, or programs with the medical or psychiatric accreditation recognized by insurers, than a disincentive to cover the treatment. A Blue Cross and Blue Shield Association study (1983) concluded that many if not most Blue plans at that time covered drug treatment under their mental and nervous disorders benefits.

The most notable evidence for the relevance of explicit policy provisions to actual coverage is the fact that the growth in private insurance reimbursements reported by treatment providers has occurred in parallel with the growth of explicit coverage.

Employees of Private Companies

Medium-sized and large companies (i.e., more than 100 employees) have increased their explicit coverage for drug treatment significantly since 1983. In 1988, 74 percent of employees in such companies had coverage, an increase from 66 percent in 1986 and 43 percent in 1983 (Morrisey and Jensen, 1988; Bureau of Labor Statistics, 1989a). The BLS 1988

Employee Benefit Survey (EBS) included much more detailed questions than any previous survey about the character of such coverage. Only sketchy statistical summaries of the responses to these items are available as yet, but these summaries are indicative of the direction of this coverage.

The 1988 EBS survey indicated that 28 million of the 31 million employees of firms sampled by the survey had employer-sponsored health insurance. Of the 31 million, 20.6 million were covered by plans that had an explicit provision for drug treatment or said that as a matter of course they would provide reimbursement for detoxification or rehabilitation charges. For the other 10 million employees of medium-sized and large firms, drug treatment episodes were excluded from their health insurance coverage.

Of the 21 million employees with drug treatment coverage, nearly all (96 percent) would be reimbursed for residential or inpatient drug detoxification—which is not drug treatment per se (referred to in this connection as "rehabilitation"), although it is certainly indicative of a drug-related diagnosis. Inpatient or residential treatment was covered for 16 million employees, and outpatient treatment was covered for 17 million. There were limitations on this coverage, however, that differed from the standard limitations in the applicable health plans.[1] For the most part, the limitations involved a differential cap on dollars or on number of days or visits, rather than different copayments, deductibles, or maximum out-of-pocket costs (Table 8-1). The most frequently imposed inpatient limit was 30 days per year; the most frequent outpatient limit was 20 or 30 visits per year. The typical inpatient limitation was based on the average chemical dependency inpatient treatment plan.

State and Local Government Employees

Insurance coverage of public employees and their dependents is relatively better documented than insurance arranged through private employers. Within the public sector, coverage for drug treatment is virtually universal for federal employees and nearly so for state and local employees. But the types of benefits are highly variable across the different plans of the thousands of state and local government entities. An estimate of this coverage is available from a BLS survey (Bureau of Labor Statistics, 1988) conducted in 1987 of benefits provided to employees of state and local governments.

Health insurance coverage for drug treatment in 1987 was more widespread among publicly employed workers than in the private sector. Among the 10.3 million full-time employees of state and local governments

---

[1] The limitations may apply to drug treatment alone, or they may apply to drug, psychiatric, and/or alcohol treatment as a group.

TABLE 8-1   Details of Drug Dependence/Abuse Benefits (percentage) for the Covered Employees of Medium-sized and Large Firms

Procedure	Any Coverage	Coverage Limitations		
		Length of Stay or Dollar Cap	Out-of-pocket Ceiling	Copayment or Deductible
Detoxification	96	0.61	0.05	0.01
Inpatient rehabilitation	77	0.58	0.05	0.01
Outpatient rehabilitation	81	0.46	0.10	0.06

Note: Of the 31 million employees of medium-sized and large firms (i.e., 100 or more employees), 90 percent have some health insurance coverage, and 74 percent of those (i.e., 20.6 million) are covered for drug detoxification or rehabilitation procedures. The first column of the table is the percentage of the 20.6 million with any coverage for a particular procedure; subsequent columns are fractions of the first column percentage to which the respective limitations apply.

Source: Bureau of Labor Statistics (1989a).

in 1987, the BLS study estimated that 94 percent had health care coverage, and of these, 94 percent had coverage for some type of inpatient hospital treatment for drug abuse; it is uncertain how much of this coverage applied only to detoxification. Outpatient coverage was conservatively estimated at 81 percent of health plan participants.

Special limitations were usually imposed on the amount of coverage for drug treatment. About 71 percent of the 94 percent with inpatient coverage were subject to special limitations on care that were different from those for other health care procedures. The most common limitation (38 percent) was a cap on payment for inpatient days of mental health, drug, and alcohol treatment. Another 22 percent of covered employees were limited in the number of days that would be covered just for treatment of drug abuse. The most common limitation (15 percent) was a maximum of 30 inpatient days; 6 percent had higher limits, and 2 percent had lower limits.

Coverage for outpatient services was more restrictive. Some form of outpatient coverage was available to at least 81 percent of employees participating in health insurance plans. Yet for only 16 percent of these was the coverage equivalent to that for other health problems. Charging benefits against mental health limits was most common—affecting 35 percent of the 81 percent with outpatient coverage. Limits on annual visits applied to 13 percent of the covered group (9 percent with 30 or fewer visits, 2 percent with 50 or more visits). There were coverage limitations on maximum dollars, or different coinsurance rates or copayments, for 18 percent of the provisions.

Federal Employees

The federal system had nearly 4 million health insurance policies in force in March 1988, covering close to 10 million current employees, retirees, and dependents.[2] The specifics of federal drug treatment benefits were closely examined by the Office of Personnel Management (OPM) in a document that outlined the pertinent benefits of all offerings within the Federal Employee Benefits Health Plan (U.S. Office of Personnel Management, 1988). Every plan was required to offer substance abuse treatment benefits; however, there were no specific coverage standards, and the nature of coverage varied widely. The common characteristic of all plans was to make no distinctions between drug and alcohol treatment benefits; in addition, their monetary values, as calculated by OPM, were all heavily weighted toward inpatient treatment. In this sense the federal plans seemed more or less to endorse chemical dependency treatment concepts, by and large tending to focus benefits on hospital-based treatment to the exclusion of nonhospital residential programs and, more importantly, to provide only minimal coverage for outpatient services.

Among the 23 fee-for-service plans available, the most common coverage package was judged to include $4,000 to $6,000 per year in potential drug treatment benefits, with significant special deductibles and copayments. There was much variation around this average: 8 plans had total annual coverage of from $2,800 to $4,000, 10 were in the $5,000 to $10,000 range, and 5 were worth $18,000 or more. In 15 policies, more than 90 percent of the value of these benefits was specifically designated for inpatient treatment in hospital-based facilities. Five fee-for-service plans offered no coverage for outpatient services, and 7 others limited such services to $250 to $400 per year. Benefits of $750 to $1,000 per year were provided by 6 plans, whereas 3 offered benefits worth $1,500 to $2,500.[3]

Health maintenance organizations (HMOs) had benefits similar in many ways to fee-for-service plans, although the major HMOs seemed to impose fewer constraints and limitations with regard to inpatient care and the same or fewer limitations with respect to covering outpatient care. Nearly all of the largest HMOs covered inpatient treatment for up to 30 days with negligible or modest copayments. Outpatient treatment was covered by all HMOs, generally to a maximum of 20 annual reimbursed

---

[2] The federal government employed 3 million persons in 1986, of which 2.6 million were full-time employees entitled to government-financed health insurance coverage. There were also an additional 1.1 million federal retirees.

[3] Nine policies included stop-loss limits (payment for any annual out-of-pocket expenditures for alcohol/drug treatment that exceeded a specific amount) ranging from $4,000 to $8,000, which were further subject to lifetime maxima. Another 9 policies specified out-of-pocket maxima of $25,000 to $50,000; 4 had no explicit lifetime maximum.

visits, which is close to, although somewhat short of, the average outpatient nonmethadone treatment plan. A significant number of plans stipulated copayments of $20 (or more) per outpatient visit, whereas about half the regional plans under one large HMO covered "all necessary outpatient counseling" at minimal copayment rates.

Employers and Coverage Decisions

Although the public sector has made a limited amount of treatment available for the past 20 years (primarily directed toward criminally active drug abusers), until recently there has been little recognition of the drug problem in the work force. Private insurance policies gave little explicit recognition to the need for this type of treatment. Drug treatment, if delivered, was reported under medical diagnoses. As recently as 1983, only 43 percent of workers in medium-sized and large private companies had explicit coverage for any kind of drug treatment (Morrisey and Jensen, 1988).

The reasons for the lack of coverage are many and varied, as are the reasons coverage has dramatically increased over the past 15 years. Not the least of the problem has been the lack of recognition or actual denial among employers that there were many or any drug-abusing and dependent individuals in their work force. Furthermore, like alcohol problems, drug problems have at best been viewed as a character flaw or personal weakness and at worst as "willful misconduct."

Another problem has been uncertainty on the part of insurers. There is uncertainty about the extent to which the benefit will be used and how much to pay for these services. It is unclear what kind or kinds of treatment should be covered—what works and what the outcomes are. This uncertainty makes it difficult for insurers to price the benefit reasonably without leaving themselves (or the self-insured entity) exposed to large potential losses if usage or cost per treatment is greater than expected. This uncertainty can motivate overpricing of the benefit until sufficient time as the benefit may be rated based on experience. Inflated pricing for a benefit may discourage employers (or individuals) from purchasing the benefit.

Implicit in the rationale for the addition of coverage for drug treatment is that drug treatment may pay for itself, either through improved worker productivity or through a "health cost offset" effect. There has been no rigorous analysis of the productivity-improving effects of chemical dependency drug treatment. However, a large and growing literature (Holder and Blose, 1986; Holder and Hallan, 1986) suggests that the cost of treating alcoholics is recovered subsequent to treatment by reducing their insurance claims for health services. The conclusions of this literature, although subject to methodological weaknesses, have by inference been applied to justify drug treatment, even though there are no studies of cost offsets with clients with primary drug abuse problems.

In the committee's view, the justification for insurance coverage for drug treatment does not and should not rest on insurance cost offsets. Most health care services are covered whether or not the treatment renders cost offsets. Many terminal or chronic illnesses might not be treated if the criteria of cost-effectiveness were applied. Advanced-stage cancer, stroke, and heart disease are primarily incident in older persons who have relatively short life expectancies even without the specific disease; they often have poor prognoses, and aggressive treatment tends to be very expensive (Hartunian et al., 1980). Similarly, organ transplants involve high costs and are undertaken with the expectation of modestly increasing life expectancy or quality of life but not necessarily of saving costs for the insurance plan. In the sense that drug treatment has no proven expectation for immediate reduction of health care expenditures and can be expensive, it is analogous to coverage of treatment for many terminal or life-threatening illnesses. There are, however, valid concerns about directing patients to the least expensive of equally effective treatments or providers. These concerns have been the most important recent trend influencing the extent of private coverage and are discussed in the next section.

TRENDS AFFECTING PRIVATE COVERAGE: COST CONTAINMENT OF HEALTH BENEFITS

The major trend that is now affecting private coverage for drug treatment is unquestionably the increasing emphasis on cost containment. There are both general and specific reasons that have led purchasers and underwriters of group policies to take long, hard looks at drug treatment benefits. Generally, the cost of health services and particularly of health insurance has grown at an uncomfortably high rate during the past two decades. Health care expenditures now make up about 11.5 percent of the U.S. gross national product, up from 7.5 percent 20 years ago. Private health insurance expenditures were $71 per capita in 1970 and $552 per capita in 1987 (Health Insurance Association of America, 1989). In the wake of these increases has come an ever-intensifying search for ways to reduce the cost of health insurance benefits by private as well as public insurance plans.

The percentage of total health insurance outlays spent on drug treatment is small. Total health care outlays by commercial insurers, Blue Cross/Blue Shield carriers, and HMOs were $140 billion in 1987. The 1987 NDATUS figure of just under $350 million for health insurance payments to all surveyed drug treatment programs amounts to just 0.25 percent of total private insurance outlays. Even if the NDATUS undercounted by as much as half, which would inflate the committee's estimate to $700 million, this figure is still only 0.5 percent of total health insurance outlays. One might further estimate, guided by reports from the public sector (see the section on detoxification in Chapter 7), that as few as one-seventh of all private detoxification episodes lead to the initiation of rehabilitation treatment. Using the ICF Incorporated (1987) report on the costs of private-tier inpatient detoxification and rehabilitation episodes as a guide, one would be led to estimate that about $700 million dollars more in health insurance dollars might be spent on drug detoxification outside of the identified treatment system. This outside figure of $1.4 billion for drug detoxification and rehabilitation is about 1 percent of total private health insurance outlays.

Of course, given the incomplete coverage of treatment, individual plans that do have adequate coverage may be expected to spend a proportion higher than this amount.[4] The committee reviewed a small number of unpublished actuarial ratings of drug treatment benefits that are typical of the 30-day/30-visit coverage seen around the country. The most careful and complete of these ratings indicated that the total costs of drug detoxification and treatment in a Blue Cross plan in one of the largest urban areas in the country were on the order of 0.7 percent of total private insurance outlays.

Nevertheless, in today's environment of general concern about health costs, insurers and funders of group plans have begun to single out for special attention the components of their insurance packages that are causing the greatest part of their payment increases. Insurance benefits for drug abuse, alcoholism, and mental health have had dramatic increases in utilization in the past five years. Although this rise in utilization would generate interest in this expenditure area under any circumstances, there have been additional concerns raised recently owing to skepticism about the cost-effectiveness—and, in some quarters, the effectiveness as such—of alcohol treatment. Close scrutiny of the evidence has led some researchers to conclude that more expensive hospital-based inpatient alcohol treatments appear to be no more effective than less expensive treatments (Saxe et al., 1983; Miller and Hester, 1986). The committee's companion Institute of Medicine (1990) panel has recently concluded that, in general, a significant

---

[4] The relationship between the degree of coverage and the claims experienced is subject to several sources of error. For example, when employee health benefit claims are processed by or available to a firm's personnel department, some individuals who would be covered for drug treatment services may be reluctant to claim the benefit for fear of jeopardizing their job standing. There is also a widespread belief among payers and providers—although no studies have been conducted or made available to support this belief—that some clinicians routinely or occasionally obfuscate the diagnosis of drug abuse or dependence (perhaps by masking it with a different diagnosis, such as depression) to increase the likelihood of reimbursement in those instances in which psychiatric diagnoses are covered but drug or alcohol diagnoses may not be.

number (about one-third) of the persons now cared for in inpatient facilities could receive appropriate care in less restrictive and less costly settings.

This finding is a problem for drug treatment because this coverage is in some sense an outgrowth of alcohol treatment coverage, and most of the private tier evolved into chemical dependency programs from an alcohol treatment focus. As the value of more expensive alcohol treatment programs has come into question, insurers have been quick to apply new limitations on coverage for alcohol treatment, largely in the form of aggressive managed care (Health Care Advisory Board, 1988; Korcok, 1988a,b; Malcolm, 1990).

Insurers, managed care companies, and employers are also increasingly critical of the lack of data on outcomes of chemical dependency treatment (cf. Chapter 5). Although increasing numbers of chemical dependency providers are compiling basic follow-up data on their clients, they do not yet have the necessary foundation in rigorously conducted outcome studies. Moreover, the outcome data compiled by and for private-tier providers (e.g., Comprehensive Care Corporation, 1988; Hoffmann and Harrison, 1988) are indicating that clients with drug problems have poorer outcomes than clients with primary alcohol problems.

In the face of increasing overall health insurance costs and doubts about the efficacy of more costly forms of alcohol treatment, the buyers of insurance, bearers of insurance risk (particularly employers), and third-party administrators have taken steps to attempt to reduce the increase in health costs. These steps have assumed the form of general policies for the entire fabric of health insurance and policies targeted specifically at drug and alcohol treatment. A prevailing hypothesis about health care costs holds that lack of competition has been responsible for a significant part of the increased costs (Fuchs, 1988; see also other articles in the same issue). It is argued that, under the old insurance plans, health services suppliers had inadequate incentives to keep the costs of services low. In fact, it has been suggested that the incentives were all in the direction of inflating health expenditures and prices (supplier-induced demand for health services). The health financing system consequently has been changing dramatically in the past decade, developing new incentives for providers and consumers as well as creating new public and private regulatory instruments.

Drug treatment has been caught up in this revolution. Supplier incentives to cut costs have been increased by encouraging capitated or prepaid health plans to develop. Health provision plans like HMOs and individual practitioner associations (IPAs) have pioneered in incorporating incentives to contain costs. Although rare at this stage, provider incentives for efficiency have been increased by the use of prospective reimbursement rates for services, like the diagnosis-related group rates established under Medicare for reimbursing hospital stays. Capitated and fee-for-service plans have been negotiating reduced-fee arrangements with preferred provider organizations (PPOs) in return for directing plan participants to these providers.

Consumer incentives to reduce costs have also been changed by modifying benefit schedules—increasing deductibles and copayment rates (Bureau of Labor Statistics, 1987). Consumers have also borne more of the visible cost of insurance through increasing employee contributions to cover the premium—in other words, by reducing salaries and wages rather than increasing fringe benefits. Changes in deductibles and copayment rates are designed not only to shift aggregate costs from the risk pool to the individual beneficiary but also to cause consumers to pay more attention to the prices of particular benefits and services.

Self-insurance administered by a third-party claims processor is an approach taken by an increasing number of private firms to reduce their health insurance bills. This strategy is designed to yield savings to the company through several avenues: avoiding state taxes on the premiums paid to commercial and Blue Cross/Blue Shield plans, giving the company control over the interest (liquidity) earned on annual premiums, avoiding payments to a financial intermediary to bear the risk associated with any kind of insurance, and avoiding expensive state mandates for insurance coverage. Self-insured companies assume the financial risk formerly born by insurers, retaining a third-party administrator to process claims.

A variety of strategies generically known as managed care have been introduced to regulate more closely the use of health services by beneficiaries or, alternatively, the supply of health services to beneficiaries by providers. These strategies include prospective certification or preadmission review (PAR) of hospital stays, utilization review during or after discharge, the use of preferred providers, and specialized high-cost case management. PAR requires that patients receive prior approval of admission to a hospital from the insurer to be entitled to full reimbursement for costs. Utilization review involves midtreatment or even retrospective review by insurers (or their managed care agents) of the "appropriateness" of services delivered, with denial of insurance reimbursement for unapproved services. Preferred providers often have contracts with the insurers about the level and nature of care to be delivered for a particular type of case. Under some contractual arrangements, managed care providers have explicit short-run financial (profit) incentives to reduce the utilization of health care services of beneficiaries under their supervision, although this arrangement is not true under fee-for-service contracts. Yet under fee-for-service contracts, a managed care contractor must eventually demonstrate success at controlling costs or risk losing the contract.

The objective of managed care strategies is to accumulate information about accepted clinical practices and the cost of these practices and to codify appropriate treatment strategies as protocols for permitting or disallowing reimbursement for particular services in particular instances. With the use of managed care, insurance carriers are attempting to address the problems of limited patient knowledge about health services and the potential for supplier-induced demand (Fuchs, 1988).

If managed care strategies for drug treatment are backed by research findings on treatment effectiveness, they can help guarantee needed access to quality treatment while containing the costs of insuring it. Under the powerful prod of negotiated services and managed care, private coverage has been moving away from its orientation toward acute inpatient care models. In this respect the private drug treatment system is repeating the earlier cycle of the public tier. Hospital-based treatment was virtually eliminated from the public drug treatment strategy in the mid-1970s when it was concluded to be no more effective than other treatment approaches but substantially more expensive (Strategy Council on Drug Abuse, 1975; Besteman, 1990). Public resources were redirected toward outpatient and nonhospital residential treatment, with the consequent ability to treat many more people for the same dollars. Managed care has the objective of identifying just such efficiencies.

On the other hand, coverage for services received from residential providers must be carefully framed. Some clients undoubtedly require residential treatment, and insurers need to recognize the distinctive value of residential providers, who may be affiliated with hospitals and even located in such settings but are disjoined from the requirements—including the financial burdens—of acute hospital care. Many insurers have in the past failed to recognize such providers as eligible for reimbursement, which may have contributed to excessive utilization of hospital inpatient treatment in the past.

As managed care strategies have matured, they have come under increasing scrutiny and criticism from alcohol and drug treatment providers following aggressive moves by managed care companies to cut the costs of treating drug and alcohol abuse. Taking cues (that is, preadmission and utilization review protocols) from the reviews by Saxe and colleagues (1983) and Miller and Hester (1986), which were entirely focused on alcohol and not drug treatment, managed care reviewers have attempted to direct all drug clients away from inpatient programs and toward outpatient services; as a result, they are certifying shorter and shorter inpatient stays. This trend is viewed with particular alarm by employee assistance program (EAP) staff, chemical dependency programs, and theapeutic communities that have received accreditation and recognition but are increasingly being asked to shorten treatment plans in ways that defy all their therapeutic experience.

Employee assistance program professionals are potentially important actors in the managed care system. There appears to be an uneasy relationship between EAP professionals and managed care providers because of the overlap of some of their respective roles. In many companies that use EAPs, the staff of the program have traditionally owned the role of "gatekeeper" to treatment, with the responsibility for assessing troubled employees, diagnosing their problems, and referring them to appropriate treatment. Because many EAP staff come from the alcoholism field and have had little professional contact with any other treatment modalities, as EAPs broadened their focus to deal with drug problems, the drug treatment of choice was by default the chemical dependency model. With the recent pressure on this model from cost-containment forces, the EAP professionals who were committed to it have, by and large, felt as though they were in a virtual state of war with managed care contractors: their referrals to treatment subject to review by external practitioners selected by the managed care firm, with fully reimbursed care available only through providers selected by that firm, with whom the EAP has had no previous relationship or knowledge of their practices.

There is clearly a significant overlap in the roles of EAPs and managed care providers, and this overlap may become a bureaucratic barrier that complicates access to needed treatment. However, EAPs are primarily charged with returning problem employees to satisfactory performance and promoting employee health over the long term. EAP personnel often establish relationships with treatment agencies to achieve these goals, sometimes with the consideration in mind of using treatment resources efficiently. Managed care personnel are primarily responsible for reducing the costs of health care episodes while ensuring that beneficiaries receive good-quality care. There are tensions between EAP responsibility for employee health and managed care accountability for cost control—often backed by contractual promises or inducements to reduce stipulated benefit payouts by specific percentage targets. Yet the tension may be a creative one if EAP and managed care personnel work together. The best relationships between EAP and managed care personnel occur when EAP staff are fundamentally involved in the adoption of managed care strategies and have a clearly delineated role in making assessments and referrals and in choosing providers. These relationships can be further improved by commitments to collecting better data on treatment processes and outcomes. The worst case seems to be when corporate benefits managers adopt managed care plans with minimal consultation of the EAP staff and no forethought about how the EAP will interface with managed care.

PRIVATE INSURANCE AND STATE MANDATES

The private tier of providers, which is linked to the corporate world of employee assistance programs, originated as and still is primarily an alcohol treatment system. Private providers have joined with the labor movement and a few underwriters and corporations in major educational efforts since about 1970 that have steadily increased the number of health plans that specifically cover alcohol and drug treatment. Also as a result of these efforts, state insurance mandates represent an important initiative relative to private coverage for drug treatment. A total of 18 states plus the District of Columbia have passed laws mandating some coverage for drug treatment. The objective has been either to require insurance plans to include coverage for this problem in their basic package of benefits or at least to require them to offer to sell such a benefit. States clearly view health insurance as a mechanism through which an increasingly costly public problem can be privatized. The mandating of drug treatment benefits began and is best seen as an offshoot of the mandation of alcohol treatment.

Access to Coverage

The first issue about the relevance of state mandates for coverage of drug treatment is whether they in fact make coverage more available to beneficiaries. As of this writing, 10 states plus the District of Columbia mandate the inclusion of drug treatment benefits in group policies. Another 8 states mandate that insurers at least offer this benefit as an optional addition to basic coverage. Each state has a similar or identical mandate for coverage of alcohol treatment.[5]

The extent of coverage (discussed earlier) for the 31 million employees (plus dependents) of medium-sized and large corporations and for 13 million public employees is much greater than would be indicated by the mandates enacted by state legislatures. States with mandates to cover or offer to cover drug treatment were home to 11.9 and 16.6 percent of the U.S. population, respectively. But in 1988, 74 percent of private employees in medium-sized and large firms that had company-sponsored health insurance had some kind of coverage for drug treatment. Among public employees the coverage rate in 1987 was 94 percent. Thus, the extent of insurance coverage for drug treatment is greater than would be indicated simply by state mandates.

A crucial issue with state insurance mandates is that private corporations that self-insure under federal ERISA (Employee Retirement Income Security Act) statutes effectively evade any insurance coverage mandates

---

[5] Another 10 states mandated provision of alcoholism coverage, and 9 more states mandated the offer of optional coverage for alcohol treatment. Altogether, 37 states plus the District of Columbia, comprising 85 percent of the U.S. population, have mandates regarding alcohol treatment coverage.

that are legislated by states. State coverage mandates are not likely to be a necessary or sufficient cause for any company to self-insure, but there is a clear tendency for self-insured companies to be less likely to cover drug treatment than companies with Blue Cross/Blue Shield coverage or employees covered under HMOs. Morrisey and Jensen (1988) found that employees of self-insured companies were much less likely to be explicitly covered for drug treatment (56 percent of employees were covered) than employees insured by a Blue Cross/Blue Shield carrier (76 percent) or an HMO[6] (88 percent). Policies with commercial insurers, however, were the least likely to offer drug treatment coverage (50 percent). A further analysis by Jensen (1988) indicates that state mandates are not significant predictors of whether a company self-insures when other characteristics of the company are examined. The important predictors of self-insurance were the size of the state tax on health insurance premiums, the nature of the industry, and the characteristics of workers of the company. Self-insured companies do so for more economically compelling reasons than to avoid coverage mandates for drug or alcohol treatment. On the other hand, an accumulation of several relatively inexpensive mandates may be expensive enough for a company to opt for self-insurance.

Adequacy of Coverage

The adequacy of mandated coverage for drug treatment is highly problematical because coverage for drug abuse is for all practical purposes an afterthought to coverage for alcohol treatment; where coverage for drug treatment is mandated, it is virtually identical to that for alcohol treatment. Only in Maryland are there different limits on coverage for drug and alcohol abuse, and in that case drug treatment has a lower minimum coverage than alcohol treatment.

Most of the state legislatures have virtually mandated only one modality, chemical dependency treatment, and made barely enough provision for a typical course of outpatient nonmethadone treatment. Of nine state drug abuse mandates that specify minimum days of inpatient coverage, six call for minimum annual coverage of 28 or 30 days; the other three call for minima of 21, 45, and 60 days.[7]

---

[6] There is a widespread belief among chemical dependency providers that HMO coverage of drug treatment is less extensive in practice than on paper. For example, providers assert that HMOs vigorously resist authorizing hospital stays, insist on group rather than individual counseling, and avoid treatment by high-cost care givers such as psychiatrists in favor of lower cost counseling professions. There is little documentary evidence on the extent of these practices or their effects on the outcomes of drug treatment of HMO clients.

[7] In a survey conducted in 1986 (ICF Incorporated, 1987), 230 chemical dependency programs charged an average of about $265 per day —about 10 percent above the average national daily

Three other state mandates cover minimum annual dollar limits for inpatient reimbursement, with values of $3,000 (per 30-day period), $4,500, and $9,000, respectively. The $9,000 coverage is for hospital-based inpatient rehabilitation treatment and is marginally or less than adequate for a 28- to 30-day stay. The lower dollar limits clearly preclude the use of most chemical dependency treatment programs at the rates typically charged. There is a great deal of evidence, however, that these rates can be drastically reduced without cutting into patient care costs by simply reducing the extraordinary rates of return that characterized these programs during the 1980s (Health Care Advisory Board, 1988). Another state mandates coverage for residential treatment "pursuant to a treatment plan" with no minimum specified for days of care or dollars. Three states mandate $1,500 to $2,000 annual coverage for outpatient treatment of drug abuse but specify no minimum coverage for inpatient services. Another three states simply require policies to offer optional coverage of an unspecified nature.

Cost Containment

State mandates recognize several mechanisms for containing the costs of drug treatment. The primary method allowed for this purpose is the use of less expensive competitive facilities for delivery of residential treatment. Alternative treatment facilities are recognized by 34 of the 35 states that have drug or alcohol abuse mandates, usually under the proviso that the facility be licensed by the state substance abuse authority or accredited by the voluntary Joint Commission on Accreditation of Healthcare Organizations (JCAHO) or the Commission on Accreditation of Rehabilitation Facilities (CARF).

Many nonhospital residential facilities have lower cost structures than hospital-based programs and charge appreciably less per day of treatment. They do not have the continuing onsite medical facilities, equipment, and personnel required for hospital licensure, but then again, these capacities are not needed for most drug treatment clients. Insurance plans thus are often given the option of covering drug treatment in lower cost facilities. A frequent criticism of health insurance plans by nonhospital treatment providers, however, is that many insurers and third-party administrators do not in fact cover treatment in nonhospital facilities, even though these

charge for a semiprivate hospital room in 1986 (Health Insurance Association of America, 1989) —for an average of 28 days in treatment, making a typical episode of treatment (if it included initial detoxification) cost approximately $7,800; with intervening health care cost inflation, that charge would now be $11,000 if no other factors intervened. Charges differed little for privately supported inpatients treated in programs located in general acute care hospitals or in freestanding (although often hospital-affiliated) settings.

facilities are licensed by the state and accredited by JCAHO or CARF for drug and/or alcohol treatment. Although it may be in the financial interest of insurers to cover treatment in these facilities, insurance plans reportedly have been reticent to do so because of uncertainty about the quality of care delivered in nonhospital-based programs.

Two state drug coverage mandates, those of North Dakota and Arkansas, specify flexibility for the policy beneficiary. In North Dakota the basic mandate is for a minimum of 60 days in a hospital plus 120 days of partial hospitalization and 20 outpatient visits. Part of the inpatient care may be exchanged for partial hospitalization care on a two-for-one basis. Arkansas mandates a minimum total value of services of $6,000 per year, delivered in hospital or nonhospital freestanding facilities or by outpatient providers. Alabama in its alcohol treatment mandate allows a trade-off of inpatient (hospital) care for treatment in a state-licensed, short-term residential alcohol treatment facility or a three-for-one exchange for outpatient treatment.

The 15 jurisdictions that mandate minimum levels of outpatient benefits range in value from $900 to $2,500 per year, or 20 to 45 visits (hours) per year. These benefits tend to have maximum copayment rates of about 20 percent.

The Value of Additional Mandates

The committee has reservations about the value of additional state mandates for drug treatment coverage. First, coverage for drug treatment is more widespread than the extensiveness of state mandates would indicate. There are clearly reasons other than mandate enactment for the spread of coverage—perhaps the increasing realization by employers that drug treatment is a valuable benefit for their employees and for the company. Second, state mandates do not apply to the growing number of companies that self-insure under the federal ERISA statutes, especially companies with more than 500 employees, of which the percentage self-insuring is now at least 60 percent. ERISA does not deal with the coverage of drug treatment services or other matters that states have attempted to address with mandates. Third, the nature of coverage mandated by many states is too much captive to the chemical dependency model, which is not the only available modality of drug treatment.

Finally, state benefit mandates are quite rigid in their structure. Only a few states permit flexibility or the trading-off of benefits of different kinds to encourage treatment purchasers and providers to seek the most cost-effective treatment choices. Typically, states mandate a minimum benefit for inpatient treatment and a minimum benefit for outpatient treatment, with no opportunities to substitute less inpatient for more outpatient or greater amounts of less expensive treatments for smaller amounts of more expensive ones. Only one state, Oregon, mandates what seems, in the committee's view, to be the most sensible option: a simple minimum dollar value of insured drug treatment coverage. If that dollar value is realistic in terms of competitive prices, it enables companies and individual beneficiaries to seek the best treatment values while using managed care strategies to guard against inappropriate use and to collect useful information about provider characteristics and performances.

CONCLUSIONS

Extent, Costs, and Trends of Coverage

The private tier of drug treatment providers is largely oriented toward treating the employed population and their family members. The majority of this population, about 140 million individuals, have specifically defined coverage for drug treatment in their health insurance plans. About 48 million others who are privately insured do not have specifically defined coverage for drug treatment, although coverage may occur de facto under general medical or psychiatric provisions. As of 1988, the health plans of about 67 percent of full-time employees of firms with 100 or more employees offered specifically defined coverage for some types of drug treatment, although the actual extent of benefits under these defined coverage provisions is uncertain.

Actuarial studies of claims experience yield rather modest estimates for the overall cost of covering drug treatment. Data about drug treatment expenditures tend to be buried under more inclusive headings and behind "horror stories" involving troubled adolescents with multiple diagnoses spending months in psychiatric facilities. Nevertheless, the committee estimates that a health plan with typical coverage now spends 1 percent or less of its total outlays for explicit drug treatment, most of it for hospital inpatient charges—with a large fraction of that cost devoted to detoxification. However, there has been a substantial apparent growth in the rate of drug treatment claims in recent years, particularly for insured adolescents. It is difficult to know how much of this increase is actually due to the replacement of psychiatric or medical diagnoses with more revealing or accurate drug problem diagnoses versus an increased demand for drug treatment in the insured population. Possibly, both processes are occurring.

Although this growth is disturbing to the degree it increases the aggregate cost of health insurance premiums, it is desirable if it means that an increased number of those who need treatment are seeking and receiving it, particularly if the treatment delivered is appropriate, effective, and reasonable in cost. Some payers, however, reacting in part to the high costs in a small number of cases and the high incidence of recidivism, have strongly questioned the value of drug treatment episodes. There is a movement at least rhetorically to view drug treatment as part of the non-medical/surgical fringe of health coverage that may be differentially limited (rather than cut back evenly with other benefits across the board) to trim increasing overall costs.

Mandating Drug Treatment Coverage

There are legislative mandates in 18 states plus the District of Columbia that require certain categories of employer-supplied group health plans to specifically cover—or offer optional coverage for—drug and alcohol treatment. (Another 19 states require some degree of coverage for alcohol treatment only.) In the committee's judgment, private coverage of drug treatment is beneficial to individuals and employers and should be included in every health package; however, legislative mandates at the state level have not necessarily proved to be an effective way, and are clearly not the only way, to induce adequate coverage. Most of those in the insured population whose plans include explicitly defined coverage for drug treatment reside in states that do not have legislative mandates for such coverage. Moreover, the political process has often produced less-than-optimal mandatory provisions that are difficult to adjust and overly rigid and that pay too much attention to limits on the length of stay and the number of visits rather than to the cost and effectiveness of treatment. Most mandatory provisions have the constraining effect of funneling people toward one particular modality of treatment by favoring inpatient stays of prespecified lengths.

The committee believes that the development of soundly derived standards for admission, care, and program performance will do more at this time to generate appropriate coverage than a further set of mandates. If mandates are to be used, efficiency and fairness dictate that they be applied to all competing insurers. Yet if the private market leaves large numbers of the insured population without coverage for drug treatment, it may be necessary for government to intervene. Such action could involve subsidies for drug treatment coverage, tax preferences for certain kinds of coverage, or mandates, with the choice dependent on judgments about the incidence, efficiency, and equity of alternative ways of financing coverage.

Optimal Coverage Provisions

Private insurance provisions (including most legislatively mandated benefits) often include financial incentives for beneficiaries to seek more expensive hospital or residential treatment. Insurance coverage until very recently has heavily favored hospital-based inpatient stays over outpatient visits and continues to encourage the "gold standard" medical model rather than more explicitly psychological or socially oriented treatment. Although residential drug treatment, including hospital treatment, often serves clinically important functions such as permitting intensive therapy, isolating the patient from an adverse environment, or treating concurrent psychiatric or medical complications, the hospital-specific components of such programs (e.g., 24-hour onsite medical coverage) do not seem to be the therapeutically important elements in the drug treatment programs that are sited there, even though the availability of these components is used to justify charging acute care hospital rates for all clients.

There is currently a movement afoot to reduce hospitalizations, mainly as a result of cost-containment measures, especially precertification, utilization review, and negotiation of preferred provider arrangements. The committee's principal response to these developments is to favor them in general, but **it specifically recommends that curbs on unit-of-service costs for inpatient care be strengthened and that payers insist on the generation of reliable performance/outcome data.** There are two reasons why it would be unwise to institute blanket denials of coverage for hospital-based drug treatment. First, in some states and localities, hospital-based programs are the only sites providing residential treatment. Second, a certain proportion of the individuals who seek drug treatment also have problems for which a course of acute hospital care is appropriate, namely, complications or co-occurring medical or psychiatric disorders.

Altogether, such cases in which it may be justifiable and necessary to initiate drug treatment services in a hospital setting may total one-fourth of privately covered clients who seek drug treatment. This figure is only guesswork, however, pending the advent of objective diagnostic assessment, systematic follow-up data collection, and systematic services research and evaluation of private treatment programs. Whatever the numbers involved, **the committee recommends that drug treatment services at hospital sites be reimbursed separately from other diagnoses or hospital services, as there appears to be no compelling reason why these services for most drug treatment patients should routinely command fees comparable to acute care rates rather than to reasonably competitive residential treatment rates.**

Insurers and employers need to become better informed about drug treatment and to structure their benefits to support controlled access to a broad range of the most appropriate, effective, and efficiently priced treatments rather than to a narrow (and expensive) band of options that are similar in form to the treatment of acute medical conditions. Private insurance, health maintenance organizations, and other health financing plans should cover appropriate, adequate, cost-effective drug treatment and

TABLE 8-2   Preferred Sites or Types of Treatment for Selected Categories
of Drug Treatment Clients

Types of Service Needed or Client Characteristic	Inpatient/Residential[a]		Outpatient/Ambulatory[a]	
	Hospital	Nonhospital	Methadone	Counseling
Drug overdose	P	X	X	X
Detoxification	X	S	P	P
Rehabilitation				
High criminality	X	P	P	S
Low criminality	X	S	P	P
Job jeopardy only	X	S	P	P
Adolescent	X	S	X	P
Domiciliary (permanent drug-induced organic brain syndrome)	X	P	X	X

[a]P = Primary site/modality of the most appropriate treatment; S = secondary or less likely site for treatment (nevertheless, for some clients this may be the primary or preferred site owing to their specific circumstances or needs); and X = generally inappropriate site/modality for this type of client.

not reimburse the cost of excessive, inappropriate treatments or charges (Table 8-2).

The committee recommends that private risk bearers, in lieu of arbitrary payment caps or exclusions, institute rigorous, independent preadmission review (where possible) and concurrent review of all hospital and residential admissions as a way to control access and utilization, ensure appropriate placement, and manage costs. Preadmission review may not be necessary for outpatient admissions, but early concurrent utilization review is important for outpatient treatment to ensure that diagnostic criteria are observed and charges are reasonable. Employee assistance programs can serve as utilization managers in cases in which their personnel have appropriate training for matching patients to treatment. Hospital utilization should be managed under the same terms as recommended for public coverage (see the section on utilization management in Chapter 7). In general, utilization management and indicators of performance are needed to meet concerns about costs and inappropriate treatment. In this area, as in other dimensions of health care, the stress should be on efficient delivery of effective care, in which responsible clinical innovation is encouraged, tested, and used when its worth is demonstrated.

The committee recommends that private payers insist that providers participate in and agree to the publication of regular, independent follow-up surveys to determine client outcomes, taking into account data on admission characteristics such as problem severity. Providers and payers should be able to compare treatment results with overall program norms to ensure that good performance is maintained and poor performance recognized when it occurs.

The committee recommends that the provisions of drug treatment benefits, including deductibles, copayments, stop-loss measures, and scheduled caps, be similar to provisions for treatment of other chronic, relapsing health problems. Except in terms of limitations on the length of stay and number of visits, such provisions are mostly the rule today. The committee believes that sound cost-containment and managed care arrangements and reliable performance and outcome measurements will in short order obviate the need for separate length-of-stay and dollar caps on coverage. Nonhospital residential and outpatient treatment delivered in state-certified treatment programs should be covered. Coverage limitations, charge schedules, and cost-containment incentives (e.g., copayment schedules) should be adjusted to reflect the findings of research on appropriate models, lengths, and costs of drug treatment—especially the recognition that longer residential and outpatient stays are strongly correlated with more beneficial results.

Coda

The best way to envision the drug problem is not as a fixed constellation but rather as a composite moving through time. As they age, each of the cohorts that constitute the U.S. population spreads across a broad continuum. At one end are lifelong abstainers, keeping a puzzled or horrified distance from illicit drugs. Partway across the continuum are light users, dabbling with newfound or occasional pleasures and, for the time being, feeling little pain. At the other extreme are devotees whose lives orbit around drug intoxication like moths worrying a flame, leaving in their wake not motes of dust but a trail of misery. Exactly who stands where on the continuum and in what numbers varies as behavior changes across time.

As a further complication, each new generation of Americans enters a transformed world. New drug technologies batten on older methods; shifting coalitions of producers and sellers maneuver for markets and profits; and social responses range from benign neglect to bruising, large-scale mobilization of force. Each new generation inserts into the picture its own quotient of social hope, morality, anger, and fear.

In this seemingly endless pharmacological and sociological diversity, treatment is both a rock of redemption and a hard place on which to secure a foothold. Treatment is designed to address the chronic, relapsing disorders of drug dependence and abuse, which characterize a minority of all illicit drug consumers but which yield probably the lion's share of the damaging consequences of drug consumption. The best treatment interventions "work"—reversing drug-seeking behavior, related criminal

298

activity, and other dysfunctions—only partially; that is, different types of treatment for these aggravated and imperfectly understood disorders work to a greater or lesser degree, and each works for only some of the people in need.

In short, success in treatment varies. It is not guaranteed and often not complete, and even if it were both, a major problem would still remain: most people who need treatment seek it only reluctantly, after failing at self-help, after much harm has been done, and after much pressure—interior and exterior—has been brought to bear. However, as with heart disease and cancer in the health domain, theft and assaultive behavior in the realm of violent crime, or homelessness and family dissolution in the area of social welfare, the absence of a panacea does not excuse society from responding with the tools at hand and to the best of its ability. The overall costs of drug problems are so high that reducing them even modestly is worthwhile. There is enough evidence to persuade this committee that a substantial proportion of the treatment available today is at least potentially capable of realizing benefits that exceed the costs of delivering it. Treatment seems to make sense on utilitarian as well as humanitarian grounds.

There are numerous managerial complications in trying to raise the level of performance of the two tiers of treatment providers—public and private—and improve the different mechanisms of funding and control that lie behind them. If there is a brief way to summarize or at least place a simple label on the recommended approaches to these complications, it is this: *the drug treatment system should do a better job of knowing itself and acting on that knowledge.* Much that was learned in the past about the elements and optimal costs of effective treatment was forgotten or brushed aside in the early and mid-1980s in the zeal to cut public spending and increase private revenues. The mechanisms that generated useful knowledge were largely disassembled or never installed in parts of the treatment system that took shape during that era.

As the 1990s begin, a different perspective is apparent with regard to issues of economy and accountability in the treatment system. There are still many obstacles to improving existing drug treatment, including inertia, vested interests, and the difficulties of finding, training, or reclaiming skilled and dedicated care givers. The weight of these obstacles should not be underestimated—but there are powerful levers to move them. Improvements are bound to fall into place, assuming that current financial trends continue, but only if the leaders of the public and private tiers bend their efforts to the modest but necessary task of making the system learn its lessons.

References

A.D. Little Co. (1975) *Social Cost of Drug Abuse*. Cambridge, Mass.: A.D. Little Co.

Allen-Hagen, B. (1988) *Public Juvenile Facilities, 1987: Children in Custody*. Juvenile Justice Bulletin. Office of Juvenile Justice and Delinquency Prevention. Washington, D.C.: U.S. Department of Justice.

Allison, M., R.L. Hubbard, and J.V. Rachal (1985) *Treatment Process in Methadone, Residential, and Outpatient Drug Free Programs*. Rockville, Md.: National Institute on Drug Abuse.

American Bar Association/American Medical Association (1961) *Drug Addiction: Crime or Disease?* Interim and Final Reports of the Joint Committee of the American Bar Association and the American Medical Association on Narcotic Drugs. Bloomington: Indiana University Press.

American Medical Association Council of Scientific Affairs (1987) Scientific issues in drug testing. *Journal of the American Medical Association* 257(22):3110-3114.

American Psychiatric Association (1987) *Diagnostic and Statistical Manual of Mental Disorders*, 3rd ed., revised. Washington, D.C.: American Psychiatric Association.

Anglin, M.D. (1988) The efficacy of civil commitment in treating narcotic addiction. Pp. 8-34 in C.G. Leukefeld and F.M. Tims, eds., *Compulsory Treatment of Drug Abuse: Research and Clinical Practice*. NIDA Research Monograph 86. Rockville, Md.: National Institute on Drug Abuse.

Anglin, M.D., and W.H. McGlothlin (1984) Outcome of narcotic addict treatment in California. Pp. 106-128 in F.M. Tims and J.P. Ludford, eds., *Drug Abuse Treatment Evaluation: Strategies, Progress, and Prospects*. NIDA Research Monograph 51. Rockville, Md.: National Institute on Drug Abuse.

Anglin, M.D., W.H. McGlothlin, and G.R. Speckart (1981) Effect of parole on methadone patient behavior. *American Journal of Drug and Alcohol Abuse* 8:153-170.

Anglin, M.D., G.R. Speckart, M.W. Booth, and T.M. Ryan (1989a) Consequences and costs of shutting off methadone. *Addictive Behaviors* 14:307-326.

Anglin, M.D., M.-L. Brecht, and E. Maddahian (1989b) Pretreatment characteristics and treatment performance of legally coerced versus voluntary methadone maintenance admissions. *Criminology* 27(3):537-557.

Attewell, P., and D. Gerstein (1979) Government policy and local practice. *American Sociological Review* 44(April):311-327.

Backer, T.E., and K. O'Hara (1988) Technical Report: Survey of Drug Abuse Services in EAPs. National Study of Workplace Drug Abuse Programs. Human Interaction Research Institute, Los Angeles.

Bale, R.N., W.W. Van Stone, J.M. Kuldau, T.J.J. Engelsing, R.M. Elashoff, and V.P. Zarcone (1980) Therapeutic communities vs methadone maintenance. A prospective controlled study of narcotic addiction treatment: design and one-year follow-up. *Archives of General Psychiatry* 37:179-193.

Ball, J.C. (1989) Unpublished data tables. Addiction Research Center, Alcohol, Drug Abuse, and Mental Health Administration, Baltimore.

Ball, J.C., H. Graff, and J.J. Sheehan, Jr. (1974) The heroin addict's view of methadone maintenance. *British Journal of Addiction* 69:89-95.

Ball, J.C., L. Rosen, J.A. Flueck, and D. Nurco (1981) The criminality of heroin addicts when addicted and when off opiates. Pp. 39-65 in J.A. Inciardi, ed., *The Drugs-Crime Connection*. Beverly Hills, Calif.: Sage Publications.

Ball, J.C., J.W. Shaffer, and D.N. Nurco (1983) The day-to-day criminality of heroin addicts in Baltimore: a study in the continuity of offense rates. *Drug and Alcohol Dependence* 12:119-142.

Ball, J.C., W.R. Lange, C.P. Meyers, and S.R. Friedman (1988) Reducing the risk of AIDS through methadone maintenance treatment. *Journal of Health and Social Behavior* 29:214-226.

Beauchamp, D.E. (1980) *Beyond Alcoholism: Alcohol and Public Health Policy*. Philadelphia: Temple University Press.

Beck, A.J., and B.E. Shipley (1989) *Recidivism of Prisoners Released in 1983*. Bureau of Justice Special Report, NCJ-116261. Washington, D.C.: U.S. Department of Justice.

Beck, A.J., S.A. Kline, and L.A. Greenfeld (1988) *Survey of Youth in Custody, 1987*. Bureau of Justice Statistics Special Report, NCJ-113365. Washington, D.C.: U.S. Department of Justice.

Beschner, G.M., B.G. Reed, and J. Mondanaro, eds. (1981) *Treatment Services for Drug Dependent Women*, Vol. 1. DHHS Pub. No. (ADM)81-1177. Rockville, Md.: National Institute on Drug Abuse.

Besteman, K.J. (1978) The NARA program. Pp. 274-280 in W.R. Martin and H. Isbell, eds., *Drug Addiction and the U.S. Public Health Service*. Proceedings of a Symposium Commemorating the 40th Anniversary of the Addiction Research Center at Lexington, Kentucky. Rockville, Md.: National Institute on Drug Abuse.

Besteman, K.J. (1990) Federal leadership in building the national drug treatment system. In D.R. Gerstein and H.J. Harwood, eds., *Treating Drug Abuse. Volume 2*. Washington, D.C.: National Academy Press.

Blaine, J.D., D.B. Thomas, G. Barnett, J.A. Whysner, and P.F. Renault (1981) Levo-alpha acetylmethadol (LAAM): clinical utility and pharmacological development. Pp. 360-388 in J.H. Lowinson and P. Ruiz, eds., *Substance Abuse: Clinical Problems and Perspectives*. Baltimore: Williams and Wilkins.

Blue Cross and Blue Shield Association (1983) *Substance Abuse Treatment Benefits: A Guide for Plans*. Chicago: Blue Cross and Blue Shield Association.

Brotman, R., and A. Freedman (1968) *A Community Mental Health Approach to Drug Addiction*. Washington, D.C.: U.S. Department of Health, Education and Welfare.

Brown, B.S., S.K. Gauvey, M.B. Meyers, and S.D. Stark (1971) In their own words: addicts' reasons for initiating and withdrawing from heroin. *The International Journal of the Addictions* 6(4):635-645.

Brown, S., ed. (1988) *Prenatal Care: Reaching Mothers, Reaching Infants*. Washington, D.C.: National Academy Press.

Bureau of Justice Assistance (1989) *Treatment Alternatives to Street Crime (TASC): Resource Catalog*. Washington, D.C.: U.S. Department of Justice.

Bureau of Labor Statistics (1987) *Employee Benefits in Medium and Large Firms, 1986*. Bulletin 2281. Washington, D.C.: U.S. Government Printing Office.

Bureau of Labor Statistics (1988) *Employee Benefits in State and Local Governments, 1987.* Bureau of Labor Statistics, Bulletin 2309. Washington, D.C.: U.S. Department of Labor.

Bureau of Labor Statistics. (1989a) *Employee Benefits in Medium and Large Firms, 1988.* Washington, D.C.: U.S. Government Printing Office.

Bureau of Labor Statistics (1989b) *Survey of Employer Anti-drug Programs.* Report 760. Washington, D.C.: U.S. Department of Labor.

Bush, G. (1990) State of the Union Message. *Congressional Record,* January 31:S632-S634.

Butynski, W., and D. Canova (1988) *State Resources and Services Related to Alcohol and Drug Abuse Problems, Fiscal Year 1987.* Washington, D.C.: National Association of State Alcohol and Drug Abuse Directors.

Butynski, W., and D. Canova (1989) *State Resources and Services Related to Alcohol and Drug Abuse Problems, Fiscal Year 1988.* Washington, D.C.: National Association of State Alcohol and Drug Abuse Directors.

Chaiken, M.R. (1989) *Prison Programs for Drug-Involved Offenders.* National Institute of Justice Research in Action, NCJ 118316. Washington, D.C.: U.S. Department of Justice.

Chasnoff, I.J. (1989) Press release, August 28. National Association for Perinatal Addiction Research and Education, Chicago.

Chasnoff, I.J., D.R. Griffith, S. MacGregor, K. Kirkes, and K.A. Burns (1989) Temporal patterns of cocaine use in pregnancy. *Journal of the American Medical Association* 261(12):1741-1744.

Chasnoff, I.J., J.J. Landress, and M.E. Barrett (1990) The prevalence of illicit-drug or alcohol use during pregnancy and discrepancies in mandatory reporting in Pinellas County, Florida. *The New England Journal of Medicine* 322(17):1202-1206.

Chavez, G.F., J. Mulinare, and J.F. Cordero (1989) Maternal cocaine use during early pregnancy as a risk factor for congenital urogenital anomalies. *Journal of the American Medical Association* 262(6):795-798.

Chollet, D. (1988) *Uninsured in the United States: The Nonelderly Population Without Health Insurance, 1986.* Washington, D.C.: Employee Benefit Research Institute.

Cole, S.G., W.E. Lehman, E.A. Cole, and A. Jones (1981) Inpatient vs outpatient treatment of alcohol and drug abusers. *American Journal of Drug and Alcohol Abuse* 8(3):329-345.

Collins, J.J., and M. Allison (1983) Legal coercion and retention in drug abuse treatment. *Hospital and Community Psychiatry* 34(12):1145-1149.

Comprehensive Care Corporation (1988) *Evaluation of Treatment Outcome.* Irvine, Calif.: Comprehensive Care Corporation.

Cook, C.C.H. (1988a) The Minnesota Model in the management of drug and alcohol dependency: miracle, method or myth? Part I. The philosophy and the programme. *British Journal of Addiction* 83:625-634.

Cook, C.C.H. (1988b) The Minnesota Model in the management of drug and alcohol dependency: miracle, method or myth? Part II. Evidence and conclusions. *British Journal of Addiction* 83:735-748.

Cook, L.F., B.A. Weinman, et al. (1988) Treatment alternatives to street crime. Pp. 99-105 in C.G. Leukefeld and F.M. Tims, eds., *Compulsory Treatment of Drug Abuse: Research and Clinical Practice.* NIDA Research Monograph 86. Rockville, Md.: National Institute on Drug Abuse.

Cooper, J.R., F. Altman, B.S. Brown, and D. Czechowicz (1983) *Research on the Treatment of Narcotic Addiction: State of the Art.* DHHS Pub. No. (ADM)83-1281. Rockville, Md.: National Institute on Drug Abuse.

Cooper, P., and D. Rice (1976) The economic costs of illness revisited. *Social Security Bulletin* 39:21-36.

Courtwright, D.T. (1982) *Dark Paradise: Opiate Addiction in America Before 1940.* Cambridge, Mass.: Harvard University Press.

Courtwright, D.T. (1990) A century of American narcotic policy. In D.R. Gerstein and H.J. Harwood, eds., *Treating Drug Abuse. Volume 2.* Washington, D.C.: National Academy Press.

Cruze, A., H. Harwood, P. Christensen, J. Collins, and D. Jones (1981) Economic Costs of Alcohol and Drug Abuse and Mental Illness—1977. Research Triangle Institute, Research Triangle Park, North Carolina.

Dackis, C., M.S. Gold, D. Sweeney et al. (1987) Single dose bromocriptine reverses cocaine craving. *Psychiatry Research* 20:261-264.

De Leon, G. (1986) The therapeutic community for substance abuse: perspective and approach. Pp. 5-18 in G. De Leon and J.T. Ziegenfuss, Jr., eds., *Therapeutic Communities for Addictions*. Springfield, Ill.: Charles C Thomas.

De Leon, G., H.K. Wexler, and N. Jainchill (1982) The therapeutic community: success and improvement rates 5 years after treatment. *The International Journal of the Addictions* 17(4):703-747.

Dole, V.P. (1971) Methadone maintenance treatment for 25,000 heroin addicts. *Journal of the American Medical Association* 215(7):1131-1134.

Dole, V.P. (1988) Implications of methadone maintenance for theories of narcotic addiction. *Journal of the American Medical Association* 260(20):3025-3029.

Dole, V.P. (1989) Methadone treatment and the acquired immunodeficiency syndrome epidemic. *Journal of the American Medical Association* 262(12):1681-1682.

Dole, V.P., and H. Joseph (1978) Long-term outcome of patients treated with methadone maintenance. *Annals of the New York Academy of Sciences* 311:181-189.

Dole, V.P., and M. Nyswander (1965) A medical treatment for diacetylmorphine (heroin) addiction: a clinical trial with methadone hydrochloride. *Journal of the American Medical Association* 193(8):80-84.

Dole, V.P., and M. Nyswander (1967) Rehabilitation of the street addict. *Archives of Environmental Health* 14:477-480.

Dole, V.P., and M.E. Nyswander (1976) Methadone maintenance treatment: a ten-year perspective. *Journal of the American Medical Association* 235(19):2117-2119.

Dole, V.P., M.E. Nyswander, and M.J. Kreek (1966) Narcotic blockage. *Archives of Internal Medicine* 118:304-309.

Dole, V.P., M.E. Nyswander, and A. Warner (1968) Successful treatment of 750 criminal addicts. *Journal of the American Medical Association* 206(12):2708-2711.

Dole, V.P., J.W. Robinson, J. Orraga, E. Towns, P. Searcy, and E. Caine (1969) Methadone treatment of randomly selected criminal addicts. *The New England Journal of Medicine* 280(25):1372-1375.

Eldred, C.A., and M.N. Washington (1976) Interpersonal relationships in heroin use by men and women and their role in treatment outcome. *The International Journal of the Addictions* 11(1):117-130.

Falkin, G.P., H.K. Wexler, and D.S. Lipton (1990) Drug treatment in state prisons. In D.R. Gerstein and H.J. Harwood, eds., *Treating Drug Abuse. Volume 2*. Washington, D.C.: National Academy Press.

Field, G. (1984) The Cornerstone program: a client outcome study. *Federal Probation* 50-55.

Field, G. (1989) The effects of intensive treatment on reducing the criminal recidivism of addicted offenders. *Federal Probation* 53(4):51-72.

Flanagan, T.J., and K.M. Jamieson, eds. (1988) *Sourcebook of Criminal Justice Statistics— 1987*. Bureau of Justice Statistics, NCJ-111612. Washington, D.C.: U.S. Department of Justice.

Friedman, A.S., N.W. Glickman, and M.R. Morrissey (1986) Prediction to successful treatment outcome by client characteristics and retention in treatment in adolescent drug treatment programs: a large-scale cross validation study. *Journal of Drug Education* 16(2):149-165.

Frohling, R. (1989) *Promising Approaches to Drug Treatment in Correctional Settings*. Washington, D.C.: National Conference of State Legislatures.

Fuchs, V.R. (1988) The "competition revolution" in health care. *Health Affairs* Summer(special issue):5-24.

Gallup, G.H. (1989) *Surveys on the Drug Crisis*. Princeton, N.J.: George H. Gallup International Foundation.

Gardiner, L.K., and R.C. Shreckengost (1987) A systems dynamics model for estimating heroin imports into the United States. *System Dynamics Review* 3(1):8-27.

Gawin, F.H., H.D. Kleber, R. Byck, B. Rounsaville, T.R. Kosten, P. Jatlow, and C. Morgan (1989a) Desipramine facilitation of initial cocaine abstinence. *Archives of General Psychiatry* 46:117-121.

Gawin, F.H., D. Allen, and B. Humblestone (1989b) Outpatient treatment of "crack" cocaine smoking with flupenthixol decanoate: a preliminary report. *Archives of General Psychiatry* 46:322-325.

Gearing, F.R. (1970) Evaluation of methadone maintenance treatment program. *The International Journal of the Addictions* 5(3):517-543.

Gearing, F.R. (1974) Methadone maintenance treatment five years later—where are they now? *American Journal of Public Health*, Supplement, 64:44-50.

Gerstein, D.R., L.L. Judd, and S.A. Rovner (1979) Career dynamics of female heroin addicts. *American Journal on Drug and Alcohol Abuse* 6(1):1-23.

Gilmore, K.M. (1985) *Hazelden Primary Residential Treatment Program: 1985. Profile and Patient Outcome.* Center City, Minn.: Hazelden.

Godshaw, G., R. Koppel, and R. Pancoast (1987) *Anti-Drug Law Enforcement Efforts and Their Impacts.* Prepared at Wharton Econometrics Forecasting Associates for the U.S. Customs Service. Washington, D.C.: U.S. Government Printing Office.

Goldschmidt, P.G. (1976) A cost-effectiveness model for evaluating health care programs: application to drug abuse treatment. *Inquiry* 13(1):29-47.

Goldstein, A. (1976) A clinical experience with LAAM. Pp. 115-117 in J.D. Blaine and P.F. Renault, eds., *Rx LAAM: 3x/Week: LAAM Alternative to Methadone.* NIDA Research Monograph 8. Rockville, Md.: National Institute on Drug Abuse.

Goldstein, A., and B. Judson (1974) Three critical issues in the management of methadone programs. Critical issue 3: can the community be protected against the hazards of take-home methadone? Pp. 140-148 in G. Bourne, ed., *Addiction.* New York: Academic Press.

Grant, M., M. Plant, and A. Williams, eds. (1983) *Economics and Alcohol: Consumption and Controls.* New York: Gardner Press.

Gray, B.H., and M.J. Field, eds. (1989) *Controlling Costs and Changing Patient Care? The Role of Utilization Management.* Washington, D.C.: National Academy Press.

Greenfeld, L.A. (1989) *Prisoners in 1988.* Bureau of Justice Statistics Bulletin, NCJ-116315. Washington, D.C.: U.S. Department of Justice.

Griffin, K.S. (1983) *The Therapeutic Community: A Cost-Benefit Analysis.* Philadelphia.: Gaudenzia.

Gunne, L., and L. Gronbladh (1984) The Swedish methadone maintenance program. Pp. 205-213 in G. Serban, ed., *The Social and Medical Aspects of Drug Abuse.* Jamaica, N.Y.: Spectrum Publications.

Gust, S.W., and J.M. Walsh (1989) Research on the prevalence, impact, and treatment of drug abuse in the workplace. Pp. 3-13 in S.W. Gust and J.M. Walsh, eds., *Drugs in the Workplace: Research and Evaluation Data.* NIDA Research Monograph 91. Rockville, Md.: National Institute on Drug Abuse.

Hargreaves, W.A. (1983) Methadone dose and duration for maintenance treatment. Pp. 19-79 in J.R. Cooper et al., eds., *Research on the Treatment of Narcotic Addiction: State of the Art.* DHHS Pub. No. (ADM)83-1281. Rockville, Md.: National Institute on Drug Abuse.

Harrison, P.A., and N.G. Hoffmann (1988) *Adult Outpatient Treatment: Perspectives on Admission and Outcome.* CATOR Report. St. Paul, Minn.: Chemical Abuse/Addiction Treatment Outcome Registry, Ramsey Clinic.

Hartunian, N.S., C.N. Smart, and M.S. Thompson (1980) The incidence and economic costs of cancer, motor vehicle injuries, coronary heart disease, and stroke: a comparative analysis. *American Journal of Public Health* 70(12):1249-1260.

Harwood, H., D.M. Napolitano, P.L. Christensen, and J.J. Collins (1984) Economic Costs to Society of Alcohol and Drug Abuse and Mental Illness: 1980. Report to Alcohol, Drug Abuse, and Mental Health Administration. Research Triangle Institute, Research Triangle Park, N.C.

Harwood, H.J., J.V. Rachal, and E. Cavanaugh (1985) *Length of Stay in Treatment for Alcohol Abuse and Alcoholism: National Estimates for Short-Term Hospitals, 1983.* Research Triangle Park, N.C.: Research Triangle Institute.

Harwood, H.J., R.L. Hubbard, J.J. Collins, and J.V. Rachal (1988) The costs of crime and the benefits of drug abuse treatment: a cost-benefit analysis using TOPS data. Pp. 209-235 in C.G. Leukefeld and F.M. Tims, eds., *Compulsory Treatment of Drug Abuse: Research and Clinical Practice.* NIDA Research Monograph 86. Rockville, Md.: National Institute on Drug Abuse.

Hawks, R.L., and C.N. Chiang, eds. (1986) *Urine Testing for Drugs of Abuse.* NIDA Research Monograph 73. Rockville, Md.: National Institute on Drug Abuse.

Health Care Advisory Board (1988) *Substance Abuse Treatment Programs: Marketing to Employers: Volume 1.* Washington, D.C.: Health Care Advisory Board.

Health Insurance Association of America (1989) *Source Book of Health Insurance Data.* Washington, D.C.: Health Insurance Association of America.

Hester, T. (1988) *Probation and Parole 1987.* Bureau of Justice Statistics Bulletin, NCJ-113948. Washington, D.C.: U.S. Department of Justice.

Hodgson, T., and N. Meiners (1979) Guidelines for Cost-of-Illness Studies in the Public Health Service. Public Health Task Force on the Cost of Illness Studies. Public Health Service, Bethesda, Md.

Hoffmann, N.G., and P.A. Harrison (1988) *Treatment Outcome: Adult Inpatients Two Years Later.* CATOR Report. St. Paul, Minn.: Chemical Abuse/Addiction Treatment Outcome Registry, Ramsey Clinic.

Holder, H.D., and J.O. Blose (1986) Alcoholism treatment and total health care utilization and costs: a four year longitudinal analysis of federal employees. *Journal of the American Medical Association* 256:1456-1460.

Holder, H.D., and J.B. Hallan (1986) Impact of alcoholism on total health care costs: a six year study. *Advances in Alcohol and Substance Abuse* 6(1):1-15.

Homer, J.D., with the UCLA Drug Abuse Research Group (1988) *A Systems Dynamics Simulation Model of Cocaine Prevalence.* Westwood, Calif.: UCLA Drug Abuse Research Group.

Hubbard, R.L., M.E. Marsden, J.V. Rachal, H.J. Harwood, E.R. Cavanaugh, and H.M. Ginzburg (1989) *Drug Abuse Treatment: A National Study of Effectiveness.* Chapel Hill: The University of North Carolina Press.

Hunt, L.G., and C.D. Chambers (1976) *The Heroin Epidemics.* Holliswood, N.Y.: Spectrum Publications.

Hunt, G.H., and M.E. Odoroff (1962) Follow-up study of narcotic drug addicts after hospitalization. *Public Health Reports* 77:41-54.

ICF Incorporated (1987) *Analysis of Treatment for Alcoholism and Drug Dependency.* Irvine, Calif.: National Association of Addiction Treatment Providers.

Inciardi, J.A. (1988) Some considerations on the clinical efficacy of compulsory treatment: reviewing the New York experience. Pp. 126-138 in C.G. Leukefeld and F.M. Tims, eds., *Compulsory Treatment of Drug Abuse: Research and Clinical Practice.* NIDA Research Monograph 86. Rockville, Md.: National Institute on Drug Abuse.

Innes, C.A. (1988) *State Prison Inmate Survey, 1986: Drug Use and Crime.* Bureau of Justice Statistics Special Report, NCJ-111940. Washington, D.C.: U.S. Department of Justice.

Institute of Medicine (1988a) *The Future of Public Health.* Committee for the Study of the Future of Public Health. Washington, D.C.: National Academy Press.

Institute of Medicine (1988b) *Homelessness, Health, and Human Needs.* Committee on Health Care for Homeless People. Washington, D.C.: National Academy Press.

Institute of Medicine (1990) *Broadening the Base of Treatment for Alcohol Problems: Report of a Study by a Committee of the Institute of Medicine, Division of Mental Health and Behavioral Medicine.* Committee for the Study of Treatment and Rehabilitation Services for Alcoholism and Alcohol Abuse. Washington, D.C.: National Academy Press.

Institute of Medicine/National Academy of Sciences (1988) *Confronting AIDS: Update 1988.* Committee for the Oversight of AIDS Activities. Washington, D.C.: National Academy Press.

Intergovernmental Health Policy Project (1989) Substance abuse testing in the workplace. *State Health Reports* 47(April):4-6.

Jacoby, J.E., and C.S. Dunn (1987) National Survey on Punishment for Criminal Offenses: Executive Summary. Paper presented at the 1987 meeting of the National Conference on Punishment for Criminal Offenders. Ann Arbor, Mich.

Jamieson, K.M., and T.J. Flanagan, eds. (1989) *Sourcebook of Criminal Justice Statistics— 1988*. Bureau of Justice Statistics, NCJ-118318. Washington, D.C.: U.S. Department of Justice.

Jensen, G.A. (1988) The Effects of State-Mandated Insurance Benefits on Employers: Preliminary Findings from Research in Progress. Unpublished manuscript prepared for the Governor's Commission on Health Plan Regulatory Reform, State of Minnesota. School of Public Health and Department of Economics, University of Illinois, Chicago.

Johnson, B.D., P.J. Goldstein, E. Preble, J. Schmeidler, D.S. Lipton, B. Spunt, and T. Miller (1985) *Taking Care of Business: The Economics of Crime by Heroin Abusers*. Lexington, Mass.: Lexington Books.

Johnston, L.D. (1985) The etiology and prevention of substance use: what can we learn from recent historical changes? Pp. 155-177 in C.L. Jones and R.J. Battjes, eds., *Etiology of Drug Abuse: Implications for Prevention*. NIDA Research Monograph 56. Rockville, Md.: National Institute on Drug Abuse.

Jones, M. (1953) *The Therapeutic Community—A New Treatment Method in Psychiatry*. New York: Basic Books.

Joseph, H. (1988) The criminal justice system and opiate addiction: a historical perspective. Pp. 106-125 in C.G. Leukefeld and F.M. Tims, eds., *Compulsory Treatment of Drug Abuse: Research and Clinical Practice*. NIDA Research Monograph 86. Rockville, Md.: National Institute on Drug Abuse.

Kandel, D.B., and D.R. Maloff (1983) Commonalities in drug use: a sociological perspective. Pp. 3-28 in P.K. Levison et al., eds., *Commonalities in Substance Abuse and Habitual Behavior*. Lexington, Mass.: Lexington Books.

Kleber, H.D. (1977) Methadone maintenance treatment—a reply. *American Journal of Drug and Alcohol Abuse* 4(2):267-272.

Kleber, H.D. (1987) Treatment of narcotic addicts. *Psychiatric Medicine* 3(4):389-418.

Kleber, H.D., and F. Slobetz (1979) Outpatient drug-free treatment. Pp. 31-38 in R.L. Dupont et al., eds., *Handbook on Drug Abuse*. Rockville, Md.: National Institute on Drug Abuse.

Kline, S. (1988) *Jail Inmates 1987*. Bureau of Justice Statistics Bulletin, NCJ-114319. Washington, D.C.: U.S. Department of Justice.

Kline, S. (1989) *Probation and Parole 1988*. Bureau of Justice Statistics Bulletin, NCJ-119970. Washington, D.C.: U.S. Department of Justice.

Korcok, M. (1988a) *Managed Care and Chemical Dependency: A Troubled Relationship*. Providence, R.I.: Manisses Communications Group.

Korcok, M. (1988b) Chemical dependency care seen lowering health costs. *American Medical News*, September 9:23-25.

Kosten, T.R., B.J. Rounsaville, and H.D. Kleber (1988) Antecedents and consequences of cocaine abuse among opioid addicts: a 2.5-year follow-up. *The Journal of Nervous and Mental Disease* 176(3):176-178.

Kozel, N.J., and E.H. Adams, eds. (1985) *Cocaine Use in America: Epidemiologic and Clinical Perspectives*. NIDA Research Monograph 61. Rockville, Md.: National Institute on Drug Abuse.

Kreek, M.J. (1983) Health consequences associated with the use of methadone. Pp. 456-482 in J.R. Cooper et al., eds., *Research on the Treatment of Narcotic Addiction: State of the Art*. NIDA Treatment Research Monograph Series. DHHS Pub. No. (ADM)83-1281. Rockville, Md.: National Institute on Drug Abuse.

Laundergan, J.C. (1982) *Easy Does It! Alcoholism Treatment Outcomes, Hazelden and the Minnesota Model*. Center City, Minn.: Hazelden.

Lemkau, P., Z. Amsel, B. Sanders, J. Amsel, and T. Seis (1974) Social and Economic Costs of Drug Abuse. Department of Mental Hygiene, School of Hygiene and Public Health, Johns Hopkins University, Baltimore.

Levin, G., E.B. Roberts, and G.B. Hirsch (1975) *The Persistent Poppy: A Computer-Aided Search for Heroin Policy.* Cambridge, Mass.: Ballinger Publishing Company.

Levison, P.K., D.R. Gerstein, and D.R. Maloff, eds. (1983) *Commonalities in Substance Abuse and Habitual Behavior.* Lexington, Mass.: Lexington Books.

Ling, W., C.J. Klett, and R.D. Gillis (1978) A cooperative clinical study of methadyl acetate. *Archives of General Psychiatry* 35:345-353.

Lipton, D.S., and H.K. Wexler (1988) The Drug Crime Connection Invests Correctional Rehabilitation With New Life. Narcotic and Drug Research, Inc., New York.

Lukoff, I.F., and P.H. Kleinman (1977) The addict life cycle and problems in treatment evaluation. In A. Schecter and S.J. Mule, eds., *Rehabilitation Aspects of Drug Dependence.* Cleveland: CRC Press.

Maddux, J. (1988) Clinical experience with civil commitment. *Journal of Drug Issues* 18(4):575-594.

Maidlow, S.T., and H. Berman (1972) The economics of heroin treatment. *American Journal of Public Health* 62(10):1397-1406.

Malcolm, R. (1990) Little battles. *Journal of the American Medical Association* 263(1):90.

Martin, W.R., and H. Isbell, eds. (1978) *Drug Addiction and the U.S. Public Health Service: Proceedings of a Symposium Commemorating the 40th Anniversary of the Addiction Research Center at Lexington, Ky.* DHEW Pub. No. (ADM)77-434. Washington, D.C.: U.S. Department of Health, Education and Welfare.

McGlothlin, W.H., and M.D. Anglin (1981) Shutting off methadone: costs and benefits. *Archives of General Psychiatry* 38:885-892.

McGlothlin, W.H., M.D. Anglin, and B.D. Wilson (1977) *An Evaluation of the California Civil Addict Program.* Services Research Monograph Series. DHEW Pub. No. (ADM)78-558. Rockville, Md.: National Institute on Drug Abuse.

McLellan, A.T., L. Luborsky, J. Cacciola, J. Griffith, P. McGahan, and C.P. O'Brien (1985) *Guide to the Addiction Severity Index: Background, Administration, and Field Testing Results.* DHHS Pub. No. (ADM)88-1419. Rockville, Md.: National Institute on Drug Abuse.

McLellan, A.T., L. Luborsky, G. Woody, and L. Goebl (1988) Counselor differences in methadone treatment. Pp. 243-250 in L.S. Harris, ed., *Problems of Drug Dependence, 1987.* Proceedings of the 49th Annual Scientific Meeting, The Committee on Problems of Drug Dependence, Inc. NIDA Research Monograph 81. Rockville, Md.: National Institute on Drug Abuse.

Mello, N.K., J.H. Mendelson, M.P. Bree, and S.E. Lukas (1989) Buprenorphine suppresses cocaine self-administration by Rhesus monkeys. *Science* 245:859-862.

Miller, H.G., C.F. Turner, and L.E. Moses (1990) *AIDS: The Second Decade.* Washington, D.C.: National Academy Press.

Miller, W.R., and R.K. Hester (1986) Inpatient alcoholism treatment: who benefits? *American Psychologist* 41:794-805.

Moffet, A.D., I.H. Soloway, and M.X. Glick (1973) Post-treatment behavior following ambulatory detoxification. Pp. 215-227 in C.D. Chambers and L. Brill, eds., *Methadone Experience and Issues.* New York: Behavioral Publications.

Moore, M.H., and D.G. Gerstein (1981) *Alcohol and Public Policy: Beyond the Shadow of Prohibition.* Washington, D.C.: National Academy Press.

Morrisey, M.A., and G.A. Jensen (1988) Employer-sponsored insurance coverage for alcoholism and drug abuse treatments. *Journal of Studies on Alcohol* 49:456-461.

Moyer, M.E. (1989) A revised look at the number of uninsured Americans. *Health Affairs* 8(2):102-110.

National Commission on Marijuana and Drug Abuse (1973) *Drug Use in America: Problem in Perspective.* Washington, D.C.: U.S. Government Printing Office.

National Institute on Drug Abuse (1976–1980) *Reports of Data from the National Drug and Alcoholism Treatment Utilization Survey.* NIDA Statistical Series F, Nos. 1, 3, 4, 6, 8, and 9. Rockville, Md.: National Institute on Drug Abuse.

National Institute on Drug Abuse (1981) *Effectiveness of Drug Abuse Treatment Programs.* DHHS Pub. No. (ADM)81-1143. Rockville, Md.: National Institute on Drug Abuse.

National Institute on Drug Abuse (1983a) *Main Findings for Drug Abuse Treatment Units, September, 1982: Data From the National Drug and Alcoholism Treatment Utilization Survey (NDATUS)*. NIDA Statistical Series F, No. 10. Rockville, Md.: National Institute on Drug Abuse.

National Institute on Drug Abuse (1983b) *Research on the Treatment of Narcotic Addiction: State of the Art*. NIDA Treatment Research Monograph Series. DHHS Pub. No. (ADM)83-1281. Rockville, Md.: National Institute on Drug Abuse.

National Institute on Drug Abuse (1987) *Topical Data from the Drug Abuse Warning Network (DAWN): Trends in Drug Abuse Related Hospital Emergency Room Episodes and Medical Examiner Cases for Selected Drugs: DAWN 1976–1985*. NIDA Statistical Series H, No. 3. DHHS Pub. No. (ADM)87-1524. Rockville, Md.: National Institute on Drug Abuse.

National Institute on Drug Abuse (1988a) *Data from the Drug Abuse Warning Network (DAWN): Annual Data, 1987*. Statistical Series I, No. 7. DHHS Pub. No. (ADM)88-1584. Rockville, Md.: National Institute on Drug Abuse.

National Institute on Drug Abuse (1988b) *National Household Survey on Drug Abuse: Main Findings 1985*. DHHS Pub. No. (ADM)88-1586. Washington, D.C.: U.S. Department of Health and Human Services.

National Institute on Drug Abuse (1989) *National Household Survey on Drug Abuse: Population Estimates 1988*. DHHS Pub. No. (ADM)89-1636. Washington, D.C.: U.S. Government Printing Office.

National Narcotics Intelligence Consumers Committee (NNICC) (1989) *The NNICC Report 1988: The Supply of Illicit Drugs to the United States*. Washington, D.C.: U.S. Drug Enforcement Agency.

National Research Council (1978) Clinical evaluation of naltrexone treatment of opiate-dependent individuals. *Archives of General Psychiatry* 35:335-340.

Newman, R.G. (1983) Critique. Pp. 168-171 in *Research on the Treatment of Narcotic Addiction: State of the Art*. NIDA Treatment Research Monograph Series. DHHS Pub. No (ADM)83-1281. Rockville, Md.: National Institute on Drug Abuse.

Newman, R.G., and W.B. Whitehill (1978) Double-blind comparison of methadone and placebo maintenance treatment of narcotic addicts in Hong Kong. *Lancet* 8141:485-488.

Nurco, D.N., I.H. Cisin, and M.B. Balter (1981a) Addict careers. I. A new typology. *The International Journal of the Addictions* 16(8):1305-1325.

Nurco, D.N., I.H. Cisin, and M.B. Balter (1981b) Addict careers. II. The first ten years. *The International Journal of the Addictions* 16(8):1327-1356.

Nurco, D.N., I.H. Cisin, and M.B. Balter (1981c) Addict careers. III. Trends across time. *The International Journal of the Addictions* 16(8):1357-1372.

Office of Drug Abuse Policy (1978) *Drug Use Patterns, Consequences and the Federal Response: A Policy Review*. Washington, D.C.: Office of Drug Abuse Policy.

Office of National Drug Control Policy (1989) *National Drug Control Strategy*. Washington, D.C.: U.S. Government Printing Office.

Office of National Drug Control Policy (1990) *National Drug Control Strategy*. Washington, D.C.: U.S. Government Printing Office.

O'Neil, J.A., E.D. Wish, and C.A. Visher (1990) Drug use forecasting (DUF) research update. Pp. 2-3 in National Institute of Justice, *Research in Action: Drug Use Forecasting, July to September 1989*. Washington, D.C.: U.S. Department of Justice.

Parent, D.G. (1989) *Shock Incarceration: An Overview of Existing Programs*. National Institute of Justice. Washington, D.C.: U.S. Department of Justice.

Petitti, D.B., and C. Coleman (1990) Cocaine and the risk of low birth weight. *American Journal of Public Health* 80(1):25-29.

Phillips, M.D. (1990) Courts, jails, and drug treatment in a California county. In D.R. Gerstein and H.J. Harwood, eds., *Treating Drug Abuse. Volume 2*. Washington, D.C.: National Academy Press.

Preble, E., and J.J. Casey, Jr. (1972) Taking care of business: the heroin user's life on the street. Pp 97-118 in D.E. Smith and G.R. Gay, eds., *It's So Good, Don't Even Try it Once: Heroin in Perspective*. Englewood Cliffs, N.J.: Prentice-Hall.

Presidential Commission on the Human Immunodeficiency Virus Epidemic (1988) *Final Report of the Presidential Commission on the Human Immunodeficiency Virus Epidemic*. Washington, D.C.: U.S. Government Printing Office.

Rawson, R.A., J.L. Obert, M.J. McCann, and A.J. Mann (1986) Cocaine treatment outcome: cocaine use following inpatient, outpatient, and no treatment. Pp. 271-277 in L.S. Harris, ed., *Problems of Drug Dependence, 1985: Proceedings of the 47th Annual Scientific Meeting*. NIDA Research Monograph 67. Rockville, Md.: National Institute on Drug Abuse.

Ray, B.A., ed. (1988) *Learning Factors in Substance Abuse*. NIDA Research Monograph 84. DHHS Pub. No. (ADM)88-1576. Rockville, Md.: National Institute on Drug Abuse.

Reed, B.G., G.M. Beschner, and J. Mondanaro, eds. (1982) *Treatment Services for Drug Dependent Women*, Vol. II. DHHS Pub. No. (ADM)87-1219. Rockville, Md.: National Institute on Drug Abuse.

Regier, D.A., J.H. Boyd, J.D. Burke, B.Z. Locke, D.S. Rae, J.K. Myers, M. Kramer, L.N. Robins, D.B. Blazer, and M. Karno (1988) One-month prevalence of mental disorders in the U.S.—based on five epidemiologic catchment area sites. *Archives of General Psychiatry* 45(11):977-986.

Resnick, R. (1983) Methadone detoxification from illicit opiates and methadone maintenance. Pp. 160-178 in *Research on the Treatment of Narcotic Addiction: State of the Art*. NIDA Treatment Research Monograph Series. DHHS Pub. No (ADM)83-1281. Rockville, Md.: National Institute on Drug Abuse.

Rice, D. (1966) *Estimating the Costs of Illness*. Division of Medical Care Administration, Public Health Service. Washington, D.C.: U.S. Department of Health, Education and Welfare.

Rice, D.P., and S. Kelman (1989) Measuring comorbidity and overlap in the hospitalization cost for alcohol and drug abuse and mental illness. *Inquiry* 26:249-260.

Rice, D.P., S. Kelman, L. Miller, and S. Dunmeyer (1990) The Economic Costs of Alcohol, Drug Abuse, and Mental Illness—1985. Institute for Health and Aging, University of California, San Francisco.

Robins, L.N. (1974) *The Vietnam Drug User Returns*. Special Action Office Monograph, Series A, Number 2. Washington, D.C.: Special Action Office for Drug Abuse Prevention, Executive Office of the President.

Robins, L.N. (1980) The natural history of drug abuse. *Acta Psychiatrica Scandinavica* 284(62):7-20.

Robins, L.N., D.H. Davis, and D.N. Nurco (1974) How permanent was Vietnam drug addiction? *American Journal of Public Health*, Supplement, 64:38-43.

Roman, P.M., and T. Blum (1987) Notes on the epidemiology of alcoholism in the U.S.A. *Journal of Drug Issues* 17:321-332.

Roman, P.M., and T.C. Blum (1990) Employee assistance and drug screening programs. In D.R. Gerstein and H.J. Harwood, eds., *Treating Drug Abuse. Volume 2*. Washington, D.C.: National Academy Press.

Romond, A.M., C.K. Forrest, and H.D. Kleber (1975) Follow-up of participants in a drug dependence therapeutic community. *Archives of General Psychiatry* 32:369-374.

Rufener, B.L., J.V. Rachal, and A.M. Cruze (1977a) *Management Effectiveness Measures for NIDA Drug Abuse Treatment Programs. Volume I: Cost Benefit Analysis*. DHEW Pub. No. (ADM)77-423. Rockville, Md.: National Institute on Drug Abuse.

Rufener, B.L., J.V. Rachal, and A.M. Cruze (1977b) *Management Effectiveness Measure for NIDA Drug Abuse Treatment Programs. Volume II: Costs to Society of Drug Abuse*. Technical paper. Rockville, Md.: National Institute on Drug Abuse.

Savage, C., E.G. Karp, S.F. Curran, T.E. Hanlon, and O.L. McCabe (1976) Methadone/LAAM maintenance: a comparison study. *Comprehensive Psychiatry* 17(3):415-424.

Saxe, L., with D. Dougherty, K. Esty, and M. Fine (1983) *The Effectiveness and Costs of Alcoholism Treatment*. Health Technology Case Study 22. Washington, D.C.: Office of Technology Assessment.

Schasre, R. (1966) Cessation patterns among neophyte heroin users. *International Journal of the Addictions* 1(2):23-32.

Sells, S.B., ed. (1974a) *Studies of the Effectiveness of Treatments for Drug Abuse. Volume 1: Evaluation of Treatments*. Cambridge, Mass.: Ballinger Publishing Company.

Sells, S.B., ed. (1974b) *Studies of the Effectiveness of Treatments for Drug Abuse. Volume 2: Research on Patients, Treatments and Outcomes*. Cambridge, Mass.: Ballinger Publishing Company.

Sells, S.B., D. Simpson, G. Joe, R. Demaree, L. Savage, and M.A. Lloyd (1976) National follow-up study to evaluate the effectiveness of drug abuse treatment: a report of cohort 1 of the DARP five years later. *American Journal of Drug and Alcohol Abuse* 3(4):545-556.

Sheffet, A., M. Quinones, M.A. Lavenhar, K. Doyle, and H. Prager (1976) An evaluation of detoxification as an initial step in the treatment of heroin addiction. *American Journal of Psychiatry* 133(3):337-340.

Shim, K.H., and M.M. DeBerry (1988) *Criminal Victimization 1987*. Bureau of Justice Statistics Bulletin, NCJ-113587. Washington, D.C.: U.S. Department of Justice.

Siegel, R.K. (1990) Cycles of cocaine. In D.R. Gerstein and H.J. Harwood, eds., *Treating Drug Abuse. Volume 2*. Washington, D.C.: National Academy Press.

Simpson, D.D. (1981) Treatment for drug abuse: follow-up outcomes and length of time spent. *Archives of General Psychiatry* 38:875-880.

Simpson, D.D., and H.J. Friend (1988) Legal status and long-term outcomes for addicts in the DARP followup project. Pp. 81-98 in C.G. Leukefeld and F.M. Tims, eds., *Compulsory Treatment of Drug Abuse: Research and Clinical Practice*. NIDA Research Monograph 86. Rockville, Md.: National Institute on Drug Abuse.

Simpson, D.D., L.J. Savage, and M.R. Lloyd (1979) Follow-up evaluation of treatment of drug abuse during 1969 to 1972. *Archives of General Psychiatry* 36:772-780.

Smith, D.E., and G.R. Gay, eds. (1972) *It's So Good, Don't Even Try it Once: Heroin in Perspective*. Englewood Cliffs, N.J.: Prentice-Hall.

Smith, J.W., and P.J. Frawley (1988) Response to the Substance Abuse Coverage Study. Schick Shadel Hospital, Santa Monica, California.

Speckart, G.R., and M.D. Anglin (1986) Narcotics and crime: a causal modeling approach. *Journal of Quantitative Criminology* 2:3-28.

State Statistical Programs Branch (1989) *Criminal Cases in Five States, 1983–86*. Bureau of Justice Statistics Special Report, NCJ-118798. Washington, D.C.: U.S. Department of Justice.

Steinberg, R.J. (1990) Markets for drug treatment. In D.R. Gerstein and H.J. Harwood, eds., *Treating Drug Abuse. Volume 2*. Washington, D.C.: National Academy Press.

Stitzer, M.L., and M.E. McCaul (1987) Criminal justice interventions with drug and alcohol abusers: the role of compulsory treatment. Pp. 331-361 in E.K. Morris and C.J. Braukmann, eds., *Behavioral Approaches to Crime and Delinquency*. New York: Plenum Publishing Corporation.

Stitzer, M.L., G.E. Bigelow, and M.E. McCaul (1983) Behavioral approaches to drug abuse. *Progress in Behavior Modification* 14:49-124.

Strategy Council on Drug Abuse (1975) *Federal Strategy for Drug Abuse and Drug Traffic Prevention*. Washington, D.C.: U.S. Government Printing Office.

Sugarman, B. (1986) Structure, variations, and context: a sociological view of the therapeutic community. Pp. 65-82 in G. De Leon and J.T. Ziegenfuss, Jr., eds., *Therapeutic Communities for Addictions*. Springfield, Ill.: Charles C Thomas.

Technical Assistance & Training Corp. (1989) *Overcoming Barriers to Drug Abuse Treatment: Market Research Report*. Report submitted to the National Institute on Drug Abuse. Washington, D.C.: Technical Assistance & Training Corp.

Tennant, F.S., Jr., and A.A. Sagherian (1987) Double-blind comparison of amantadine and bromocriptine for ambulatory withdrawal for cocaine dependence. *Archives of Internal Medicine* 147:109-112.

Toborg, M.A., and M.P. Kirby (1984) Drug use and pretrial crime in the District of Columbia. *Research in Brief*, October. Washington, D.C.: National Institute of Justice.

Trice, H.M. (1966) *Alcoholism in America*. New York: McGraw-Hill.

U.S. Department of Commerce (1988) *Statistical Abstract of the United States: 1989*, 109th ed. Bureau of the Census. Washington, D.C.: U.S. Government Printing Office.

U.S. General Accounting Office (1988) *Employee Drug Testing: Information on Private Sector Programs.* GAO/GGD-88-32. Washington, D.C.: U.S. General Accounting Office.

U.S. General Accounting Office (1990) *Methadone Maintenance: Some Treatment Programs Are Not Effective; Greater Federal Oversight Needed.* GAO/HRD-90-104. Washington, D.C.: U.S. General Accounting Office.

U.S. Office of Personnel Management (1988) *A Guide to Substance Abuse Treatment Benefits Under the Federal Employees Health Benefits Programs for 1989.* Washington, D.C.: U.S. Government Printing Office.

Vaillant, G.E. (1966a) A twelve-year follow-up of New York narcotic addicts: I. The relation of treatment to outcome. *American Journal of Psychiatry* 122:727-737.

Vaillant, G.E. (1966b) Twelve-year follow-up of New York narcotic addicts: II. The natural history of a chronic disease. *The New England Journal of Medicine* 275(23):1282-1288.

Vaillant, G.E. (1966c) A 12-year follow-up of New York narcotic addicts: III. Some social and psychiatric characteristics. *Archives of General Psychiatry* 15:599-609.

Vaillant, G.E. (1973) A 20-year follow-up of New York narcotic addicts. *Archives of General Psychiatry* 29:237-241.

Vaillant, G.E. (1988) What can long-term follow-up teach us about relapse and prevention of relapse in addiction? *British Journal of Addiction* 83:1147-1157.

Vocational Rehabilitation Administration (1966) *Rehabilitating the Narcotic Addict.* Washington, D.C.: U.S. Department of Health, Education and Welfare.

Waldorf, D. (1973) *Careers in Dope.* Englewood Cliffs, N.J.: Prentice-Hall.

Wesson, D.R., and D.E. Smith (1985) Cocaine: treatment perspectives. Pp. 193-203 in N.J. Kozel and E.H. Adams, eds., *Cocaine Use in America: Epidemiologic and Clinical Perspectives.* NIDA Research Monograph 61. Rockville, Md.: National Institute on Drug Abuse.

Wexler, M.K., G.P. Falkin, and D.S. Lipton (1988) *A Model Prison Rehabilitation Program. An Evaluation of the Stay'n Out Therapeutic Community.* New York: Narcotic and Drug Research, Inc.

White, H.R. (1988) Longitudinal patterns of cocaine use among adolescents. *American Journal of Drug and Alcohol Abuse* 14(1):1-15.

White House Office of Public Affairs (1988) The Reagan Record on the Crusade for a Drug-Free America. Mimeo, June 6. White House Office of Public Affairs, Washington, D.C.

Wiener, C. (1981) *The Politics of Alcoholism.* New Brunswick, N.J.: Transaction Books.

Winick, C. (1962) Maturing out of narcotic addiction. *U.N. Bulletin on Narcotics* 14:1-7.

Wish, E.D., and J.A. O'Neil (1989) Drug use forecasting (DUF) research update. Pp. 2-8 in National Institute of Justice, *Research in Action: Drug Use Forecasting, January to March 1989.* Washington, D.C.: U.S. Department of Justice.

World Health Organization (in press) *International Statistical Classification of Diseases, Injuries, and Causes of Death,* 10th ed. Geneva: World Health Organization.

Yablonsky (1965) *Synanon: The Tunnel Back.* Baltimore: Penguin.

Zuckerman, B., D.A. Frank, R. Hingson et al. (1989) Effects of maternal marijuana and cocaine use on fetal growth. *The New England Journal of Medicine* 320(12):762-768.

Biographical Sketches
of Committee Members and Staff

LAWRENCE S. LEWIN, chair of the Committee for the Substance Abuse Coverage Study, is president of the Lewin/ICF Health Group, a Washington-based health policy management consulting firm founded in 1970. He has directed a wide range of health policy and strategic planning studies for federal, state, and local governments; academic health centers; hospitals; nursing homes; public foundations; health maintenance organizations; insurance companies; and suppliers of services and products to the health care industry. He has also conducted more than 50 workshops for senior state and local health officials, state legislators, and business coalition members on a variety of health policy issues. He has helped develop and evaluate programs in the fields of aging, child development, education, and community development. He has chaired and staffed a variety of task forces, including the Task Force on Medicaid and Related Programs, of which he was vice chair, and gubernatorial task forces on health care issues in several states. He is a member of the Institute of Medicine. He received a B.A. from the Woodrow Wilson School of Public and International Affairs, Princeton University, and an M.B.A. from Harvard University.

RAUL CAETANO is a psychiatrist and epidemiologist with the Alcohol Research Group, Institute of Epidemiology and Behavioral Medicine, Medical Research Institute of San Francisco at Pacific Presbyterian Medical Center, and associate professor in the Department of Social and Administrative Health Sciences, School of Public Health, University of California,

Berkeley. He was previously the recipient of fellowships from the Brazilian Ministry of Education, the Pan American Health Organization, and the Medical Council on Alcoholism Research. He has been involved in a wide range of epidemiological studies in the psychiatric and substance abuse fields. His research has focused on the relationship between ethnicity and substance abuse, especially among U.S. Hispanics, and on conceptual issues associated with the diagnosis of alcohol dependence. He has been an adviser to the Pan American Health Organization and university and government institutions throughout Latin America. He is a member of the American College of Epidemiology, the American Public Health Association, and the Brazilian Psychiatric Association. He received an M.D. from the School of Medicine, Rio de Janeiro State University, and an M.P.H. and Ph.D. from the School of Public Health, University of California, Berkeley.

DAVID T. COURTWRIGHT is professor and chair of the Department of History at the University of North Florida. He has also been a faculty member at the University of Hartford, the University of Connecticut Health Center, and the University of Texas School of Public Health. He has received fellowships from the University of Texas Medical Branch, the Samuel E. Ziegler Educational Foundation, and the National Endowment for the Humanities. He is a member of the American Historical Association and the Organization of American Historians. His publications include *Dark Paradise: Opiate Addiction in America Before 1940* and *Addicts Who Survived: An Oral History of Narcotic Use in America, 1923–1965*. He received a B.A. from the University of Kansas and a Ph.D. from Rice University.

DAVID A. DEITCH, a clinical and social psychologist, is vice president and chief executive officer for field operations at Daytop Village, Inc., a nonprofit drug and alcohol treatment agency with facilities in New York, California, and Texas. He is also director of clinical and organizational consultation, Pacific Institute for Clinical Training, Education, and Consultation, Berkeley, California. He was previously executive director and cofounder of Daytop Village, senior vice president and chief clinical officer of Phoenix House Foundation, and chief of substance abuse services, University of California, San Francisco. He has also been a clinical faculty member in departments of psychiatry at the University of California, San Diego; the University of Chicago; and Temple University. He was chairman of the White House Task Force on Prevention, a consultant to the Presidential Commission for the Study of Crime and Juvenile Delinquency and the National Commission on Marijuana and Drug Abuse, and a member of the Pennsylvania Governor's Council on Alcohol and Drug Abuse. He received the state of California award for outstanding contributions in the drug abuse field. He received his M.S. and Ph.D. from the Wright Institute, Berkeley, California.

DOUGLAS A. FRASER is professor of labor studies at Wayne State University. He was the Jerry Wurf Fellow and Lecturer at the John F. Kennedy School of Government, Harvard University. He is retired from the United Auto Workers, where he served as vice president and president. First appointed to the staff of the UAW in 1947, he concentrated much of his energy on negotiating and implementing employee benefit programs. He was responsible for the union's early retirement program, restrictions on compulsory overtime, a comprehensive health and safety program, dental care benefits, reduced work time, and improvements in the cost-of-living allowance formula. He has served as cochair of the Michigan Governor's Commission on Jobs and Economic Development and as a member of the board of trustees of the Aspen Institute for Humanistic Studies and the Executive Committee of the Leadership Conference on Civil Rights and as a member of the board of governors of the United Way.

JAMES G. HAUGHTON is medical director of the Martin Luther King, Jr./Charles R. Drew Medical Center of the Los Angeles County Department of Health Services. After serving in leading public health positions with the New York City Health and Welfare Departments, he served for nine years as the executive director for the Health and Hospitals Governing Commission in Chicago and subsequently as director of the Department of Health and Human Services, City of Houston. He is currently a member of the advisory board of the Robert Wood Johnson Foundation AIDS health service programs and the board of directors of the Alan Guttmacher Institute. He has received awards from the National Association of Health Services Executives, the March of Dimes, and the Los Angeles Board of Supervisors. He is a fellow of the American College of Preventive Medicine and the American Public Health Association, and a member of the American Medical Association, National Medical Association, Southern Medical Association, Texas Medical Association, United States Conference of Human Services Officials, and the United States Conference of Local Health Officials. He is a member of the Institute of Medicine. He received a B.A. from Pacific Union College, an M.D. from Loma Linda University, and an M.P.H. from Columbia University School of Public Health and Administrative Medicine.

ROBERT L. HUBBARD is a social psychologist and program director for alcohol and drug abuse research in the Center for Social Research and Policy Analysis, Research Triangle Institute, North Carolina. He was principal investigator for the Treatment Outcome Prospective Study follow-up of a large multicity sample of drug treatment clients, and he is the lead author of *Drug Abuse Treatment*. He has completed studies on adult and teenage drug use epidemiology; the relationships among drug use, employment, and crime; assessment of vocational services in drug treatment programs; and management styles and occupational programs in industry. He is currently directing a study of substance abuse prevention for high-risk youth and a methodological study of client self-reports after treatment, among other drug research studies at the Research Triangle Institute. He was previously at the Survey Research Center, University of Michigan. He is a member of the American Association for Public Opinion Research, American Psychological Association, American Public Health Association, American Society of Criminology, American Sociological Association, and the American Statistical Association. He received a B.A. from Ohio University, a Ph.D. from the University of Michigan, and an M.B.A. from the Fuqua School of Business, Duke University.

JAMES D. ISBISTER is president of Pharmavene, Inc. His career in government from 1962 to 1977 included service as the administrator of the Alcohol, Drug Abuse, and Mental Health Administration. He has been vice president of the Orkand Corporation, associate director for management of the International Communication Agency, senior vice president of the Blue Cross and Blue Shield Association, and president of Combined Technologies, Inc. He has received the William A. Jump Foundation Award for exemplary achievement in public administration, the Arthur S. Flemming Award, and numerous other commendations. He received a B.A. from the University of Michigan and an M.A. from George Washington University.

HERBERT D. KLEBER is on leave as professor of psychiatry at Yale University School of Medicine where he is founding director of the Substance Abuse Treatment Unit at the Connecticut Mental Health Center. He is also director of Yale's Center for Opioid and Cocaine Abuse Treatment Research and chief executive officer of APT Foundation, Inc. He served on the Governor's Drug Advisory Council (Connecticut) and cochaired the Mayor's Task Force on Drugs (New Haven). He has received the American Psychiatric Association Gold Award, the Foundations Fund Award for Research, and the Founders Award of the American Academy of Psychiatrists in Alcoholism and Addiction (AAPAA). He previously served on the national advisory councils of the National Institute on Drug Abuse and the National Institute of Mental Health. He is a fellow of the American Psychiatric Association and the American College of Neuropsychopharmacology, a member of the American Medical Association, and a founding member of AAPAA. He received a B.A. from Dartmouth College and an M.D. from Jefferson Medical College, serving a psychiatric residency at Yale. In

August 1989 he was confirmed by the U.S. Senate as deputy director for demand reduction in the Office of National Drug Control Policy.

JUDITH R. LAVE is professor of health economics at the Graduate School of Public Health, University of Pittsburgh. She has also taught economics and urban affairs at Carnegie Mellon University and was director of the Office of Research, Health Care Financing Administration, U.S. Department of Health and Human Services. She is a member of the American Economic Association, the American Public Health Association, and the Association for Health Services Research, which she served as president. She is a member of the Institute of Medicine. She received a B.A. from Queen's University and an M.A. and Ph.D. from Harvard University.

DAVID J. MACTAS, a certified addictions specialist and social worker, is president of Marathon, Inc., a nonprofit drug and alcohol treatment and research agency based in Providence, Rhode Island. He was previously on the staff of the Morris J. Bernstein Institute, St. Vincent's Medical Center, and the Vera Institute of Justice, all in New York City, and he served as assistant commissioner of the New York City Addiction Services Agency. He has taught at Rhode Island College and New England Institute of Technology. He served as president of Therapeutic Communities of America and is a board member of the World Federation of Therapeutic Communities. He received a B.A. from City College of New York and an M.A. from the New School for Social Research.

DONALD J. McCONNELL is executive director of the Connecticut Alcohol and Drug Abuse Commission. He has previously been a priest with the Archdiocese of Newark, New Jersey; an educational consultant with the Institutes for Rural Education, Santiago, Chile; director of Latin American Studies at Seton Hall University; director of education and training, State of New Jersey Drug Abuse Project; and director of addiction services, Connecticut Department of Corrections. He was the recipient of the National Association of State Alcohol and Drug Abuse Directors' award for outstanding leadership and dedication, the Alcohol and Drug Problems Association award for outstanding achievement for an individual, the Nyswander/Dole award for contributions to the field of methadone maintenance, and the Connecticut Hispanic Addiction Commission award for dedication to the recovery of Latino substance abusers. He is a member of the Alcohol and Drug Problems Association; the Advisory Council on AIDS of the National Institute on Drug Abuse; and the National Association of State Alcohol and Drug Abuse Directors, which he has served as president. He received a B.A. from Seton Hall University, an M.Div.

from Immaculate Conception Seminary, and two M.A. degrees and a Ph.D. candidate certificate from the University of Wisconsin at Madison.

JOHN H. MOXLEY III is vice president and partner at Korn/Ferry International, where he conducts nationwide searches for physician executives sought by organizations in the private and public sectors. Before joining Korn/Ferry, he had his own consulting practice focusing on organizational issues in health care. His prior experience includes positions as senior vice president of American Medical International, Inc.; assistant secretary of defense for health affairs in the Department of Defense; vice chancellor and dean of medicine at the University of California, San Diego; dean of the University of Maryland School of Medicine; and assistant to the dean of Harvard Medical School. In 1984, he served as director of Polyclinic Health Services for the XXIII Olympics. He has served on the board of trustees of the American Hospital Association and chaired the scientific board and served on the governing council of the California Medical Association. He currently serves on the board of the National Fund for Medical Education and the Henry M. Jackson Foundation for the Advancement of Military Medicine. He is board-certified in internal medicine and is a fellow of the American College of Physicians and a distinguished fellow of the American College of Physician Executives. He is a member of the Association of American Medical Colleges, the Society of Medical Administrators, and the American Society of Clinical Oncology. He is a member of the Institute of Medicine. He received an A.B. from Williams College and an M.D. from the University of Colorado.

PETER S. O'DONNELL is a partner and cofounder of the KEREN Group, a health care management and marketing firm based in Princeton, New Jersey. He has previously been the president and chief executive officer of a regional managed care health plan with more than 20,000 members and 1,400 physicians under contract. Prior to that he was senior vice president of ALTA Health Strategies, Inc., a major third-party administrator of health benefits, where he developed and implemented utilization review programs and related managed care programs. He was previously director of employee benefits for the RCA Corporation; a consultant for the Wm. Mercer Company, a national health benefits consulting firm; senior health adviser to the governor of Florida; staff associate with the National Governors' Association; and a member of the staff of the Advisory Commission on Intergovernmental Relations. He is a member of the editorial board of Managed Care Outlook and serves on the board of the Alpha Center and the Foundation for Health Services Research. He received a B.A. from the Pennsylvania State University and an M.A. from Rutgers University.

MARK V. PAULY is professor of health care systems and public management at the Wharton School, director of research of the Leonard Davis Institute of Health Economics, and professor of economics at the University of Pennsylvania. His major interests are public finance, collective decision making, insurance regulation, and medical economics. He serves on the health advisory board of the American Enterprise Institute, where he has been an adjunct scholar, and he has also been a board member of the Association for Health Services Research. He has held fellowships at the International Institute of Management (Berlin) and the International Institute for Applied Systems Analysis (Vienna). He has been a faculty research fellow at the National Bureau of Economic Research, professor of economics at Northwestern University, and a research associate with the U.S. Public Health Service. He is a member of the American Economic Association and the Association for Health Services Research. He is a member of the Institute of Medicine. He received an A.B. from Xavier University, an M.A. from the University of Delaware, and a Ph.D. from the University of Virginia.

HAROLD A. RICHMAN is director of Chapin Hall Center for Children and Hermon Dunlap Smith Professor in the School of Social Service Administration, University of Chicago. His earlier positions at the University of Chicago include dean of the School of Social Service Administration, founding chairman of the Committee on Public Policy Studies, and codirector of the children's policy research project. He was previously a White House fellow and special assistant to the secretary of labor. He is currently on the board of the University of Chicago Laboratory Schools and is a member of the executive management committee, National Opinion Research Center. He chairs the research advisory committee on youth of the Lilly Endowment, Inc., and the Children's Program Committee of the Edna McConnell Clark Foundation; he is also a member of numerous nonprofit boards and advisory committees. He received an A.B. from Harvard College and a Ph.D. in social welfare policy from the University of Chicago.

MAXINE L. STITZER is associate professor of behavioral biology in the Department of Psychiatry and Behavioral Sciences, Johns Hopkins University School of Medicine, and associate director of the drug abuse treatment research unit at Francis Scott Key Medical Center. She has been active in drug abuse research with areas of specialization in human behavioral pharmacology and substance abuse treatment evaluation. She serves as editorial consultant for several scientific journals and was previously a member of the clinical/behavioral research review committee of the National Institute on Drug Abuse. She is a fellow of the American Psychological Association and a member of the Behavioral Pharmacology Society, American Public Health Association, and Society for Behavioral Medicine. She received a

B.A. from the University of California, Berkeley, and an M.S. and Ph.D. from the University of Michigan.

DEAN R. GERSTEIN, a sociologist, is a study director at the Institute of Medicine and National Research Council of the National Academy of Sciences, where his earlier studies include *Alcohol and Public Policy: Beyond the Shadow of Prohibition, Commonalities in Substance Abuse and Habitual Behavior, Guidelines for Studies on Substance Abuse Treatment,* and *The Behavioral and Social Sciences: Achievements and Opportunities.* He has done research on addiction careers, drug treatment programs, alcohol and highway crashes, smoking and mortality, and the development of social theory and held editorial positions with *Contemporary Drug Problems* and *Sociological Theory.* Previously, he was at the University of California, Los Angeles, the University of California, San Diego, and the Veterans Administration Medical Center, La Jolla. He is a member of the American Sociological Association, the American Public Health Association, the Kettil Bruun Society for Sociological and Epidemiological Research on Alcohol, and the Alcohol and Drug Study Group of the American Anthropological Association. He received a B.A. from Reed College and a Ph.D. from Harvard University.

HENRICK J. HARWOOD, an economist, served as associate study director for the Substance Abuse Coverage Study. Prior to joining the staff of the Institute of Medicine, he was at the Research Triangle Institute in North Carolina, where he was the principal author of *Economic Costs of Alcohol and Drug Abuse and Mental Illness—1980* and contributed the economic analyses used in the Department of Health and Human Services' report to Congress, *Toward a National Plan to Combat Alcohol Abuse and Alcoholism.* He has done research on the impact of alcohol and drug consumption on productivity in the work force, the crime-related costs and benefits of different modalities of drug treatment, and the provision of employment services and vocational services in drug treatment programs. He has held adjunct faculty appointments at Erasmus University in Rotterdam, the Netherlands, and Duke University. He received a B.A. from Stetson University and performed graduate studies in economics at the University of North Carolina, Chapel Hill. In December 1989 he accepted the position of senior policy analyst in the Office of National Drug Control Policy.

Index

A

Abstinence
  as central goal of drug treatment, 8, 129
  full, partial, and nonrecovery, 126-127
  goals of chemical dependency programs,
    170–171
  individual drug history, 62
Accreditation, Medicaid and drug
  treatment programs, 26
Acquired immune deficiency syndrome
  (AIDS)
  Anti-Drug Abuse Act of 1988, 55
  epidemic and national drug policy, 4
  goals of drug treatment, 11, 105
  health costs of drug problem, 104
  Medicaid coverage, 271–272
  methadone programs, 14
  transmission by injection, 68 n.2
Addiction Severity Index, 110
Admissions, residential treatment
  committee recommendations on optimal
    private coverage provisions, 31
  elimination of waiting lists, 232
  utilization management and review, 28,
    251
Adolescents
  additional policy questions, 37–38
  age of drug use onset, 68, 69
  aggregate need for drug treatment, 7
  estimating extent of need for drug
    treatment, 80
  patterns of drug consumption, 4–5
  research recommendations, 21, 198–199
Adults
  aggregate need for drug treatment, 7–8
  arrests for drug crimes, 114
  committee findings and
    recommendations, 37
  estimating extent of need for drug
    treatment, 80
  patterns of drug consumption, 4
  treatment research statistics, 20–21
Aftercare, chemical dependency programs,
  171
Age
  aggregate need for drug treatment, 7
  individual drug history, 68–69
  patterns of drug consumption, 4–5
  treatment research statistics, 20–21
Aid to Families with Dependent Children
  (AFDC), 198, 268
Alabama, state drug coverage mandates,
  292

Alcohol and alcoholism
  Addiction Severity Index, 110
  chemical dependency programs, 16, 275
  cost-effectiveness of treatment, 284–285
  employee assistance programs, 121, 288
  employers and private coverage
    decisions, 282–283
  extension of treatment capacity to drug
    treatment, 218
  partial legality, 62
  pregnant women, 85
  private insurance coverage, 278
  recovery and relapse compared to
    heroin, 73
  state mandates regarding treatment
    coverage, 289 n.5
  therapeutic communities, 162
  trends in provider characteristics,
    208–209
Alcohol, Drug Abuse, and Mental Health
  Administration (ADAMHA)
  block grant administration, 241
  emergency appropriation for FY 1990,
    216
  health services research programs, 195
  strategic planning for drug treatment,
    235
  trends in federal funding, 214
Alcoholics Anonymous
  chemical dependency programs, 16, 53,
    170, 171, 190
  drug treatment programs, 135
Amantadine, 175
Ambivalence, client
  incentives and motivation, 224
  spectrum of recovery, 125–130
Anslinger, Harry, 48·
Anti-Drug Abuse Act of 1986
  call for independent study of substance
    abuse treatment coverage, 1, 33
  emphasis on enforcement and
    interdiction, 55
  federal support of research, 192
  federal support of treatment, 104, 202
    n.1, 216, 244
  TASC programs, 116
Anti-Drug Abuse Act of 1988
  federal policy and treatment, 55, 216,
    245
  federal support of research, 192
  TASC programs, 116
  waiting list reduction, 232
Arkansas, state drug coverage mandates,
  292

321

Arrests, law enforcement and drug crimes, 114
Attitudes
full, partial, and nonrecovery, 128
normative, 62, 64
Attrition, client, 126

B

Barbiturates, detoxification, 174 n.21
Benefits (*see* Cost/benefit analysis, Insurance)
Bennett, William, 55
Block grants
federal role in 1980s, 241–245
management and federal funding, 246
reduction in federal funding, 202 n.1
research on women, 198
sources of treatment dollars, 212
Blue Cross/Blue Shield, 278, 284
Boot camps, effectiveness of correctional treatment programs, 17, 183–184
Brain
effects of opiates, 138–139
effects of psychoactive drugs, 64
Bromocriptine, 175
Budget (*see* Financing)
Buprenorphine, 175
Bureau of Narcotics and Dangerous Drugs, 51

C

California
Civil Addict Program, 180–183
Medicaid and AIDS, 271–272
Medicaid and drug treatment, 267–268
methadone maintenance programs, 144, 146, 151–152
CareUnit system, 173
Certification
performance and public support, 29, 252
Chemical Abuse/Addiction Treatment Outcome Registry (CATOR), 123, 173
Chemical dependency programs
average daily charges, 290–291 n.7
description of modality, 170–172
effectiveness of, 16, 172–173
private coverage and effectiveness data, 275
research on treatment effectiveness, 20, 186, 285
research recommendations, 197
rise of modern treatment, 53
state-mandated coverage, 290

summary of committee findings, 190
variations in effectiveness, 173–174
Child care, mothers and drug treatment, 198, 234
Children (*see also* Adolescents, Pregnant Women)
age of drug use onset, 68
external costs of drug abuse, 229, 233–234
patterns of drug consumption, 4
women and therapeutic communities, 198
Civil Addict Program (CAP), 146, 180–183
Civil rights
concern for drug-dependent individuals, 108
economic status of clients, 127
Class
chemical dependency program clients, 53
criminal and medical views of drug addiction, 48
employee assistance programs, 121
opium addiction and medical idea, 46, 47
Client-Oriented Data Acquisition Process (CODAP), 164, 240
Clients, drug treatment
chemical dependency programs and therapeutic communities compared, 172
individual goals, 129–130
parties involved in treatment, 107
public and private tiers, 205–206
trends in numbers and provider characteristics, 206–210
Clinical trials, research on major modalities of drug treatment, 18 n.2
detoxification, 175–176
methadone maintenance, 142–145, 149
therapeutic communities, 158–160
Cocaine
detoxification, 175, 176
drug sequencing, 69
emergency room and medical examiner cases, 77
employee assistance programs, 122
federal policy emphasis on enforcement, 55
history of use, 66–67
improvement of public coverage, 233
methadone programs, 14
need for expansion of public tier, 219
normative attitudes, 62
patterns of drug consumption, 5
patterns of drug treatment motivation, 111 n.2
positive tests among arrestees, 100

pregnant women, 85
research recommendations, 20, 197–198
state prison inmates, 82, 83
therapeutic communities, 14, 154, 162
urinalysis, 99
Collective bargaining, employer-sponsored
health insurance, 273
Colorado, Medicaid funding of drug
treatment, 271
Community-based treatment
Alcoholics Anonymous methods, 135 n.2
criminal justice system referrals, 10, 120
goals of drug treatment, 108
origins of, 50–52, 133
Community Mental Health Centers Act,
52
Consumer price index (CPI), 210 n.2
Contracts, direct program financing of
public tier, 25
Copayments, treatment needs and cost
concerns, 299 n.2
Cornerstone program, effectiveness of
correctional treatment programs,
178, 180
Correctional treatment programs
effectiveness, 176–178, 180–185
summary of committee findings, 191
trends in client numbers, 207
Cost/benefit analysis
effectiveness of drug treatment
programs, 18
methadone treatment, 151–152, 188
outpatient nonmethadone programs, 170,
189–190
therapeutic communities, 165–166, 189
Costs
balancing concerns with treatment needs,
228–230
baseline comparison values, 256–257
committee recommendations for private
coverage, 296
comprehensive strategy option, 260–262
core strategy option, 238, 257–260
estimation for drug problems, 102–104
external costs and logic of mandating
private insurance coverage of drug
treatment, 276
external costs and public intervention,
222–225
goals of drug treatment, 129
intermediate strategy option, 263–265
management and health care issues, 275
offsets and private coverage of drug
treatment, 282–283
private and public tiers, 218

private coverage and drug treatment,
293–294
private coverage and health benefits,
283–288
quantification of societal, 88–90
state mandates and private coverage, 291
utilization management, 28, 251
Counseling and counselors
improvement of public coverage, 232–233
methadone maintenance, 141–142
private versus public tiers, 204
Courts, criminal justice
prison overcrowding and referrals to
treatment, 120
referrals to private programs, 112
referrals to treatment, 114, 116–117
Courtwright, David, 34
Crime
effectiveness of Stay'n Out program, 178
estimating costs of drug problems, 102,
103
methadone clients, 13, 143, 153
outpatient nonmethadone programs, 170
reduction as goal of drug treatment, 11,
108, 129
societal costs of drug abuse, 89
type and probable need for treatment,
100
therapeutic communities, 162, 166
Criminal idea
classic era of narcotics control, 48–49
drug policy, 3, 47–48, 55, 57, 218
evolution of governmental roles, 53–56
external costs and public intervention,
223
Criminal justice system (*see also* Law
enforcement, Parole, Probation)
Addiction Severity Index, 110
additional policy questions, 38
agencies as parties in drug treatment,
108
comprehensive strategy option, 238–239
estimating extent of need for treatment,
81–84, 88
estimating need for treatment among
arrestees, 99–102
federal drug policy, 215
goals of drug treatment, 10–11, 106,
113–114, 116–120, 131
health services research, 196
implications of involvement in admissions
to drug programs, 112–113
inducing more clients to accept
treatment, 235
reasons for seeking treatment, 112

D

Data and data systems
  federal role in 1980s, 244, 245
  health services research, 197–198
  performance standards, 247
  private coverage and sources, 274
  utilization management, 28–29, 252
Daytop Village
  early success stories, 157
  therapeutic community approach to
    treatment, 51
Deaths, heroin recovery and relapse, 74
Dederich, Charles, 51
Defense, Department of (DoD), 266 n.5
Demography
  populations of different modalities, 134
  therapeutic community population, 154
  treatment research statistics, 20–21
Demonstration grants, health services
    research, 196–197
Depression, emotional, 112
Depression, Great, 49
Desipramine hydrochloride, 175
Deterrance
  prisons and criminological thought, 49
Detoxification
  cross-dependence, 138–139
  effectiveness, 16, 174–176
  indications for hospital-based inpatient,
    28, 251–252
  recovery and relapse, 6
  summary of committee findings, 190–191
Diagnosis, individual need for drug
    treatment, 7, 69–72
*Diagnostic and Statistical Manual of Mental
    Disorders* (DSM-III-R), 70, 71, 76
Dole, Vincent, 50–51
Drug abuse and dependence
  complexity of problem and estimation of
    need for treatment, 90–92
  diagnostic critiera, 69–72
  diagnosis and detoxification, 174 n.20
  individual drug history, 59–75
  quantification of societal costs, 88-90
Drug Abuse Forecasting (DUF) system,
    99, 100, 101, 196
Drug Abuse Reporting Program (DARP)
  evaluation of effectiveness of OPNMs,
    168, 170
  research on effectiveness of drug
    treatment, 12, 134, 196
  study of effectiveness of therapeutic
    communities, 160–163, 165–166
Drug Abuse Treatment Outcome Study
    (DATOS), 12, 134, 196

Drug Abuse Warning Network (DAWN)
  cocaine consumption, 67
  data systems and research, 196
Drug consumption
  estimation of need for treatment, 90–91
  goals of drug treatment, 129
  individual drug history, 60–61
  level of use and criminality, 119
  methadone dosage levels, 150
  patterns and need for drug treatment,
    4–5, 59
  use, abuse, and dependence stages,
    61–62
"Drug czar," 55
Drug dependence (*see* Drug abuse and
    dependence)
Drug-Free Workplace Act of 1988, 123
Drug history, individual
  age of onset and drug sequencing, 68–69
  learning and drug experience, 64–66
  model and overview of individual, 59–62
  social environment, 66–67
Drug screening programs
  availability to workers, 121 n.4
  employers and goals of treatment, 123,
    124
Drug sequencing, individual drug history,
    68–69
Drug testing, employee
  libertarian ideas, 45
  private treatment programs and goals of
    drug treatment, 108–109
Drug trade
  crime control resources, 102–103
  homicide, 102
Drug treatment (*see also* Chemical
    dependency programs, Correctional
    treatment programs, Detoxification,
    Methadone maintenance, Private
    tier, Public tier, Therapeutic
    communities)
  balancing needs and cost concerns,
    228–230
  changing nature of drug problems,
    298–299
  determining individual need, 7, 69–72
  diverse interests and goals, 106–109
  effectiveness, 11–21, 32, 132–199
  employers and goals, 120–125
  erosion of after 1976, 215–216
  estimating extent of need for, 7–8,
    76–86, 88
  estimating need for among arrestees,
    99–102
  estimating need for in criminal justice
    populations, 76–80

estimating need for in homeless population, 84
estimating need for in household population, 77–80, 92–94, 96–99
evaluation of effectiveness and untreated recovery rate, 75–76
goals, 8–11, 130–131
growth of national system, 206–216
health insurance cost outlays, 283–284
improvement as priority of public coverage, 232–233
modeling future treatment needs and effects, 265–266
overall tendencies of effectiveness, 134–135
as principle of public intervention, 227–228
reasons for seeking, 109–113
recommendations for research on services and methods, 192–199
research on effectiveness, 133–134
rise of modern, 49–56
role of in federal anti-drug abuse strategy, 214–215
state Medicaid coverage for specific services, 271
two-tiered system, 21–22
DuPont, Robert, 55

E

Economics (*see also* Indigency; Poverty)
client assets and motivation for recovery, 127
quantification of societal costs, 88–90
Education
chemical dependency programs, 171, 172
goals of drug treatment, 129
Effectiveness (*see* Drug treatment)
Elderly, concern about abuse and dependence, 68
Emergency rooms, estimating extent of need for treatment, 76–77
Employee assistance programs (EAPs)
defining goals of treatment, 121–123
employee drug testing, 124
managed care system, 287–288
Employee Retirement Income Security Act (ERISA), 289–290
Employers
drug screening programs, 123
extent and nature of insurance coverage for drug treatment, 273, 282–283
federal government and drug treatment coverage, 281–282
goals of drug treatment, 120–125, 131

parties involved in drug treatment, 108
private companies and drug treatment coverage, 278–279
reasons for seeking treatment, 112
state and local government and drug treatment coverage, 279–280
Employment
Addiction Severity Index, 110
aggregate need for drug treatment, 8
cost/benefit ratio of methadone maintenance, 153
cost/benefit ratio of outpatient nonmethadone programs, 170
goals of drug treatment, 10, 129
therapeutic communities and treatment retention, 162

F

Facilities, improvement of public coverage, 233
Families
Addiction Severity Index, 110
chemical dependency programs, 171
criminal view of drug problem, 47–48
goals of drug treatment, 129
parties involved in drug treatment, 107, 108 n.1
reasons for seeking treatment, 112
therapeutic communities, 156
Federal Employee Benefits Health Plan, 281
Financing
amounts needed to meet priority objectives, 255
differences between private and public tiers, 202–204
private coverage, 29–32, 273–300
public care, 21–29, 220–272
sources of treatment dollars, 211–214
trends in federal funding, 214–216
trends in funding base, 210–211
Flupenthixol decanoate, 175
Food and Drug Administration
Dole-Nyswander model of methadone maintenance, 51
LAAM, 139 n.6
Function impairments, recovery process, 6

G

Gatekeepers
employee assistance program staff, 288
utilization management, 27, 28, 250
Gaudenzia House, 166

Goals
    criminal justice agencies, 113–114,
        116–120
    detoxification, 176
    diverse interests, 106–109
    drug treatment, 8–11, 130–131
    employers, 120–125
    full, partial, and nonrecovery from drug
        problems, 126–128
    methadone maintenance, 137
    operational for programs, 105
    and priorities of public coverage, 22–24
    reasons for seeking treatment, 109–113
    setting realistic, 128–130
Government, federal
    crime control resources, 102–103
    employees and drug treatment coverage,
        281–282
    financing of public tier, 21, 24–25
    libertarian ideology, 44–45
    Medicaid and matching dollars, 267
    national drug policy, 3–4
    role in the 1990s, 240–241, 245–248, 256
    support for drug research, 192
    trends in funding, 214–216
Government, local
    crime control resources, 103
    employees and drug treatment coverage,
        279–280
    sources of treatment dollars, 211–212,
        213–214
Government, state (see also States, and
        individual states)
    crime control resources, 103
    employees and drug treatment coverage,
        279–280
    financing of public tier, 21, 24–25,
        211–212, 213–214
    responsibility for public tier in 1980s,
        244, 256
    role in the 1990s, 240–241, 245–248
Grants (see also Block grants;
        Demonstration grants)
    direct program financing of public tier,
        25
    matching and maintenance-of-effort
        requirements, 26, 249
Great Britain, methadone maintenance,
        137
"Great Society," 3

H

Harrison Act of 1914, 48
Hazelden Foundation, 53, 173

Health (see also Public health)
    Addiction Severity Index, 110
    estimating costs of drug problems, 104
    methadone clients, 13
Health Maintenance Organizations
        (HMOs), 281–282, 290 n.6
Health services
    cost offsets, 283
    research and treatment systems, 19–20
    research recommendations, 195–197
Heart infections, transmission by injection,
        68 n.2
Hepatitis, transmission by injection, 68 n.2
Heroin
    detoxification and relapse, 138–139, 176
    Dole-Nyswander research on methadone
        maintenance, 50–51
    effects compared to methadone, 140
    emergency room and medical examiner
        cases, 77
    literature on dependence and recovery,
        73–74
    literature on patterns of drug treatment
        motivation, 111 n.2
    Nixon administration "War on Drugs,"
        53–54
    research and problem of noncompliance,
        157–158 n.14
    state prison inmates, 82–83
    therapeutic communities, 14, 154, 162
Homeless, estimating extent of need for
        treatment, 84–85, 88
Homicide, drug trafficking, 102
Hong Kong, study of methadone
        maintenance, 144 n.8
Hospitals
    chemical dependency programs, 16, 190
    committee recommendations on optimal
        private coverage provisions, 30–31
    cost control and utilization management,
        28
    drug detoxification, 16, 175, 190–191
    optimal private coverage provisions,
        294–295
    prescription of methadone, 141
    trends in drug treatment client numbers,
        207–208
    utilization management and public tier,
        251–252
Household population, estimating extent
        of need for treatment, 77–80, 92–94,
        96–99
Human immunodeficiency virus (HIV) (see
        also Acquired immune deficiency
        syndrome)
    methadone programs, 14

I

Ideas
  character of governing, 41–42
  drug treatment policy, 2–4, 56
  rise of modern drug treatment, 49–56
  spectrum of about drugs, 42–49
Illinois Drug Abuse Program, 52
Incapacitation, prisons and criminological
    thought, 49
Incentives
  external costs and public intervention,
    224
  private providers and efficiency, 285–286
  staff performance, 233
Income
  constraints and public support of
    treatment, 225–227
  employee productivity losses, 103–104
  estimating extent of need for drug
    treatment, 80
  as index of external costs, 229
  private tier and insurance coverage, 277
  sensitivity of drug abusers to price of
    treatment, 276
Indigency, committee estimates of and
    public coverage, 23, 227, 254–255
Infants (*see* Pregnant women)
Injection, transmission of disease, 68 n.2
Insurance, health (*see also* Financing,
    Medicaid, Private coverage, Public
    coverage)
  employer-sponsored and unions, 273
  and income constraints, 225–227
  mandates, 30, 275–276, 288–293, 294
*International Statistical Classification of
    Diseases, Injuries, and Causes of
    Death* (ICD-10), 70, 71

J

Jaffe, Jerome, 52
Jails, compared to prisons, 82 n.5
Job applicants, drug screening programs,
    123
Johnson Institute, 53
*Journal of the American Medical
    Association*, 50
Justice Assistance Act of 1984, 116

L

Law enforcement (*see also* Crime,
    Criminal justice system)
  additional policy questions, 38
  arrests for drug crimes, 114

  crime control resources, 102–103
  societal costs of drug abuse, 89
Learning
  drug consumption behavior, 69
  individual drug history, 64–66
Legalization, illicit drugs, 265
Legislation (*see also* specific acts:
    Anti-Drug Abuse, Drug-Free
    Workplace, Employee Retirement
    Income Security, Harrison, Justice
    Assistance, Narcotic Addiction
    Rehabilitation, Omnibus Budget
    Reconciliation)
  early anti-drug, 45
  federal and Medicaid, 248, 271
  federal anti-drug and expansion of
    public tier, 22
  state-mandated private coverage, 30,
    275–276, 288–293, 294
Levo-alpha-acetylmethadyl (LAAM), 139
    n.6, 158 n.14
Libertarian ideas
  drug policy, 3, 44–46, 56, 57
  influence on nation's collective thinking,
    223

M

Managed care
  employee assistance program personnel,
    288
  health insurance and cost containment,
    286–287
Marijuana
  drug sequencing, 69
  emergency room reports, 77
  employee assistance programs, 122
  normative attitutes, 62
  patterns of drug consumption, 5
  positive tests among arrestees, 100
  state prison inmates, 82, 83
  urinalysis, 99–100
Marketing, chemical dependency
    programs, 20, 197
Maryland, state-mandated drug treatment
    coverage, 290
Medicaid
  federal contribution, 212
  federal legislation and drug treatment
    needs, 248–250
  public tier funding of treatment services,
    26–27, 256, 265–272
  transitional steps toward the year 2000,
    249
Medical idea
  classic era of narcotics control, 48

drug policy, 3, 46–47, 48, 56, 57
  evolution of governmental roles, 53–56
  influence on nation's collective thinking,
    223
  private treatment programs and goals of
    drug treatment, 108
Medical price index (MPI), 210 n.2
Medicare
  nursing home care and Medicaid, 268
  population served and treatment needs,
    266
  public coverage and income constraints,
    225–227
Men
  aggregate need for drug treatment, 7
  estimating extent of need for drug
    treatment, 80
  married and reasons for seeking
    treatment, 112
  treatment research statistics, 20–21
Meperidine, 136 n.3
Methadone
  compared to naltrexone and LAAM, 158
    n.14
  effects compared to heroin, 140
  opiate detoxification, 174
  types of narcotic analgesics, 136 n.3
Methadone maintenance
  characteristics of long-term clients, 160
  Civil Addict Program supervision,
    182–183
  clinical behavioral strategy, 140–142
  compared to outpatient nonmethadone
    programs, 15, 168, 169, 170
  compared to therapeutic communities,
    166
  cost/benefit ratio, 18, 151–152
  criminal justice system and reasons for
    seeking treatment, 112
  description of modality, 136–137
  effectiveness, 12–14, 142–144, 146,
    152–154
  excess capacity, 206
  expansion of private tier, 218
  goals of treatment, 137
  incentives to continue treatment,
    224–225
  need for expansion of public tier, 219
  negative beliefs among public and policy
    makers, 136 n.4
  prevalence of repeat admissions, 111
  research on expenditures and
    effectiveness, 18, 19
  research on treatment effectiveness,
    185–186
  rise in modern treatment, 50–51, 133

significant private demand not subsidized
    by private insurance reimbursements,
    277
  substitution, 138–140
  summary of committee finding, 187–188
  trends in client numbers, 206–207
  variations in effectiveness, 17, 147–150
Modeling, future treatment needs and
    effects, 265–266
Mothers (*see also* Pregnant women)
  additional policy questions, 37
  priorities of public coverage, 233–234
  research recommendations, 21, 198
Motivations, client
  ambivalence and spectrum of recovery,
    126
  full, partial, and nonrecovery, 126–128
  goals of drug treatment, 9–10, 106
  reasons for seeking drug treatment,
    109–113

N

Naltrexone
  compared with methadone, 158 n.14
  incentives to continue treatment,
    224–225
Narcotic Addiction Rehabilitation Act
    (NARA) of 1966, 52
National Academy of Sciences, 33–34
National Association of State Alcohol and
    Drug Abuse Directors (NASADAD),
    232
National Drug and Alcoholism Treatment
    Utilization Survey (NDATUS)
  baseline comparison values, 256–257
  data on client numbers and provider
    characteristics, 206
  data on provider insurance receipts, 274
  health insurance and cost of drug
    treatment, 283–284
  public and private tiers, 202, 216–219
  women and special services, 198
National Drug Control Strategy
    (September 1988), 76, 235–236
National Forum on the Future of Children
    and Families, 38
National Household Survey of Drug
    Abuse (1988), 92
National Institute of Justice, 77, 99
National Institute on Drug Abuse (NIDA)
  evolution of government roles, 54–55
  health services research programs, 195
  household survey data and estimation of
    extent of need for treatment, 76, 77,
    77–78

research on treatment services and
methods, 193–194
research recommended on adolescents,
pregnant women, and mothers, 21,
199
research responsibilities, 19
sponsor of report, 33
transfer of authority from SAODAP, 241
transition of role to research and
educational functions, 241
zoning and "not in my backyard"
problem, 197
New York
Dole-Nyswander research and
methadone treatment programs, 51
early trials of methadone maintenance,
142–143, 147–148
Medicaid policies, 267, 270, 271
study of heroin recovery and relapse, 74
Nicotine, partial legality, 62
Nixon, Richard, administration and drug
policy, 3, 53–54
Normative attitudes, individual drug
history, 62, 64
North Dakota, state drug coverage
mandates, 292
"Not in my backyard" (NIMBY) problem,
197
Nursing homes, Medicare and Medicaid,
268
Nyswander, Marie, 50–51

O

Office of Economic Opportunity, 52
Office of National Drug Control Policy
establishment and federal drug policy,
55–56, 245
inconsistencies among federal programs,
27
strategic planning for drug treatment,
235
Office of Personnel Management, 278, 281
Office of Treatment Improvement, 195,
235
Omnibus Budget Reconciliation Act
(OBRA), 241
Opiates (*see also* Buprenorphine, Heroin,
LAAM, Methadone, Naltrexone)
addiction in nineteenth century, 46
effects on brain, 138–139
pharmacological agents and
detoxification, 174
pharmacological properties of, 139
positive tests among arrestees, 100
urinalysis, 99

Opium
early anti-drug legislation, 45
nineteenth-century addiction and medical
idea, 46–47
types of narcotic analgesics, 136 n.3
Oregon, state drug coverage mandates,
293
Outpatient nonmethadone programs
(OPNMs)
cost/benefit ratio, 18, 170
cost effectiveness compared to
therapeutic communities, 166
description of modality, 167–168
effectiveness of drug treatment, 15,
168–169
prison treatment programs, 17
private coverage and effectiveness data,
275
research on treatment effectiveness,
18–19, 185–186
rise in modern treatment, 52, 133
summary of committee finding, 189–190
trends in client numbers, 206
variations in effectiveness, 169
Oxford House, 135

P

Parole (*see also* Civil Addict Program,
Criminal justice system)
community-based treatment programs, 10
estimating extent of need for treatment,
84
implications of criminal justice
involvement in admissions to drug
treatment, 113
reasons for seeking treatment, 112
state prison inmates and revocation, 82
n.6
Pennsylvania, Medicaid and drug
treatment, 267, 271
Performance
certification and public support, 29
committee recommendations on optimal
private coverage provsions, 31,
296–297
states and data systems, 247
utilization management, 250
Phillips, Mary Dana, 35
Phoenix House, 161
Pleasure seeking, methadone as effective
analgesic, 140
Policy, national drug
effect of alternative scenarios on need
for treatment, 265–266
fundamental questions, 220-221

ideas governing, 2–4, 56–57
questions for additional study, 2, 37–39
rise of modern drug treatment, 49–56
rule of simple ideas, 41–42
spending patterns, 213
spectrum of ideas about drugs, 42–44
Population studies, estimating extent of
    need for treatment, 76
Poverty (*see also* Indigency)
    external costs and treatment needs, 229
Preferred provider organizations (PPOs),
    286
Pregnant women (*see also* Children,
    Mothers)
    comprehensive strategy option, 239
    core strategy option, 238
    estimating extent of need for treatment,
        85–86, 234
    Medicaid coverage, 272
    research recommendations, 21, 198
Presidential Commission on the Human
    Immunodeficiency Virus Epidemic
    (1988), 76
Price, sensitivity of drug abusers to cost of
    treatment, 276, 277
Prison-hospitals
    classic era of narcotics control, 48
    rise of modern treatment, 49–50
Prisons
    compared to jails, 82 n.5
    effectiveness of drug treatment, 17,
        176–185, 191
    external costs and public intervention,
        223
    motivations for treatment, 127
    overcrowding and criminal justice
        referrals to treatment, 10, 120
    populations and estimating extent of
        need for treatment, 81–84
    referrals to treatment, 117–119
Private coverage
    committee recommendations, 293–297
    cost containment of health benefits,
        283–288, 291–292
    extent, 277–283
    logic of mandating coverage of drug
        treatment, 276–277
    state mandates, 288–293
Private tier
    clients compared to public tier, 205, 206
    defined, 201–202
    drug treatment coverage, 29–32, 277–283
    drug treatment supply system, 216–217,
        217–218
    excess capacity, 206, 218–219
    expansion in 1980s, 215, 218

financing, 21–22, 202–203
goals of drug treatment, 108–109
overview, 273–276
ownership of programs, 209
ratio of drug treatment expenditures,
    203–204
referrals from criminal justice system,
    112
sources of treatment dollars, 21
Probation (*see also* Criminal justice
    system)
    community-based treatment programs, 10
    estimating extent of need for treatment,
        84
    implications of criminal justice
        involvement in admissions to drug
        treatment, 113
    outpatient nonmethadone treatment, 167
    prisons and criminological thought, 49
    reasons for seeking treatment, 112
Productivity
    employers and drug treatment, 124, 282
    estimating costs of drug problems,
        103–104
    goals of drug treatment, 106
    societal costs of drug abuse, 89
Profit, growth of drug treatment industry
    in 1980s, 277
Psychoactive drugs (*see also* Heroin;
    Methadone; Opiates)
    effects on brain, 64
    federal and state codes, 62
    medical and social uses and fundamental
        ideas about drugs, 40
    outpatient nonmethadone programs, 167
Psychotherapy, clinical rigor, 126
Public health
    goals of drug treatment, 11
    policy role of treatment, 56–57
    societal costs of drug abuse, 89
    street sales of methadone, 137 n.5
Public Health Service, 199
Public coverage
    adequacy of present means for
        managing, 221
    committee recommendations, 248–252,
        254–256
    federal and state roles, 239–248
    Medicaid, 248–250, 265–272
    principles of coverage, 221–230
    priorities, 230–235
    strategy options, 235–239, 256–264
    veterans, 252–254
Public tier
    ambulatory treatment, 209
    capacity and need for expansion, 219

clients compared to private tier, 205–206
criminal justice referrals, 112
defined, 201
drug treatment supply system, 216, 217
erosion after 1976, 215–216, 218
excess capacity, 206
financing, 21, 25–27
goals and priorities, 22–24
ratio of drug treatment expenditures, 203–204
selective expansion and resource intensity, 22

experimental evaluation of effectiveness of therapeutic communities, 158–160
needs and priorities for treatment services and methods, 19–21, 192–199
optimal private coverage provisions, 32
Retention
therapeutic communities, 189
treatment effectiveness, 187–188 n.26
Rice, Dorothy, 89

R

Race/ethnicity
criminal and medical views of drug addiction, 48
libertarian view of drug use, 45
therapeutic community clients, 154 n.12
Reagan, Ronald
administration and drug policy, 55
California and Civil Addict Program, 181
Recidivism
drug consumption and criminality, 119
length of imprisonment and drug involvement, 118
Recommendations (*see* Policy, national drug; Private coverage; Public coverage; Research, needs and priorities)
Recovery
ambivalence and spectrum of, 125–130
drug dependence, 6–7
full, partial, and nonrecovery, 126–128
goals of drug treatment, 106, 131
individual drug history, 73–76
Rehabilitation, prisons and criminological thought, 49
Reimbursers, third-party and drug treatment, 107
Relapse
detoxification, 16, 138–189
drug dependence, 5–6
individual drug history, 73–76
Remission, term compared to recovery, 73 n.3
Research
animal models, 64
character of nonexperimental evaluations, 156–157
on effectiveness and expenditures for major treatment modalities, 18–19
on effectiveness of drug treatment, 12, 185–186

S

Self-recovery, relapse, 6–7
Sentences, criminal justice
law enforcement and drug crimes, 114
varying lengths and prison populations, 82 n.6
Shock incarceration (SI), effectiveness of correctional treatment programs, 17, 183–184
Social change, fundamental ideas about drugs, 40
Social services
improvement of public coverage, 233
outpatient nonmethadone programs, 167–168
Society
ethical position on income constraints, 225
external costs and private coverage, 276
external costs and public intervention, 223
Socioeconomic environment
additional policy questions, 38–39
drug dependence, 5
individual drug history, 66–67
recovery and relapse, 6, 75
Special Action Office for Drug Abuse Prevention (SAODAP), 54, 240–241, 250
Staff
chemical dependency programs and therapeutic communities compared, 172
composition of in 1982 NDATUS, 210 n.1
differential effectiveness of treatment programs, 24
improvement of public coverage, 233
requirements of public tier programs, 206
variations in treatment effectiveness, 150, 164, 185

States (*see also* Government, state)
  drug problems among prison inmates,
    82, 83 n.7
  mandates of private coverage of drug
    treatment, 30, 275–276, 288-293, 294
  medical/criminal ideas and evolution of
    governmental roles, 54, 55
  use of Medicaid to fund treatment, 267
Statistics, sample size and standard error,
  98–99
Stay'n Out, effectiveness of correctional
  treatment programs, 177–178, 180
Stereotypes
  individual drug history, 60
  pleasure user and ethnicity, 45
Supplemental Security Income, 268
Supreme Court, criminal idea and drug
  policy formation, 48
Sweden, methadone maintenance, 143–144
Synanon
  early success stories, 157
  therapeutic community approach to
    treatment, 52, 133

                    T

Technology, libertarian view of drug use,
  45
Therapeutic communities
  compared to chemical dependency
    programs, 171–172
  compared to outpatient nonmethadone
    programs, 15, 168, 169, 170
  cost/benefit ratio, 18, 165–166
  description of modality, 154–156
  effectiveness of drug treatment, 14–15,
    156–163, 166–167
  origins and development, 133
  prison treatment programs, 17, 180
  research on expenditures and
    effectiveness, 18
  research on treatment effectiveness,
    185–186
  rise in modern treatment, 51–52
  summary of committee findings, 188–189
  variations in effectiveness, 163–165
Tobacco
  partial legality, 62
  pregnant women, 85
Treatment Alternatives to Street Crime
  (TASC), 114, 116–117, 157
Treatment Outcome Prospective Study
  (TOPS)
  cost/benefit analyses, 152
  effectiveness of drug treatment, 12, 35,
    134, 196
  effectiveness of OPNMs, 168–169, 170

  effectiveness of therapeutic communities,
    160, 162–163, 166
  veterans as clients, 253
  TASC referrals, 116
  variations in effectiveness of methadone
    maintenance programs, 148–149
  veterans and drug treatment programs,
    253

                    U

Unemployment
  aggregate need for drug treatment, 8
  estimating extent of need for drug
    treatment, 80
  goals of drug treatment, 10
Unions, employer-sponsored health
  insurance, 273
Urban neighborhoods, goals of drug
  treatment, 108
Urinalysis
  clinical rigor, 125–126
  estimating need for treatment among
    arrestees, 99–100
Utilization management
  optimal private coverage provisions, 31
  public financing of drug treatment, 27–29
  public intervention in the 1990s, 250–252

                    V

Veterans, as special case of public
  coverage, 25, 252–254, 256
Veterans Affairs, Department of, 252–254,
  266 n.5
Vietnam War, 253

                    W

Waiting lists
  elimination as priority of public
    coverage, 232
  reduction and core strategy option, 238
Willmar State Hospital, 53
Withdrawal, methadone and symptoms of
  heroin, 140
Women (*see also* Mothers; Pregnant
  women)
  opiate addiction in nineteenth century,
    46
  reasons for seeking treatment, 112
  research recommendations, 198, 199
  self-esteem, and treatment, 198
  Stay'n Out program, 178
  therapeutic communities and graduation
    rates, 161 n.17
World War II, decline in drug problem, 49

                    Z

Zoning, drug treatment programs, 197